Fetal and Hybrid Procedures in Congenital Heart Diseases

Gianfranco Butera • John Cheatham
Carlos A.C. Pedra • Dietmar Schranz
Gerald Tulzer
Editors

Fetal and Hybrid Procedures in Congenital Heart Diseases

Springer

Editors
Gianfranco Butera
IRCCS Policlinico San Donato
San Donato Milanese
Italy

John Cheatham
Pediatric Cardiology
Nationwide Children's Hospital
Columbus, Ohio
USA

Carlos A.C. Pedra
Hospital do Coraçao
Instituto D. Pazzanese de Cardiolog
Sao Paulo
Brazil

Dietmar Schranz
Justus Liebig University Hospital
Giessen
Hessen
Germany

Gerald Tulzer
Kepler University Hospital
Linz
Austria

ISBN 978-3-319-40086-0 ISBN 978-3-319-40088-4 (eBook)
DOI 10.1007/978-3-319-40088-4

Library of Congress Control Number: 2016953296

Printed on acid-free paper

This Springer imprint is published by Springer Nature
The registered company is Springer International Publishing AG Switzerland

Preface

The field of congenital heart disease has dramatically changed over the past years as a consequence of significant advances in imaging, understanding of disease mechanisms, and treatments through surgical and/or transcatheter techniques.

Among all, two fields have had interesting and significant evolutions: the development of fetal transcatheter treatments and the hybrid approach to therapy of congenital heart disease.

The idea of performing a therapy during fetal life has the aim to modify the natural history of some congenital heart diseases as aortic or pulmonary stenosis and the restrictive interatrial septum. The development of these techniques has opened new hopes. However, there are still many debated issues. All these aspects are developed throughout the book by world-renowned experts in the field.

The hybrid concept refers to the effort of joining the knowledge and the skills from both the interventionalists and the surgeons in order to minimize risks and optimize results. Furthermore, undergoing these procedures, patients may have a quicker recovery, a shorter hospital stay, and a better quality of life.

These techniques require not only a specific training but also need a tight collaboration within the team which includes pediatric interventionist, echocardiographer, surgeon and anesthesiologist. Almost all the leaders of the field collaborated to the book providing a complete overview of technique and results.

This book is the result of the collaboration of 40 world-renowned experts and gives plenty of details, tips, and tricks on 48 different topics. It provides the state of the art in the fetal interventional and the hybrid fields. To the reader the effort to develop new ideas in order to improve lives of our small patients.

San Donato Milanese, Italy — Gianfranco Butera
Columbus, OH, USA — John Cheatham
Sao Paulo, Brazil — Carlos A.C. Pedra
Giessen, Hessen, Germany — Dietmar Schranz
Linz, Austria — Gerald Tulzer

Contents

Part I

Introductory Aspects in Fetal Procedures

Ethical Aspects of Fetal Heart Interventions

1

Patrizia Salice, Nicola Persico, Carlo Casalone, Salvatore Natoli, and Federico Lombardi

The treatment of fetuses with altered cardiovascular physiology due to critical valvular stenosis or atresia is a complex clinical situation involving several ethical issues.

In contemporary clinical practice, a prenatal diagnosis of these pathological situations usually leads to the termination of pregnancy (TOP), that is offered, according to the different legal issues in different countries. It must be kept in mind and eventually discussed with the patient that, in early diagnosis, legal constraints on gestational age limit for TOP together with the development of defensive medicine may lead to an increasing number of women opting for TOP [1]. Fetal heart interventions (FHI), under these circumstances, are an alternative to TOP, offering to women the choice to continue their pregnancies and to more babies to reach birth with an acceptable outcome.

There are no laws forcing a pregnant woman to undergo invasive fetal treatment outside mainly historical legal orders of performing caesarean section for fetal distress [2]. Embarking on fetal invasive therapy or surgery is a demanding

P. Salice, MD (✉)
Perinatal and Pediatric Cardiology, Cardiovascular Disease Area, Fondazione Policlinico IRCCS, Via Commenda 12, Milan, Italy
e-mail: patrizia.salice@policlinico.mi.it

N. Persico, MD
Interventional Foetal Unit, Obstetric Clinic Mangiagalli Fondazione Policlinico IRCCS, Milan, Italy

C. Casalone, MD
Theological Ethics, Pontifical Theological Faculty, Southern Italy, Naples, Italy

S. Natoli, PHD
Theoretical Philosophy and Social Ethics, University of Milan Bicocca, Milan, Italy

F. Lombardi, MN
Cardiology, Fondazione Policlinico IRCCS, University of Milan, Milan, Italy

G. Butera et al. (eds.), *Fetal and Hybrid Procedures in Congenital Heart Diseases*, DOI 10.1007/978-3-319-40088-4_1

commitment, not only for the heaviness of the immediate treatment but also for the long-term consequences, encompassing perinatal care, postnatal management, and follow-up, including medical and social aspects, which cannot be successful without the full and active cooperation of the pregnant woman.

Given the complexity, the risks (for both woman and fetus), and the long-lasting effects of this specific interventional treatment, particular care must be paid to the practice of informed consent (IC). Moreover, it is mandatory for the ethical standard of any medical act to be aware of its shortcomings. Autonomy and human dignity are respected and promoted in the IC through accurate and complete information on the medical act, with all the benefits, side effects, and risks that it implies. The IC refers to the clinical perspective of a physician who performs his job with responsibility, fairness, and conscience, through the evidence-based medicine. The main aim has always been the patient's interest.

In order to avoid possible conflict of interests, a third person should ideally be in charge of the IC procedure. Nevertheless, when this is not possible and the information is provided by the same operator, the potential conflict must be disclosed and handled with particular care. It is also important to keep in mind that words such as child, baby, mother, and parents have important emotional impact. It must be considered if it is worthwhile to avoid them, using more neutral terms such as fetus, womb, and pregnancy, whose connotation is anatomical or functional. It is not only a linguistic choice but also an ethical one [3–4].

It is important for the IC:

1. To clarify that the aim is to increase the chances of biventricular repair [5–7], to underline fetal risks (pro and cons) either in case the FHI would be performed or in case the procedure wouldn't be performed, and to report, from most recent data, what is the clinical success rate [8–14]
2. To explain to the mother and the couple how the FHI will be held, detailing the steps of the procedure and the anesthesia for both mother and child and to deeply take into consideration both physical and psychological mother risks [15]
3. To remind that this is not a stand-alone intervention and patients will require a combination of repeated balloon aortic valvuloplasty, coarctation repair, endocardial fibroelastosis resection, and mitral or aortic valvuloplasty

The limit of the IC in this field is the paucity of data and the lack of:

(a) Data on progression of the lesions to determine whether outcome would be favorable or unfavorable. *There is a conflict of timing particularly in the diagnosis and treatment of critical aortic stenosis (AS) and intact atrial septum. On the one hand, it seems logical that earlier fetal intervention could reverse pathophysiology at least in case of AS. On the other hand, the earlier the decision is made to intervene, the less confidence the physicians have that the defect will ultimately progress to hypoplastic left heart syndrome* [16].
(b) Randomized studies on real utility of the procedure. Many argue that only a properly designed, adequately powered, and meticulously conducted

prospective trial, ideally randomized, would sufficiently overcome bias. The counteragument is that available data [8] allow to differentiate, in well selected cases, what patients were highly likely to evolve toward hypoplastic left heart syndrome and what were born with a nearly normal-sized left ventricle after fetal valvuloplasty.

Because of these reasons, women's request for treatment while refusing to enter a trial is not a rare situation. Finally, nowadays, it is preferable to take the stance of a controlled trial with possible crossover, in case of worsening of fetal conditions, being the only way to access treatment, even if TOP is then requested when treatment cannot be offered.

IC is only a part of the communication and counseling. It is very important to build a multidisciplinary team to overcome the possible difference from clinical background of different practitioners. In fact, for example, fetal cardiologists and pediatricians accord somewhat less weight to maternal decision-making than obstetrics and shift the focus of care to the fetus and perhaps privilege the interests and claims of the fetus over those of the pregnant woman [17, 18].

Ethical issues specifically related to fetal therapy articulate to a large extent around the transition between experimentation, therapeutic innovation, and standard of care. Our ability to diagnose and treat several fetal conditions has developed more rapidly than our understanding of their short-term and, even more so, long-term outcome in both treated and untreated cases.

Enthusiasm for fetal intervention must be tempered by mindfulness of the interests of the mother and her family, by careful study of the natural history of the disease in untreated human fetuses, and by willingness to abandon therapy that does not prove effective and safe, in properly performed trials.

To date, clinical results of maternal/fetal intervention for AS are based on comparisons with historical controls and address efficacy (Technè) rather than safety (Praxis) [19, 20].

In conclusion, interventional fetal cardiology is a model where ethical considerations must guide decisions, aimed to minimize damages and to increase success rate of proposed interventions. Such opportunity of applied ethics has to produce the right choice to realize the beneficence of the mother, fetus, and future child.

References

1. Feess E. Malpractice liability, technology choice and negative defensive medicine. Eur J Health Econ. 2011;13(2):157–67.
2. Lescale KB, Inglis SR, Eddleman KA, Peeper EQ, Chervenak FA, McCullough LB. Conflicts between physicians and patients in non-elective cesarean delivery: incidence and the adequacy of informed consent. Am J Perinatol. 1996;13(3):171–6.
3. Chervenak F, McCullough L. Ethics of fetal surgery. Clin Perinatol. 2009;36(2):237–46.
4. Boltanski L. The foetal condition: a sociology of engendering and abortion. Malden: Polity Press; 2013, chapt. 5.
5. Gadiner HM. The case for fetal cardiac intervention. Heart. 2009;95:1648–52.

6. Bacha E. Impact of fetal cardiac intervention on congenital heart surgery. Semin Thorac Cardiovasc Surg Pediatr Card Surg Ann. 2012;14:35–7.
7. McElhinney DB, Marshall AC, Wilkins-Haug LE, et al. Predictors of technical success and postnatal biventricular outcome after in utero aortic valvuloplasty for aortic stenosis with evolving hypoplastic left heart syndrome. Circulation. 2009;120:1482–90.
8. Schidlow DN, Tworetzky W, Wilkins-Haug LE. Percutaneous fetal cardiac interventions for structural heart disease. Am J Perinatol. 2014;31(7):629–36.
9. Moon-Grady AJ, Belfort M. International fetal cardiac intervention registry. JACC. 2015;66:388–99.
10. Pedra SR, Peralta CF, Crema L, Jatene IB, da Costa RN, Pedra CA. Fetal interventions for congenital heart disease in Brazil. Pediatr Cardiol. 2014;35:399–405.
11. Kalish BT, Tworetzky W, Benson CB, et al. Technical challenges of atrial septal stent placement in fetuses with hypoplastic left heart syndrome and intact atrial septum. Catheter Cardiovasc Interv. 2014;84:77–85.
12. Gomez-Montes E, Herraiz I, Mendoza A, Albert L, Hernandez-Garcia JM, Galindo A. Pulmonary atresia/critical stenosis with intact ventricular septum: prediction of outcome in the second trimester of pregnancy. Prenat Diagn. 2011;31:372–9.
13. Kovacevic A, Roughton M, Mellander M, et al. Fetal aortic valvuloplasty: investigating institutional bias in surgical decision-making. Ultrasound Obstet Gynecol. 2014;44(5):538–44.
14. Gitter R, Tulzer G. Intrauterine aortic valvuloplasty in fetuses with critical aortic stenosis: experience and results of 24 procedures. Ultrasound Obstet Gynecol. 2011;37:689–95.
15. Wohlmuth C, Tulzer G, Arzt W, Gitter R, Wertaschnigg D. Maternal aspects of fetal cardiac intervention. Ultrasound Obstet Gynecol. 2014;44(5):532–7.
16. Mavroudis CD. Foetal cardiac intervention: an ethical perspective. Cardiol Young. 2011;21:1467–7.
17. Ville Y. Fetal therapy: practical ethical considerations. Prenat Diagn. 2011;31:621–7.
18. Brown SD, Truog RD, Johnson JD, Ecker JL. Do Differences in the American Academy of Pediatrics and the American College of Obstetricians and Gynecologists Positions on the Ethics of Maternal–Fetal Interventions Reflect Subtly Divergent Professional Sensitivities to Pregnant Women and Fetuses? Pediatrics. 2006;117:1382–7.
19. Arzt W, Wertaschnigg D, Veit I, Klement F,Gitter R, Tulzer G. Intrauterine aortic valvuloplasty in fetuses with critical aortic stenosis: experience and results of 24 procedures. Ultrasound ObstetGynecol 2011;37:689–95
20. McElhinney DB, Marshall AC, Wilkins-Haug LE,et al. Predictors of technical success and postnatal biventricular outcome after in utero aortic valvuloplasty for aortic stenosis with evolving hypoplastic left heart syndrome. Circulation 2009;120:1482–90.

Tools in Fetal Heart Procedures

2

Cleisson Fábio Andrioli Peralta, Simone Rolim Fernandes Fontes Pedra, and Carlos Augusto Cardoso Pedra

2.1 Introduction

Fetal cardiac interventions have gained acceptance in the fetal medicine and cardiology fields as their efficacy and safety have been demonstrated throughout the world [1–13]. Some of the tools used in these procedures deserve comments.

In order to guarantee a successful intervention by a multidisciplinary team, an adequate case selection and some technical aspects should be respected [12, 13].

Despite slight variations exist in the assessment of different congenital heart abnormalities, the main instruments used for these procedures are basically the same. We shall comment about some details of maternal and fetal perioperative care, as well as about the main tools used during and after the fetal procedure [12, 13].

2.2 Maternal and Fetal Perioperative Care

Maternal fasting should start about 8 h before the procedure, which is performed under spinal blockage. We do not recommend general anesthesia because it could impede fetal positioning, which is more easily accomplished with an active fetus. Local anesthesia could eventually be an option; however, most patients do not tolerate well the external manipulation of the uterus. Depending on maternal anxiety, conscious sedation can be used after the fetus is properly positioned [12, 13].

For uterine relaxation, several options can be considered. In our unit, oral nifedipine (20 mg TID) is started about 12 h before the procedure, with two additional doses after the intervention. Other options are terbutaline (intravenous or subcutaneous) and atosiban (intravenous) during the procedure, followed by two additional doses of nifedipine [12, 13].

C.F.A. Peralta (✉) • S.R.F.F. Pedra • C.A.C. Pedra
Fetal Cardiology Unit, Heart Hospital, Sao Paulo, Brazil
e-mail: cfaperalta@gmail.com

G. Butera et al. (eds.), *Fetal and Hybrid Procedures in Congenital Heart Diseases*, DOI 10.1007/978-3-319-40088-4_2

After the mother is anesthetized and the fetus is well positioned, fetal anesthesia is given either by intramuscular or intravenous injection of pancuronium (20 μg/Kg), fentanyl (10 μg/Kg), and atropine (20 μg/Kg) using a 15-cm-long 20-gauge Chiba needle. If polyhydramnios is present, it is imperative that it is drained before the access to the fetal heart, so that the deepest vertical pocket of amniotic fluid does not exceed 8 cm. This process avoids passive fetal dislodgement during the heart intervention [12, 13].

2.3 Main Tools Used During Fetal Intervention

All steps from external version of the fetus to the heart procedure are performed under continuous ultrasound guidance using high-resolution ultrasound devices equipped with convex 2–6 MHz transducers.

As previously described, in our institution, a 15-cm-long 17–18-gauge Chiba needle (Fig. 2.1) is advanced through the maternal abdomen, uterine wall, and fetal chest wall and into the cardiac chamber (left or right ventricles or right atrium) [12, 13]. Other groups have described the use of cannulas with diamond-tipped stylet needle instead of the sharp-tipped Chiba needle [1–11]. There is no need for open surgery to expose the uterus in these procedures, as long as the fetal medicine specialist is familiar enough with the external manipulation of the fetus. Adjustments in the imaging plane are continuously done to include both the whole needle and the target cardiac chamber in the same field of view. The entry through the apex of the left or right ventricles is achieved as the tip of the needle is directed to the stenotic or atretic semilunar valves. The needle may occasionally need to traverse the placenta or the fetal liver. Pre-marked systems with rapid exchange 6–10-mm-long coronary balloons pre-mounted over cutoff 0.014-in. floppy-tip guidewires are used (Fig. 2.1). Clear visualization of the guidewire in the ascending aorta for aortic valvuloplasty or across the ductus for pulmonary valvuloplasty is recommended before balloon inflation. The coronary balloons are inflated up to two to four times with a pressure gauge device to reach diameters that are 20–30 % larger than the valve annulus. In our unit, the fetal medicine specialist is responsible for the external

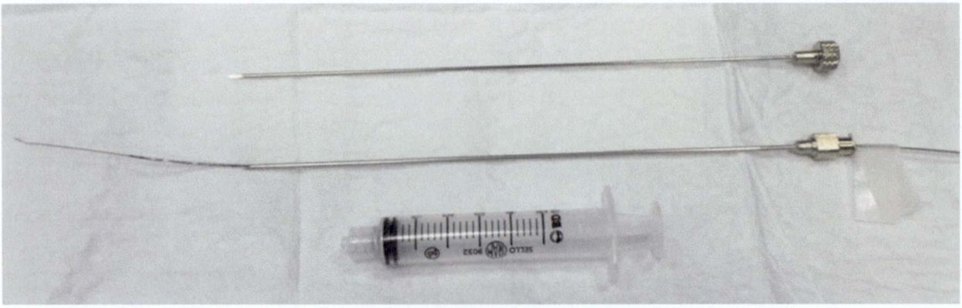

Fig. 2.1 Chiba needle (17 gauge, 15 cm long) and pre-marked system with rapid exchange 10-mm-long coronary balloon pre-mounted over a cutoff 0.014-in. floppy-tip guidewire

version of the fetus, as well as the ultrasound self-guided needle steps, and the interventionist manipulates the catheters and wires. After valve or interatrial septum dilatation, the whole system (needle + balloon + wire) is pulled out of the fetal heart and maternal body as a unit to avoid shearing off the balloon from the catheter shaft. No attempts should be made to recapture the balloon through the sharp tip of the needle. In cases of tamponade, the pericardium is promptly punctured for drainage using a 15-cm-long 20-gauge needle. If severe and persistent fetal bradycardia occurs, epinephrine (1–10 μg/kg) and atropine are injected directly into the ventricle [12, 13].

The use of stents and special catheters instead of coronary balloons is an option for interatrial septum procedures, although our team does not have experience with this technique.

2.4 Main Tools Used After Fetal Intervention

After the main steps of fetal cardiac intervention are finished, fetal monitoring is performed by ultrasound. Apart from an initial evaluation of the success of the procedure, umbilical and cerebral Doppler can be used to reassure fetal hemodynamic stability. Middle cerebral artery peak systolic velocity is measured to detect fetal anemia, usually the day after the procedure, in cases of excessive fetal bleeding (subjective evaluation) [14].

Magnetic resonance imaging is also a useful tool that can be used especially in cases of severe fetal bleeding and tamponade followed by persistent bradycardia and/or heart arrest. It allows the detection of acute and recent fetal brain damage, through the evaluation of water diffusion restriction, and it can be performed right after the cardiac intervention until 7–10 days after the procedure [15, 16].

In summary, the tools used for fetal cardiac interventions nowadays are relatively simple and widely available. Despite new instruments, as catheters and dilating devices, are welcome and may help to improve results in the future, it seems that the success of fetal cardiac intervention relies mainly on the expertise of a dedicated multidisciplinary team.

References

1. Maxwell D, Allan L, Tynan MJ. Balloon dilation of the aortic valve in the fetus: a report of two cases. Br Heart J. 1991;65(5):256–8.
2. Kohl T, Sharland G, Allan LD, Gembruch U, Chaoui R, Lopes LM, et al. World experience of percutaneous ultrasound- guided balloon valvuloplasty in human fetuses with severe aortic valve obstruction. Am J Cardiol. 2000;85(10):1230–3.
3. Tworetzky W, Wilkins-Haug L, Jennings RW, van der Velde ME, Marshall AC, Marx GR, et al. Balloon dilation of severe aortic stenosis in the fetus: potential for prevention of hypoplastic left heart syndrome: candidate selection, technique, and results of successful intervention. Circulation. 2004;110(15):2125–31.

4. Marshall AC, Tworetzky W, Bergersen L, McElhinney DB, Benson CB, Jennings RW, et al. Aortic valvuloplasty in the fetus: technical characteristics of successful balloon dilation. J Pediatr. 2005;147(4):535–9.
5. Wilkins-Haug LE, Tworetzky W, Benson CB, Marshall AC, Jennings RW, Lock JE. Factors affecting technical success of fetal aortic valve dilation. Ultrasound Obstet Gynecol. 2006;28(1):47–52.
6. Arzt W, Werttaschnigg D, Veit I, Klement F, Gitter R, Tulzer G. Intrauterine aortic valvuloplasty in fetuses with critical aortic stenosis: experience and results of 24 procedures. Ultrasound Obstet Gynecol. 2011;37(6):689–95.
7. Marshall AC, Levine J, Morash D, Silva V, Lock JE, Benson CB, et al. Results of in utero atrial septoplasty in fetuses with hypoplastic left heart syndrome. Prenat Diagn. 2008;28(11):1023–8.
8. Tulzer G, Arzt W, Franklin RC, Loughna PV, Mair R, Gardiner HM. Fetal pulmonary valvuloplasty for critical pulmonary stenosis or atresia with intact septum. Lancet. 2002;360(9345):1567–8.
9. Arzt W, Tulzer G, Aigner M, Mair R, Hafner E. Invasive intrauterine treatment of pulmonary atresia/intact ventricular septum with heart failure. Ultrasound Obstet Gynecol. 2003;21(2):186–8.
10. Galindo A, Gutierrez-Larraya F, Velasco JM, de la Fuente P. Pulmonary balloon valvuloplasty in a fetus with critical pulmonary stenosis/atresia with intact ventricular septum and heart failure. Fetal Diagn Ther. 2006;21(1):100–4.
11. Tworetzky W, McElhinney DB, Marx GR, Benson CB, Brusseau R, Morash D, et al. In utero valvuloplasty for pulmonary atresia with hypoplastic right ventricle: techniques and outcomes. Pediatrics. 2009;124(3):e510–8.
12. Pedra SF, Peralta CF, Pedra CAC. Future directions of fetal interventions in congenital heart disease. Intervent Cardiol Clin. 2013;2:1–10.
13. Pedra SR, Peralta CF, Crema L, Jatene IB, da Costa RN, Pedra CA. Fetal interventions for congenital heart disease in Brazil. Pediatr Cardiol. 2014;35(3):399–405.
14. Tavares NM, Ferreira SG, Bennini JR, Marussi EF, Barini R, Peralta CF. Longitudinal reference intervals of maternal-fetal Doppler parameters. Rev Bras Ginecol Obstet. 2013;35(1):33–8.
15. Gomes Neto O, Marins M, Botelho RD, Nivoloni RC, Saura GE, Vessoni Arias A, Barini R, Peralta CF. Feasibility and reproducibility of diffusion-weighted magnetic resonance imaging of the fetal brain in twin-twin transfusion syndrome. Prenat Diagn. 2014;34(12):1182–8.
16. Luminoso D, Figueira CO, Marins M, Peralta CF. Fetal brain lesion associated with spontaneous twin anemia-polycythemia sequence. Ultrasound Obstet Gynecol. 2013;42(6):721–2.

3 Role of Multicenter Registries to Assess Outcomes of Fetal Interventions

Daud Lodin, Tara Karamlou, and Anita J. Moon-Grady

3.1 Introduction to Congenital Heart Registries

3.1.1 What Are Health Registries?

Health registries are databases that are managed by an organized network of centers that contribute clinical data for research purposes. Within these registries, analysts, researchers, and physicians work together to generate new knowledge from pooled data that may improve treatments, outcomes, and systems of care. By combining cases from multiple sources, health registries create larger pools of study data without the added expense of clinical trials. They provide sample populations that have superior variability and therefore may have better representation of larger populations. Because registries utilize aggregate data, they are ideal for studying rare diseases, complications, or adverse effects. Registries also provide a unique source of collaboration for the research community, as the creation of these multicenter partnerships requires extensive participation from experts across many disciplines.

D. Lodin • T. Karamlou, MD
Division of Pediatric Cardiac Surgery, Department of Surgery, University of California, San Francisco, CA, USA

A.J. Moon-Grady, MD (✉)
Fetal Cardiovascular Program and Fetal Treatment Center, UCSF Benioff Children's Hospital, University of California San Francisco, 550 16th Street 5th Floor, Box 0544, San Francisco, CA 94158, USA

Division of Cardiology, Department of Pediatrics, University of California San Francisco, San Francisco, CA, USA
e-mail: anita.moongrady@ucsf.edu

G. Butera et al. (eds.), *Fetal and Hybrid Procedures in Congenital Heart Diseases*, DOI 10.1007/978-3-319-40088-4_3

3.1.2 Fetal and Congenital Heart Registries

Currently, three major registries of infant, children, and adult case data exist internationally that contribute to the body of knowledge for the treatment of congenital heart diseases (CHD). The Society of Thoracic Surgeons (STS) was the first organization to develop databases in the United States (US) for the sole purpose of tracking heart disorders requiring surgical intervention [1]. The STS Adult Cardiac Surgery Database and the STS Congenital Heart Surgery Database (CHSD) contain over five million surgical cases, with data from approximately 90 % of all cases occurring nationally [1]. Two other major cardiac health registries, the European Association for Cardio-Thoracic Surgery (EACTS) database [2] and the Japanese Congenital Cardiovascular Surgery Database (JCCVSD) [3], both obtain similar data on patients undergoing surgery for cardiac disease. Though none of these registries currently collect data specifically on prenatal intervention, the STS-CHSD will ascertain prenatal intervention and many prenatal and maternal variables in the next upgrade.

Although lacking the sponsorship of major congenital heart organizations, the necessity for more in-depth data is what initially drove the creation of a small collection of fetal intervention centers to join together to create the first global registry. The International Fetal Cardiac Intervention Registry (IFCIR) was created in 2010 to collect data and monitor the state of rare congenital heart cases that were referred for or received fetal cardiac interventions (FCI) [4]. The IFCIR is a collective of 35 fetal surgery centers worldwide, working to collect data on all cases. While currently in its infancy, the registry has collected over 450 FCI cases over its 5-year existence and was the subject of a recent report detailing the results that have been cultivated so far [5]. Preliminary reports of the registry's efforts have shown promise and may well pave the way in improving aspects regarding FCI.

3.2 Overview of Registry Structure and Standards

The creation of a reliable and well-functioning registry requires a high level of standardization and quality control in order for it to serve as an effective tool for identifying risk factors and advances in care. The development and use of a common nomenclature, standardized data collection procedures, and a network for long-term validation of data from participating sites contribute to the success of health registries. Understanding these concepts as they pertain to multicenter health databases will help elucidate the complexities of registries describing fetal and hybrid pediatric cardiac surgery.

3.2.1 Registry Structure

The first step in developing a registry is the creation of a network of data collection centers that may require cooperation from participating medical centers, state health departments, and potentially national organizations, depending on the scope of variables included. Data progresses from these smaller centers and is shuttled to larger, overseeing centers, responsible for collating, correcting, and analyzing the complete dataset. As an example of this structural balance, the STS recommends that each center utilizes a dedicated data manager to enter data for local cases and send them to a central data warehouse, the Duke Clinical Research Institute, DCRI, for concatenation, quality assurance, and data verification [1]. For developing registries, the importance of establishing structure relies on the coordination and recruitment of new centers. For IFCIR, operations began in 2011 with four centers contributing case data [3]. At its current size of 35 centers across 15 countries, the organization will require greater infrastructure to handle the complexity and bureaucratic aspects of their growing registry. Moon-Grady and colleagues discussed the program's preliminary experience in a 2015 publication, detailing the work they had done since their inception [5]. The authors explained the importance of establishing an FCI registry and elucidated many of the shortcomings in the initial iteration of the dataset. Noncompliance from institutions, the need for individual institutional/ethics review board approval, the legal implications of local regulations, and variations on what information centers were able to divulge all contributed to limitations in the data collection process. The IFCIR has potential to overcome these shortcomings, as the registry adapts to handle these expansions. As was the case with the establishment of the STS national databases, harnessing the support of national organizations and personnel may facilitate growth of the registry with fewer complications and greater data accuracy.

3.2.2 Common Coding and Nomenclature

A common system of nomenclature and health coding must be established in which diseases, outcomes, interventions, and anatomy consistently have the same code, description, name, and characterization for successful high-quality data collection. In 1998, the EACTS and the STS worked together to develop the International Congenital Heart Surgery Nomenclature and Database Project (ICHSNDP) [6]. The project worked to combine the knowledge of both organizations in order to form a standardized, internationally accepted, CHD nomenclature. The end result of the three entities' roles was the creation of the International Pediatric and Congenital Cardiac Code (IPCCC), a standardized code on the web (http://www.IPCCC.net) that offers standardized lists of CHD code [6]. The establishment of these standardized codes, as well as the presence of committees dedicated to ensuring its integrity, is paramount to ensuring the quality of CHD data being collected is at a high standard and that bias from data errors and misclassification is minimized.

From the standpoint of fetal cardiac intervention, however, several unique issues regarding nomenclature exist. For example, what "diagnosis" should the fetus with evolving heart disease seen in the midtrimester (or in some cases as early as the late first trimester) be assigned? Aortic stenosis clearly may evolve to hypoplastic left heart syndrome [7], but pulmonary stenosis may or may not become pulmonary atresia after birth; currently, the IFCIR utilizes an overall classification scheme coupled with key echo-derived anatomic and physiologic descriptors rather than a set nomenclature system. This issue regards the natural versus the “unnatural” history of disease evolution, when prenatal intervention may change the postnatal diagnosis substantially. This concern needs to be resolved before fetal cardiac registries can be integrated into the existing registry efforts mentioned previously.

3.2.3 Data Collection and Variables of Interest

The selection of variables to be collected is a paramount step in establishing a basis for both new and growing registries. Different study designs from all aspects of the field in question will require an assortment of diverse variables, allowing for several hypotheses be tested longitudinally and cross-sectionally. Variable categories that may be of interest in FCI registries are included in the table (Table 3.1).

Table 3.1 Fetal cardiac intervention variable categories and examples

Variable category	Example variables
Demographics (maternal)	Age, race, gender, obstetric history, gravity, parity, pregnancy dating
Noncardiac congenital abnormalities (fetus)	List of congenital disorders in the fetus (diaphragmatic hernia, brain abnormalities, omphalocele, etc.)
Chromosome abnormalities (fetus and infant)	Trisomies, monosomies, or chromosomal deletions detected by invasive or noninvasive means
Syndromes (fetus and infant)	List of syndromes (DiGeorge, Noonan, etc.)
Hospitalization (maternal and infant)	Hospital location, insurance information, admission and procedure date
Preoperative factors (fetus/infant/child)	List of factors (hydrops, atrioventricular block, etc.)
Diagnoses (fetus)	Aortic valve abnormalities, atrial septal restriction, pulmonary valve abnormalities, mitral valve abnormalities, arrhythmias
Procedures (maternal/fetal)	List of procedures for each diagnosis
Anesthesia (maternal and fetal)	Anesthetic used, adverse events
Operative factors (maternal, infant/child)	Procedure type, surgeon, procedure duration, anatomic and access factors, i.e., placental location, technical components, medications, and resuscitative measures
Postoperative factors (maternal)	Blood products utilized, tocolysis
Complications (maternal and fetal)	List of complications (intraoperative death, preterm rupture of membranes or labor, late intrauterine death, etc.)
Discharge and outcomes	Date of birth, operations, discharge, readmission, mortality
Adult factors	Smoking status, history of chronic disease, family history, operations, and complications

Intended as illustrative, not necessarily comprehensive

3.2.4 Quality Assurance and Data Verification

Quality assurance and data verification go hand in hand to address issues with duplicate records, incorrectly entered data, and missing entries. There are several ways in which checks and balances can be implemented to ensure complete data and the reduction of errors. Depending on the infrastructure, the size of the registry, and the number of data entry points, evaluations and audits at each level are required to ensure high data integrity. As one model, in the STS National Database, each center participating in the registry receives a data quality report of their own data after each bulk submission [8, 9]. These reports include information on the raw data they submitted, changes to this data, completeness issues, and a percent missing itemized list of missing variables [8, 9]. They allow centers to audit their own records, as well as confirm or correct the changes made by STS in their database. Their annual national report also presents an opportunity to benchmark individual center results compared to the aggregate using composite quality ratings. Voluntary public reporting for in-hospital mortality is currently an option using a center's own STS data. Such national initiatives may improve quality, by facilitating transparency regarding outcomes. The current FCI database represented by IFCIR relies on intermittent data quality review and manual query and data verification. Clearly, a more rigorous model for data verification will be necessary, as the registry matures and before the information can be made publicly available.

3.2.5 Risk Adjustment Modeling and the Goal of Registry-Based Data

Because global benchmarks and goals must be set for fetal cardiac centers in order to reduce complications and mortality, registry data is likely to play an increasingly important role. One of the analytical tools that registries utilize is a risk-adjusted model, an analysis method that collectively examines several associations to a single outcome. Risk-adjusted models rely on comparing the effect of multiple relevant variables together, ensuring that false association is not made and that a proper description of vulnerable populations can be determined. Continuing with the STS-CHSD as an example for CHD case analysis, the organization's most recent risk adjustment models had excellent discrimination regarding in-hospital mortality and clearly identified several predictor variables that increased the risk of in-hospital death. The analysis was conducted comparing mortality in 54,224 patients in over 80 centers. Demographic, diagnostic, surgical, and clinical characteristics were examined first individually for their effect, then by an examination of their collective effect on mortality. The final risk-adjusted model included primary procedure, patient age, weight, and several other important comorbidities [10, 11]. This complete model effectively identified which patient populations are at a greater risk for adverse surgical outcomes, as well as which disorders and procedures carry a greater risk for death, thereby allowing clinicians to discuss and set goals to improve care for these specific populations. As changes are made to the management of care and interventions, future multivariate analyses will help determine if these improvements have ultimately led to better outcomes. Risk-adjusted models serve as an important tool for registries to determine areas of improvement and to examine the efficacy of clinical and procedural developments.

3.2.6 Limitations to Multicenter and Registry-Based Studies

There are certain limitations to multicenter and registry studies that must be addressed to better understand their strengths and weakness. Studies associated with health registries are not randomized or blind and may not include a proper control group. Many registries are voluntary, and therefore the data may not be extrapolatable or representative [12, 13]. Misclassification from coding inaccuracies, duplicated records, or missing values may introduce important bias [12]. Additionally, selection bias can occur from institutions or individuals, who may have a financial or other stake in these studies [12]. Smaller, poorly performing, or low-resource medical facilities may abstain from participating in registry data collection, introducing another important source of bias and further limiting generalizability [12, 13]. One additional limitation unique to the field of fetal cardiac intervention regards the potential linkage of fetal data from maternal records with postnatal databases, as there is a potential for data lost due to case data not being recorded separately or included solely in maternal records. In particular, some fetuses may not survive to live birth and thus may be present only in maternal records, creating a situation that could cause the loss of records on patients that undergo any interventions prenatally.

3.3 Public Health Implications of Registry Data

3.3.1 Data Linkage: Challenges and Advantages to Registry Collaboration

As congenital and fetal registries begin to grow in size, a standard for data collection and patient recruitment will require the collaboration of multiple centers and registries in order to properly collect case data and present important results. Creating a linkage between these registries will be important for examining the efficacy of FCI and has been an important topic for CHD databases over the past few years. The STS-CHSD has worked on linking their data with two other major registries. The Congenital Heart Surgeons' Society (CHSS) and the Pediatric Health Information System (PHIS) are two organizations whose databases have separate yet important focuses and intentions for CHD data [14–16]. Certain analyses, such as longitudinal and Medicare-based studies, could never have been conducted by the STS without the combined effort of these organizations [14–16]. Linkage also identified gaps, misclassifications, and errors within databases, highlighting the importance of cross-examining patient information and increasing the sample size for conducting analyses [14–16]. Lastly, combining population data allows these registries to examine the overall representative nature of the study pool with the rest of the population, improving statistical adjustments to state and nationwide statistics [14–16]. As registries begin to expand to include data on FCI, collaboration through data linkage will help to expand the effort in regard to improving the field and creating long-term benefits for patients while capitalizing on the efforts of these larger organizations and minimizing duplication of effort in data collection and storage.

3.3.2 Fetal Registries and New Discoveries

The overarching purpose of multicenter FCI registries is to provide large databases for use in discovering rare associations and ultimately improving care and interventional techniques [12, 17]. The increased statistical power of multicenter studies is extremely beneficial to studying rarer diseases and their treatments [12, 17]. This concept has been proven important in the field of CHD, as several multicenter studies have successfully shown unique traits and characteristics associated with cardiac interventions and disorders. Research on FCI will benefit immensely from the development of new and current registry systems. In only the recent few decades, fetal interventions have gone from an experimental aspect of cardiology to a viable opportunity to address congenital malformations before birth. Intervention data globally has been scarce, however, as IFCIR has collected less than 500 cases over the past 5 years [5]. The organization's most recent analysis showed the importance of this small data pool with regard to three major cardiac procedures: aortic valvuloplasty, pulmonary valvuloplasty, and atrial septal interventions [5]. The highlight of their 2015 report showed that fetal patients with CHD who underwent these interventions were more likely to have improved cardiac physiology upon discharge than patients that had no intervention [5]. The results of this publication are a small step forward in the right direction for furthering FCI efficacy. While the IFCIR has grown slowly since its debut, developments to the size of their network have been impressive and will be paramount to the future of the registry. The number of centers associated with IFCIR has grown to almost ten times its initial size in 2011, and ongoing progress and participation will be essential to its success.

3.3.3 The "Public" View: Awareness, Transparency, and Accountability

In the context of FCI, the US Affordable Care Act (ACA) emphasizes the right to equity and access to care for all, including mothers and their fetuses [18]. While this declaration ensures that there will be support for FCI, its ascension into a common medical practice will not arrive without scientific scrutiny. The need to progress and justify the efficacy of these procedures will be paramount in developing public perception of the field, as well as provide reasoning for conducting them.

Beyond creating transparency and building public perception, the role that multicenter studies have had on healthcare payers will ultimately play a part in the success of whether FCI will be a viable and accepted healthcare option. For instance, one prominent health agency offering insurance in the Unites States recently released a policy brief explaining their rationale for coverage of only certain fetal surgical procedures [19]. Effective May of 2015, the cost of repair procedures for six noncardiac fetal diagnoses will be covered. The company's published brief stated that there was sufficient evidence associated with specific repair techniques that proved the scientific efficacy. However, fetal interventional techniques associated with congenital heart disease were listed as a non-coverable medical expense. According to the agency, study evidence was found inadequate to verify the efficacy of any FCI. The studies cited, however, were all single site, utilizing only small datasets that would have created little study power to prove the usefulness of FCI on the whole, let alone for individual procedures [19]. The lack of large-scale viable studies for use in verifying procedures will be a challenge for the field to overcome as it develops. The use of FCI multicenter or registry studies may well be the stepping stone necessary for organizations and the public to embrace FCI as a medically and financially safe form of healthcare.

3.3.4 Challenges to Fetal Registries: Politics, Ethics, and Fetal Data

While bias and systematic limitations are a threat to the integrity of registry data, social and political aspects present unique challenges in the context of FCI and their registries. As was stated earlier, the ACA in the United States mandated access to healthcare for all, including the consignment of this right to a fetus. But does that necessarily mean that a fetus may have other rights? What about the right to privacy or the respect for autonomy? Stem cell research brought these questions into light several years ago, as politicians and the public debated whether the benefits of research superseded a fetus' right to life [20]. The debate regarding fetal rights created a stigma that has since divided the nation and been detrimental to advancements in fetal and stem cell research in the United States. Prenatal studies have and will come under greater scrutiny from governmental and institutional officials. Such hurdles present themselves for new and ongoing fetal databases to overcome in order to survive and flourish in the current political climate.

Within the realm of medical ethics, several vulnerable subpopulations have been identified, including minors, seniors, prisoners, and the mentally disabled [21]. These groups are fortunate enough to have the protection of certain laws and regulations that prevent coercion and manipulation [21]. A continuing international debate on fetal rights, however, has not established similar criteria for fetuses. Guidelines on intrauterine fetal research generally only condone work done where there is minimal (or no) risk to the fetus and that proper consent is documented from the parents [22]. These guidelines also restrict research procedures that would possibly cause harm to the pregnancy, regardless of the benefits of study outcomes or if the mother had decided upon pregnancy termination prior to enrollment [22]. There is, however, no mention within ethics board guidelines of long-term privacy or dissemination of the patient data. As FCI databases develop and research begins to investigate outcomes that extend into early child or adulthood, the private data of a fetus will instead become associated with a born individual. A barrier that fetal cardiac registries will need to consider is the right to hold maternal and/or fetal data for long-term use. Regulation may need to be developed for adults, who successfully survived fetal cardiac intervention, to be informed of their status in registry participation and be given the option to have their data kept or removed.

3.4 The Future: Fetal Intervention Registries and Advocating for a Global Database for All Congenital Heart Disorders

The focus of this chapter was to discuss the means, rationale, and hurdles for the creation and maintenance of FCI registries, looking at current and non-FCI models to explain the many facets of registry and multicenter studies. It must be made clear that the future of FCI registries will rely on the collective effort of established CHD registries and will also require the extensive cooperation from their large governing bodies. While IFCIR currently serves as the largest FCI database on a global scale, their outreach is limited, as the organization does not carry any major infrastructural or collaborative support from larger organizations such as STS or EACTS. The prospects of improving FCIs lie in the joint organization of several major international bodies, working together to gather data and help build the field. In 2010, Jacobs and colleagues published a summative report on the feasibility of producing an international system of data collection for a global CHD registry [6]. Citing consensus between international standards for nomenclature, interagency cooperation, data quality, and verification, the authors provided evidence showing that this large-scale endeavor was achievable. They also underlined two important points for future development. First, registries relying on multidisciplinary collaboration would be the key in ensuring the database's success [6]. This field-wide rule would include specialists of FCI, helping to bring awareness and expansion for the field. Second, they made clear that a new system of data collection was not necessary and that a global system could simply be integrated into the current infrastructure of each major organization [6]. The field would benefit greatly from the fruition of a global CHD system and receive greater attention and support for improving FCI.

Conclusion

Registry and multicenter studies benefit the field of FCIs by providing aggregate data for analysis and support for further innovation and by providing a potential source of advertising for participating centers. There are important limitations inherent in voluntary registry data that must be recognized in order to avoid the threats of chance, bias, and confounding. Moreover, several political, ethical, and social barriers exist that will create obstacles in further progress with fetal registries. However, the benefits of creating a unified system of data collection are likely to advance care, increase education initiatives and patient access, and ultimately improve maternal and fetal outcomes worldwide.

References

1. Grover FL, et al. The STS national database. Ann Thorac Surg. 2014;97(1):S48–54.
2. Head SJ, et al. The European association for cardio-thoracic surgery (EACTS) database: an introduction. Eur J Cardiothorac Surg. 2013;44(3):e175–80.
3. Murakami A, et al. The national clinical database as an initiative for quality improvement in Japan. Korean J Thorac Cardiovasc Surg. 2014;47(5):437–43.
4. Moon-Grady AJ, et al. Outcomes after in-utero cardiac interventions: a preliminary report of the collaborative international fetal cardiac intervention registry. Circulation. 2014;130 Suppl 2:A16469.
5. Moon-Grady AJ, et al. International fetal cardiac intervention registry: a worldwide collaborative description and preliminary outcomes. J Am Coll Cardiol. 2015;66(4):388–99.
6. Jacobs JP, et al. Congenital heart surgery databases around the world: do we need a global database? In: Seminars in thoracic and cardiovascular surgery: pediatric cardiac surgery annual. 2010. Elsevier.
7. Makikallio K, et al. Fetal aortic valve stenosis and the evolution of hypoplastic left heart syndrome: patient selection for fetal intervention. Circulation. 2006;113(11):1401–5.
8. Clarke DR, et al. Verification of data in congenital cardiac surgery. Cardiol Young. 2008;18 Suppl 2:177–87.
9. Shahian DM, et al. The society of thoracic surgeons national database. Heart. 2013;99(20):1494–501.
10. O'Brien SM, et al. The society of thoracic surgeons congenital heart surgery database mortality risk model: part 1-statistical methodology. Ann Thorac Surg. 2015;100(3):1054–62.
11. Jacobs JP, et al. The society of thoracic surgeons congenital heart surgery database mortality risk model: part 2-clinical application. Ann Thorac Surg. 2015;100(3):1063–8.
12. Welke KF, Diggs BS, Karamlou T. Chance, bias, and confounding: threats to valid measurement of quality in the context of pediatric cardiac surgery. Semin Thorac Cardiovasc Surg Pediatr Card Surg Annu. 2010;13(1):79–83.
13. Mavroudis CD, et al. Ethical issues confronting outcomes analysis and quality assurance. In: Pediatric and congenital cardiac care. London: Springer; 2015. p. 295–303.
14. Pasquali SK, et al. Linking clinical registry data with administrative data using indirect identifiers: implementation and validation in the congenital heart surgery population. Am Heart J. 2010;160(6):1099–104.
15. Jacobs JP, et al. Linking the congenital heart surgery databases of the Society of Thoracic Surgeons and the Congenital Heart Surgeons' Society: part 1 – rationale and methodology. World J Pediatr Congenit Heart Surg. 2014;5(2):256–71.
16. Jacobs JP, et al. Linking the congenital heart surgery databases of the Society of Thoracic Surgeons and the Congenital Heart Surgeons' Society: part 2 – lessons learned and implications. World J Pediatr Congenit Heart Surg. 2014;5(2):272–82.
17. Donofrio MT. The power is in the numbers: using collaboration and a data registry to answer our burning questions regarding fetal cardiac intervention. J Am Coll Cardiol. 2015;66(4):400–2.
18. Representatives U.S.H.o. Patient protection and affordable care act. Public Law. 2010:111–48.
19. United Healthcare. In utero fetal surgery. Medical Policy, 2015;2015T0035N:16.

20. Nisbet MC, Brossard D, Kroepsch A. Framing science the stem cell controversy in an age of press/politics. Int J Press/Politics. 2003;8(2):36–70.
21. Sciences C.f.I.O.o.M. International ethical guidelines for biomedical research involving human subjects. Bulletin of medical ethics. 2002(182):17.
22. Drane JF. Medical ethics and maternal-fetal conflicts. Pa Med. 1992;95(7):12–6.

4 Role of Counseling in Fetal Congenital Heart Diseases

Maria Giovanna Russo, Fiorella Fratta, Beniamino Tormettino, and Nicola Colacurci

Counseling is a profession that helps individual, family, or group through the relationship between the professional and client. Counseling facilitates the processes of change and improves the quality of life, enhancing both the resources and the relationships with the environment surrounding. The fetal echocardiography is a technique born in the late 1980s, when the improvement of ultrasound technology has made it possible to highlight the characteristics of the fetal heart. Huhta JC, one of the fathers of this method, wondered immediately if, without the possibility of dealing with in utero congenital heart disease, it was useful or advisable to diagnose before birth. Numerous studies have now clearly demonstrated that a team consisting of a gynaecologist and a cardiologist pediatrician can diagnose with very high accuracy a number of congenital heart defects in the fetal stage; so, the spectrum of the anomalies discovered in the uterus is almost superimposed on the heart disease observed at birth. Nowadays, high attention to the anatomy of the fetal heart is associated with an equally close attention to the psychological aspect of the matter: in practice it is not always possible to deal adequately with the counseling prospective parents.

In the last years, thanks to the ultrasound equipment and to the skills of the perinatologists, the prenatal diagnosis of fetal malformation is improved, and it's now possible to detect or suspect a fetal malformation from the mid-gestation. This is for sure an important improvement in the field of the fetal medicine, but it resulted in another issue, the ones related to the counseling, the ethical and psychological aspect of the problem. These aspects are of great important as we can see by the large and growing scientific literature on this argument [1–4]. As a consequence of

M.G. Russo (✉) • F. Fratta
Pediatric Cardiology Unit, Second University of Studies of Naples – Monaldi Hospital, Naples, Italy
e-mail: mgiovannarusso@hotmail.com

B. Tormettino • N. Colacurci
Department of Woman, Child and of General and Specialized Surgery, Second University of Studies of Naples, Naples, Italy

G. Butera et al. (eds.), *Fetal and Hybrid Procedures in Congenital Heart Diseases*, DOI 10.1007/978-3-319-40088-4_4

these observations, many authors [5, 6] state that it is mandatory a multidisciplinary counseling comprise the obstetrician, the cardiologist, the pediatric surgeon, and the psychologist, in order to provide a comprehensive information to the parents. This raises the question of whether or not repeated consultations during the follow-up of the mother and the fetus, on the one hand, could improve the emotional side of parents, but according to others, this approach would worsen the anxiety. At present the literature did not arrive at conclusions supported by evidence [7, 8]. There is evidence that prospective parents may be able to face up with anxiety with a psychological support; therefore, in these cases a single consultation may be inadequate.

4.1 Invasive Fetal Cardiac Intervention (FCI)

The outcome of fetuses with congenital heart disease, developing a postnatal univentricular heart despite improvements in neonatal surgical care and development of dedicated follow-up programs, remains poor. This case has become the main indication for antenatal intervention. Postnatal surgery, which results in a far from optimal single-ventricle Fontan-type circulation [9], has a considerable mortality rate, leading to a total long-term survival of less than 65 % [10]. Numerous studies have been published documenting the natural history of congenital heart defects in utero and the potential of prenatal progression [11, 12]. A well-functioning biventricular heart may develop into a univentricular heart, or it may acquire myocardial damage, which can lead to congestive heart failure, arrhythmias, hydrops, and intrauterine death. Pulmonary development may be also affected. It would therefore seem logical that a fetal intracardiac intervention at the right time and in the right fetus should be able to improve or even normalize hemodynamics and to prevent secondary damage to the fetal heart and lungs [13]. Recently, technological advances in fetal cardiac imaging have given us a window into the womb, creating the field of fetal cardiology, where the fetus is considered an individual patient from the time of diagnosis. One of the challenges we face as fetal caregivers is that we must strive to understand the "prequel" of what we already know: the natural history and progression of congenital heart disease in utero. More than 25 years ago, researchers reported that structural heart disease, specifically aortic stenosis, evolves in utero [11]. Fetal therapy, either by catheter intervention or surgery, is based on the fundamental principle that intervention will alter the natural history of the disease process. To prove that this is true, we must first gain an understanding of the unaltered progression of heart disease in utero. Referral centers have shown that fetal cardiac intervention can be performed successfully, with minimal risk to the mother and encouraging outcomes for fetuses, particularly in those with aortic stenoses evolving to HLHS hypoplastic left heart syndrome (HLHS).

4.2 Counseling in Fetal Cardiac Intervention

In recent years, several advances have been made in the fetal cardiac intervention of congenital heart disease. All these advances are accompanied by the need to be prepared for the best to be able to explain clearly to parents what are these procedures and the risks associated with them. Indeed counseling with parents regarding these procedures really becomes a very delicate process. It must not only be accurate in the technical description of the procedure, but list all of the risks and complications and less common and finally also understand the emotional side. Counseling is both multidisciplinary and multistage. Of primary importance is the story of the mother, the presence of diseases and allergies, or taking drugs. A careful consultation should be carried out with the consultant physicians. The counseling should be carried out in the presence of both parents and possibly all members of the family who may support the decision.

The duration varies from case to case; it is necessary to be sure that parents have understood all the risks associated with the procedure and all the possible complications postprocedure. Only after being sure that counseling has been comprehensive, you may ask the parents to sign written informed consent. If it is assumed that the parents do not demonstrate a clear understanding of the benefits and risks of the procedure, it is a contraindication to the same.

Parents are counseled extensively about the maternal and fetal risks.

4.2.1 Maternal Risk

The mother's safety, health, and future reproductive potential remain the priorities when undertaking fetal therapy. A comprehensive preprocedure workup is performed to exclude maternal contraindications for the procedure. Nevertheless, complications related to the anesthesia, laparotomy, and uterine manipulation can occur. In addition, a sick or hydropic fetus can lead to premature labor or the maternal mirror syndrome, a preeclampsia-like syndrome for which the only therapy is the delivery of the sick fetus. Given appropriate technique, maternal morbidity is rare, except when uterine exposure is needed or when fetal deterioration requires immediate abdominal delivery [14]. The interventions remain invasive, as the amniotic cavity has to be entered transabdominally with an 18- or 19-gauge needle; there are inevitable risks for the mother such as prelabou preterm rupture of the membranes, premature labor, placental abruption, bleeding, or infection. The quoted pPROM rates 2–7 % [15, 16]. Long-term outcomes are not yet available. The precise number of procedures and types of personnel needed for a successful center has yet to be determined, but analysis of registry data, including that in the International Fetal Cardiac Intervention Registry (IFCIR), may help us gain insight into the learning curve and the minimum number of cases needed to obtain initial, and maintain ongoing, proficiency.

4.2.2 Fetal Risk

Fetal death during the procedure is not uncommon (11 %) and occurred across all procedure types. Additionally, early postprocedural (<48 h) fetal demise was an issue in this dataset. These rates, which are higher than those previously published in single-center experiences with fetal cardiac surgery, likely represent a combination of different learning curves combined with the known complications of any invasive intervention in a compromised fetus [17]. Fetal intraprocedural complication rates remain high, with bradycardia and hemopericardium occurring in a significant number of cases and across all procedure types, underlining the need for a team of experienced maternal/fetal and pediatric cardiologist and surgical practitioners whenever these cases are performed. Fetal bradycardia is common, occurring in about 50 % of cases in which there was needle access to a ventricle. Fetal bradycardia has not been experienced with access to the right atrium. The bradycardia is treated by discontinuing manipulation and either intramuscular or direct intracardiac administration of epinephrine. Small pericardial effusions are common, and moderate to large ones can occur and can be drained successfully. Thrombus formation within a ventricle can occur but usually resolves within days without treatment. Fetal aortic valve dilation may leave significant aortic regurgitation, which usually is well tolerated and improves or even disappears until the term. The rate of complications is definitely dependent on the experience of the operating team: fetal positioning, imaging, choice of the right instruments, correct diameter of the balloon, technique of balloon withdrawal, and management of complications have an impact and are subject to a learning curve [18].

Conclusions

During pregnancy there is a tendency to idealization of the unborn and attributed qualities, feelings, and abilities that he would like to possess. The child already has a fantastic space. The birth of a child with a birth defect is the loss of the imagined child. The new parents have to put together new indications. Considering that most of the diagnoses of fetal congenital heart disease are made after the 18th week of gestation, when the mother has already warned the first fetal movements. For these reasons gynaecologist and pediatric fetal cardiologist must have counseling skills, and a psychological support should be provided to the couple. The prognosis is a communicative event and not only an informative event. To follow the patient through difficult choices is one aspect of the medical profession as important as the diagnostic and therapeutic competence. Building and maintaining a relationship require a prerequisite: the empathy which is the imaginary reconstruction of the experience of the other. The counseling skills can be summarized in being able to maintain "the right distance" from the couple. It is important to learn to recognize our emotions and not to minimize the couple's emotions. On the other hand, it is mandatory to avoid behavior of fusion like excessive familiarity with the couple.

In conclusion, it is necessary that those involved in counseling of the interventional procedures (cardiologists, gynaecologist, anesthesiologists, and parents) speak "the same language," both in technical terms (avoiding language too complex) and, above all, in psychological terms. The needs of the couple must be put in the first place, and the pair is ridden without constraints in the difficult path that leads to the taking care of a fetus with a congenital heart disease. The words of Jean-Claude Fouron "We cannot run the Fetal echocardiography ignoring the consequences of our act" [19] enclosed all the complexity of this matter.

References

1. Caniano A, Baylis F. Ethical considerations in prenatal surgical consultation. Pediatr Surg Int. 1999;15:303–9.
2. Flake AW. Prenatal intervention: ethical considerations for life-threatening and non-life threatening anomalies. Seminars Pediatr Surg. 2001;10:212–21.
3. Aite L, Trucchi A, Nahom A, Zaccara A, La Sala E, Bagolan P. Antenatal diagnosis of surgically correctable anomalies: effects of repeated consultations on parental anxiety. J Perinatol. 2003;23(8):652–4.
4. Di Giusto M, Lazzari R, Giorgetti T, Paesano R, Pachi A. Psychological aspects of therapeutic abortion after early prenatal diagnosis. Clin Exp Obstet Gynecol. 1991;18:169–73.
5. Lorenz R, Kuhn M. Multidisciplinary team counselling for fetal anomalies. Am J Obstet Gynecol. 1989;161:263–6.
6. Dallaire L, Lortie G, Des Rochers M, Clermont R, Vachon C. Parental reaction and adaptability to the prenatal diagnosis of fetal defect or genetic disease leading to pregnancy interruption. Prenat Diagn. 1995;15:249–59.
7. Gotzmann L, Schonholzer S, Kolbe N, et al. Suspected fetal malformation in ultrasound examination: effects on the psychological well-being of pregnant women. Ultraschall Med. 2002;81:33–40.
8. Hunfield J, Agterberg G, Wladimiroff JW, Passchier J. Quality of life and anxiety in pregnancy after late pregnancy loss: a case–control study. Prenat Diagn. 1996;16:783–90.
9. Gewillig M. The Fontan circulation. Heart. 2005;91:839–46.
10. Rychik J, Szwast A, Natarajan S, et al. Perinatal and early surgical outcome for the fetus with hypoplastic left heart syndrome: a 5-year single institutional experience. Ultrasound Obstet Gynecol. 2009;36:465.
11. Allan LD. Development of congenital lesions in mid or late gestation. Int J Cardiol. 1988;19:361e2.
12. Yagel S, Weissman A, Rotstein Z, et al. Congenital heart defects: natural course and in utero development. Circulation. 1997;96:550e5.
13. Arzt W, Tulzer G. Fetal surgery for cardiac lesions. Prenat Diagn. 2011;31:695e8.
14. Golombeck K, Ball RH, Lee H, et al. Maternal morbidity after maternal-fetal surgery. Am J Obstet Gynecol. 2006;194:834–9.
15. Oepkes D, Moon-Grady AJ, Wilkins-Haug L, et al. 2010 Report from the ISPD Special Interest Group fetal therapy: fetal cardiac interventions. Prenat Diagn. 2011;31:249–51.
16. Gardiner HM, Kumar S. Fetal cardiac interventions. Clin Obstet Gynecol. 2005;48:956–63.
17. McElhinney DB, Tworetzky W, Lock JE. Current status of fetal cardiac intervention. Circulation. 2010;121:1256–63.
18. Mizrahi-Arnaud A, Tworetzky W, McElhinney DB, Marshall AC. Pathophysiology, management, and outcomes of fetal hemodynamic instability during prenatal cardiac intervention. Pediatr Res. 2007;62:325–30.
19. Fouron JC. The changing and complex relationship between paediatric cardiologists and life. Cardiol Young. 2000;10:551–6.

Part II

Aortic Valve Disease

Fetal Anatomy: The Aortic Valve in Fetal Aortic Valve Diseases

5

Annalisa Angelini, Marny Fedrigo, Carla Frescura, and Gaetano Thiene

5.1 Introduction

As in the adults, also in the fetus, the pathology of aortic valve diseases can manifest at subvalvular, valvular, or supravalvular level [1–4]. Fetal supravalvular aortic stenosis is very rare, while subvalvular stenosis is encountered more often in the setting of complex congenital defect, like posterior malalignment of conal septum, subaortic conus, or mitral valve tissue [5]. The most common fetal aortic valve diseases are represented by atresia or valvular stenosis.

5.2 Morphological features

Aortic valvular stenosis is often characterized by restricted cusps excursion and post-stenotic dilatation of the ascending aorta. In aortic atresia an imperforate membrane is guarding the aortic severe hypoplastic annulus and ascending aorta (Fig. 5.1).

Congenital aortic stenosis is a very rare condition falling in the spectrum of congenital left heart obstructions, encompassing a wide range of morphological features, from tricuspid aortic valve dysplasia or asymptomatic bicuspid aortic valve to unicuspid, severely stenotic valve to complete atresia and can be part of the hypoplastic left heart syndrome [1, 2, 6–9].

As in critical pulmonary valve stenosis, also in critical aortic valve stenosis, the blood flow and pressure during gestation impact on the remodeling cardiac process

A. Angelini (✉) • M. Fedrigo • C. Frescura • G. Thiene
Department of Cardiac, Thoracic and Vascular Sciences, University of Padua, Padua, Italy
e-mail: annalisa.angelini@unipd.it

G. Butera et al. (eds.), *Fetal and Hybrid Procedures in Congenital Heart Diseases*, DOI 10.1007/978-3-319-40088-4_5

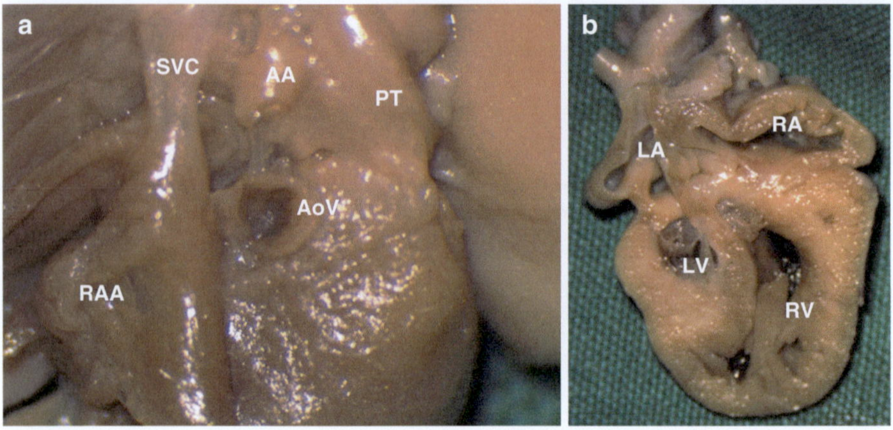

Fig. 5.1 Aortic valve atresia with imperforate valve. (**a**) View of the imperforate valve from above, after sectioning of the ascending aorta. Three well-formed commissures are still identifiable. (**b**) Four-chamber cut of the heart, showing the well-formed right ventricle reaching the apex and the dilated right atrium. Note the severe hypoplasia of the left ventricle, with hypertrophic free wall and minute mitral valve. *AA* ascending aorta, *AoV* aortic valve, *LA* left atrium, *RA* right atrium, *RAA* right atrial appendage, *RV* right ventricle, *SVC* superior vena cava, *PT* pulmonary trunk

and can lead to hypoplastic left heart syndrome (HLHS) due to impairment in left ventricle and aortic arch growth [10, 11].

HLHS with mitral and aortic stenosis manifests with severe aortic stenosis and left ventricular remodeling of different degree: at midtrimester of gestation, with hypoplasia, or dilatation, if associated to mitral valve incompetence; later in the gestational period, critical aortic stenosis can occur with a borderline left ventricle or even a relatively normal ventricle. In some setting the dimensions of the left ventricle remain unchanged throughout the gestational period [12–14].

Critical aortic valve stenosis can be due to an anomaly in the number of cusps, namely, unicuspid, bicuspid, or even quadricuspid, and/or to dysplasia of the cusps. The structure of the cusp is composed by the fibrosa covered by the ventricularis and the arterialis and by the spongiosa located on the ventricular side between the fibrosa and the ventricularis. In the setting of dysplasia, the structure is altered with loss of fibrosa integrity and mucoid degeneration and nodular thickening. The dysplastic cusps are usually thicker and rigid than the normal ones.

In the setting of unicuspid valve, there are one commissure with an eccentric intrinsically stenotic commissural orifice, only one well-formed interleaflet triangle, and a small aortic annulus and dysplastic cusp with myxoid nodular excrescences usually located on the ventricular aspect of the valve (Figs. 5.2 and 5.3). Two raphes can be identified as remnants of the commissures indicating lack of cusp separation or fusion. Bicuspid aortic valve is usually non-stenotic, and stenosis is usually present when there is associated dysplasia of the cusps (Fig. 5.4). Even tricuspid valve can be stenotic due to cusp dysplasia. The ascending aorta and aortic arch can be hypoplastic to a different extent. The left cavities can present with different patterns:

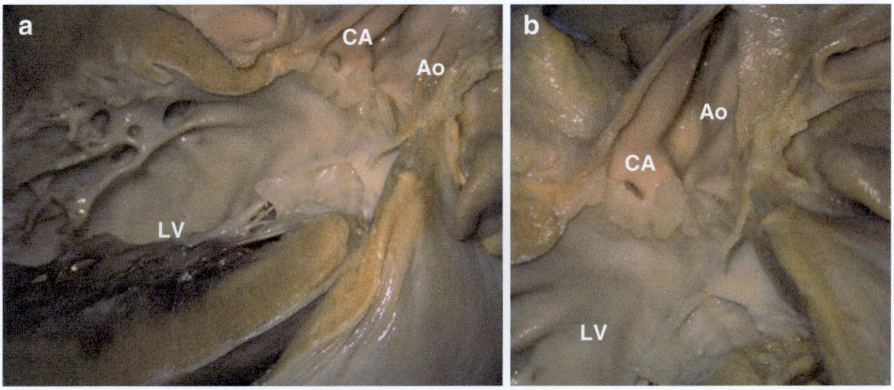

Fig. 5.2 Critical aortic valve stenosis with dysplastic valve. (**a**) View of the left ventricle and the aorta: note the unicuspid valve with severe dysplastic thickening and one identifiable commissure and the left ventricle with whitish thickened endocardium suggestive of endocardial fibroelastosis. (**b**) Close-up of the same specimen showing the hypoplasia of the annulus and the origin of the right coronary artery. *Ao* aorta, *CA* coronary artery, *LV* left ventricle

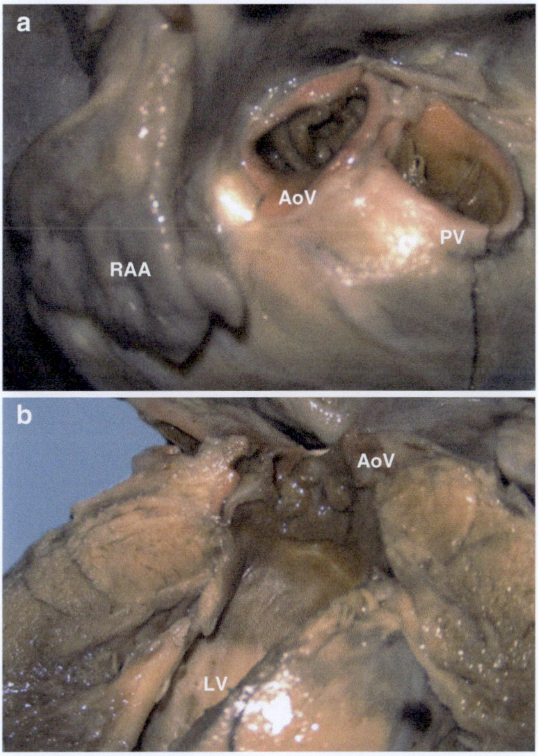

Fig. 5.3 Critical aortic valve stenosis with unicuspid dysplastic valve. (**a**) Right lateral view of the great arteries and of the right atrial appendage: the aortic valve present hypoplasia of the anulus and an eccentric orifice. (**b**) View from the left outflow tract showing the dysplastic cusp with nodular thickening. *AoV* aortic valve, *PV* pulmonary valve, *RAA* right atrial appendage

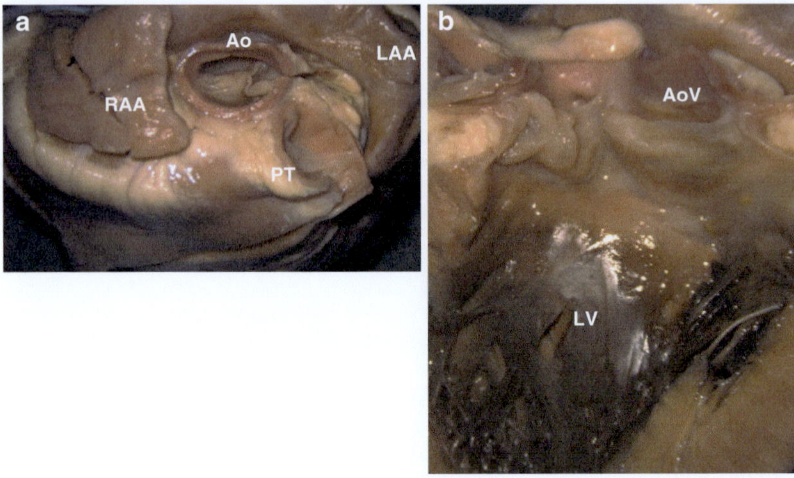

Fig. 5.4 Aortic valve stenosis with bicuspid valve. (**a**) View from the above of the great arteries and of the right and left atrial appendages two well formed interleaflets triangles and one aborted triangle in relation to the raphe are present. (**b**) View from the left outflow tract showing the two cusps, the anterior one with the raphe and dysplasia of the cusp. *AAo* ascending aorta, *LV* left ventricle

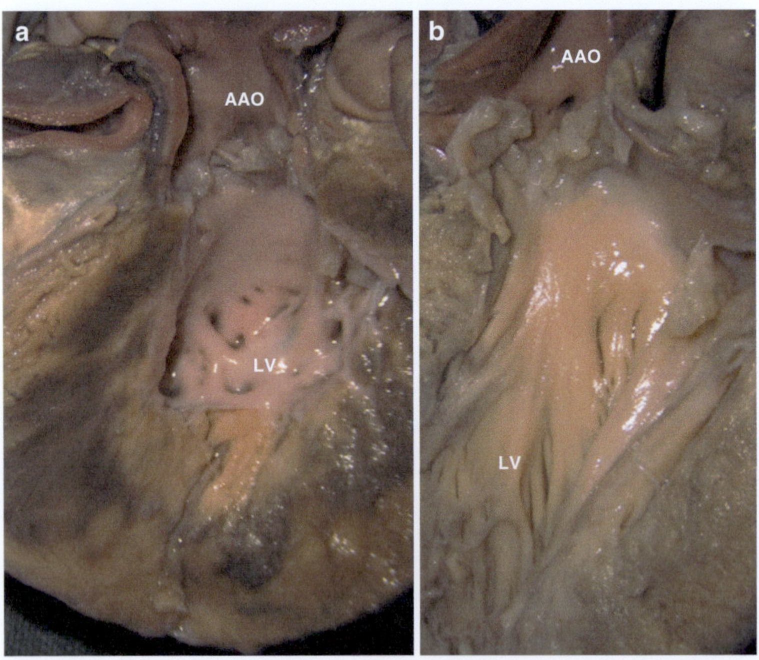

Fig. 5.5 Critical aortic valve stenosis with unicuspid valve. (**a**) View from the left outflow tract showing the dysplasia of the cusp and the small left ventricle with hypertrophy of the parietal wall and severe diffuse endocardial fibroelastosis. (**b**) View from the left outflow tract showing the dysplasia of the cusp and a more developed left ventricle and less severe endocardial fibroelastosis confined to the lateral wall. *RAA* right atrial appendage, *LAA* left atrial appendage, *Ao* aorta, *PT* pulmonary trunk, *AoV* aortic valve, *LV* left ventricle

Critical aortic stenosis and HLHS can be associated to severely restricted or intact atrial septum. With left heart obstructive lesions, there is left atrial hypertension leading to severe pulmonary vein dilatation and altered blood flow, which can produce dilated lymphatics and arterialization of the pulmonary veins.

Valve stenosis is due, in the majority of cases, not only to the fusion of the cusps with the presence of rudimentary commissures but also (sometimes mainly) to irregular cups thickening. These excrescences protrude into valve orifice and hamper its opening. Endocardial fibroelastosis is usually associated with critical aortic stenosis and can be focal, involving the papillary muscle or the septum, or can be diffuse to all the ventricular cavity with, at macroscopic evaluation, whitish appearance of the endocardium and severe thickening due to fibroelastic fiber endocardial deposition [15] (Fig. 5.5). There is no association between the severity of the endocardial fibroelastosis and size of the aortic valve and leaflet.

Conclusions

Aortic valve disease can present with a wide spectrum of abnormalities, at subvalvular, valvular or supravalvular level. Heterogeneity affects the number of cusps, grade of dysplasia of the cusp, and is associated with aortic annular hypoplasia. This is directed related to the number of cusps. Critical aortic valve stenosis or atresia is associated to hypoplasia of the left ventricle, mitral valve involvement and usually endocardial fibroelastosis. If mitral valve incompetence is present the left ventricle can be dilated with thin parietal wall and giant left atrium.

References

1. Frescura C, Ho SY, Thiene G. La collezione anatomica di cardiopatie congenite dell'Università di Padova. Cleup, Padova 1996.
2. Anderson RH, Devine WA, Ho SY, Smith A, McKay R. The myth of the aortic annulus: the anatomy of the subaortic outflow tract. Ann Thorac Surg. 1991;52:640–6. J Heart Valve Dis. 5 Suppl 3:S272-5.
3. Ho SY. Structure and anatomy of the aortic root. Eur J Echocardiogr. 2009;10:i3–10.
4. Sievers HH, Hemmer W, Beyersdorf F, Moritz A, Moosdorf R, Lichtenberg A, Misfeld M, Charitos EI, Working Group for Aortic Valve Surgery of German Society of Thoracic and Cardiovascular Surgery. The everyday used nomenclature of the aortic root components: the tower of Babel? (2012). Eur J Cardiothorac Surg. 2012;41:478–82.
5. Yamamoto Yand Hornberger LK. Progression of outflow tract obstruction in the fetus. Early Hum Dev. 2012;88:279–85.
6. Angelini A, Ho SY, Anderson RH, Devine WA, Zuberbuhler JR, Becker AE, Davies MJ. The morphology of the normal aortic valve as compared with the aortic valve having two leaflets. J Thorac Cardiovasc Surg. 1989;98:362–7.
7. Duran AC, Frescura C, Sans-Coma V, Angelini A, Basso C, Thiene G. Bicuspid aortic valves in hearts with other congenital heart disease. J Heart Valve Dis. 1995;4:581–90.
8. Frescura C, Thiene G. Small aortic root in neonates. J Heart Valve Dis. 1996;Suppl 3:S272–5.
9. Maizza AF, Ho SY, Anderson RH. Obstruction of the left ventricular outflow tract: anatomical observations and surgical implications. J Heart Valve Dis. 1993;2:66–79.
10. Arzt W, Wertaschnigg D, Veit I, Klement F, Gitter R, Tulzer G. Intrauterine aortic valvuloplasty in fetuses with critical aortic stenosis: experience and results of 24 procedures. Ultrasound Obstet Gynecol. 2011;37:689–95.

11. Freud LR, McElhinney DB, Marshall AC, Marx GR, Friedman KG, del Nido PJ, Emani SM, Lafranchi T, Silva V, Wilkins-Haug LE, Benson CB, Lock JE, Tworetzky W. Fetal aortic valvuloplasty for evolving hypoplastic left heart syndrome: postnatal outcomes of the first 100 patients. Circulation. 2014;130:638–45.
12. Marantz P, Grinenco S. Fetal intervention for critical aortic stenosis: advances, research and postnatal follow-up. Curr Opin Cardiol. 2015;30:89–94.
13. Maskatia SA, Ing FF, Justin H, Crystal MA, Mullins CE, Mattamal RJ, O'Brian Smith E, Petit CJ. Twenty-five year experience with balloon aortic valvuloplasty for congenital aortic stenosis. Am J Cardiol. 2011;108:1024–8.
14. McKay R, Smith A, Leung MP, Arnold R, Anderson RH. Morphology of the ventriculoaortic junction in critical aortic stenosis. Implication for hemodynamic function and clinical management. J Thorac Cardiovasc Surg. 1992;104:434–2.
15. McElhinney DB, Vogel M, Benson CB, Marshall AC, Wilkins-Haug LE, Silva V, Tworetzky W. Assessment of left ventricular endocardial fibroelastosis in fetuses with aortic stenosis and evolving hypoplastic left heart syndrome. Am J Cardiol. 2010;106:1792–7.

Fetal Aortic Stenosis: Natural History and Echocardiographic Evaluation

6

David Black and Gurleen Sharland

6.1 Introduction

Aortic stenosis encompasses a spectrum of abnormality ranging from mild to critical forms. Antenatal diagnosis of aortic stenosis can be made in the full range of the spectrum, but it is the more severe cases that are dominant in the fetal series, as these are more easily detected during obstetric screening scans. The progressive nature of obstructive lesions detected in the fetus has been well described, and this type of progression was first described in a case of fetal aortic stenosis [1]. In this chapter, we discuss the echocardiographic features, natural history, and progression of fetal aortic stenosis in relation to the degree and timing of aortic obstruction.

Congenital aortic stenosis occurs in 0.2–0.5 per 1000 live births [2]. In a series from a large tertiary referral center, aortic stenosis was diagnosed in 2 % of cases with fetal congenital heart disease, with 91 % of cases being critical aortic stenosis [3].

6.2 Fetal Echocardiographic Features

The usual form of obstruction to the left ventricular outflow in the fetus is valvar. Diagnosis is based on echocardiographic visualization of a stenotic dysplastic aortic valve with reduced excursion or an increased Doppler velocity across the valve or both. Impaired left ventricular function which may be associated with left ventricular dilatation is a feature seen in cases at the severe end of the spectrum.

Fetal aortic stenosis results in restricted movement of the aortic valve. The valve leaflets will appear thickened and the aortic annulus may be hypoplastic. There is

D. Black (✉) • G. Sharland
Department of Congenital Heart Disease, Evelina London Children's Hospital, London, UK
e-mail: David.Black@uhs.nhs.uk

G. Butera et al. (eds.), *Fetal and Hybrid Procedures in Congenital Heart Diseases*, DOI 10.1007/978-3-319-40088-4_6

often an association with a bicuspid aortic valve which is more commonly identified postnatally, though the valve may be tricuspid or unicuspid.

The Doppler velocity across the aortic valve in the normal fetal heart changes with advancing gestation. The peak velocity is around 30–40 cm/s at 14 weeks, increasing to 1–1.2 m/s at term. The peak velocity in the aorta is usually slightly higher than in the pulmonary artery. In cases of aortic stenosis, an increased Doppler velocity may be detected depending on the function of the left ventricle (see below).

The fetal echocardiographic features will be influenced by the degree and timing of obstruction.

6.3 Degree of Obstruction

6.3.1 Mild to Moderate

The echocardiographic appearance of the four-chamber view in these cases is usually normal. The size and function of the left ventricle are preserved. The dimension of the aortic valve and aorta is also normal. The aortic valve may appear mildly thickened or echobright with restrictive movement. Occasionally there may be associated post-stenotic dilatation of the ascending aorta. The Doppler velocity across the aortic valve will be mildly elevated in the range of 1.2–2 m/s.

6.3.2 Moderate to Severe

In the four-chamber view, the left ventricle may appear normal with preserved function. There may however be evidence of left ventricular hypertrophy (Fig. 6.1). The aortic root and aorta are of a normal size but may become smaller with advancing gestation. The aortic valve annulus is often normal although the valve itself will appear dysplastic and doming (Fig. 6.2). The Doppler velocity across the valve will be increased, and in cases with preserved function, velocities in the range of 2–4 m/s may be observed (Fig. 6.3). Color flow demonstrates turbulent flow across the valve and occasionally in the aortic arch.

6.3.3 Critical Cases

At least four different kinds of pathophysiology have been described in fetal critical aortic stenosis [4]:

(i) Early left ventricular hypoplasia with markedly reduced left ventricular size and volume in the first or early second trimester
(ii) Left ventricular dilatation with endocardial fibroelastosis and myocardial dysfunction which is likely to evolve to hypoplastic left heart syndrome
(iii) Left ventricular dilation and dysfunction with fetal hydrops

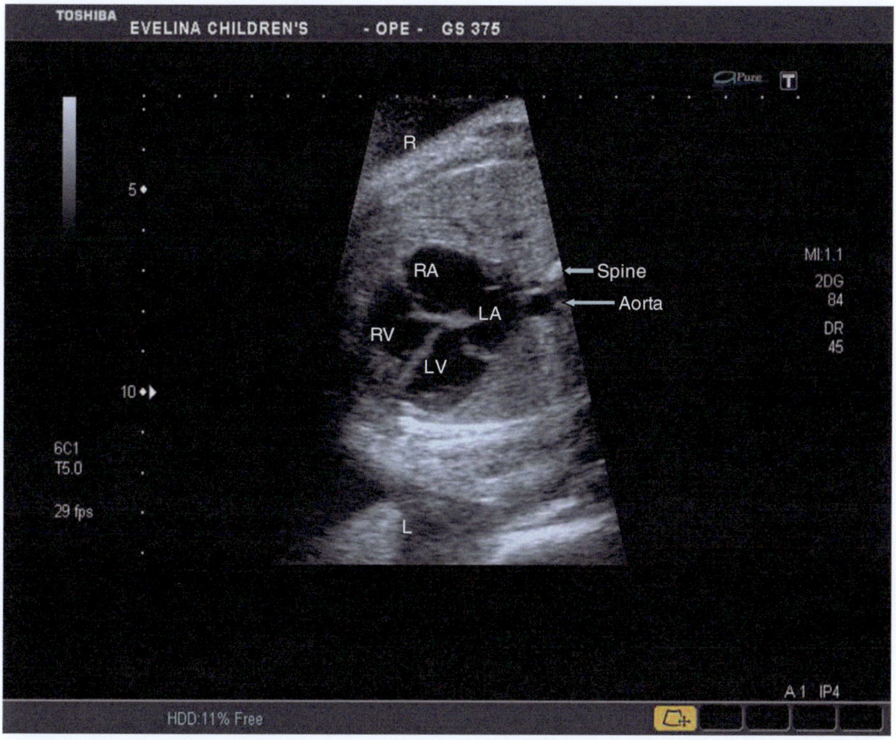

Fig. 6.1 Four-chamber view in a fetus with moderate aortic stenosis. In these cases there is often preservation of left ventricle function and size. *RA* right atrium, *LA* left atrium, *RV* right ventricle, *LV* left ventricle

(iv) Left ventricular dilatation and dysfunction with severe mitral regurgitation and an enlarged left atrium

It is not possible to predict which pathophysiology will be the predominant feature in a given case. In fetal lamb studies of left ventricular outflow tract obstruction during which the aorta was banded, the fetal hearts responded in different ways with some dilating and others becoming hypoplastic as gestation progressed. Interestingly in this study, endocardial fibroelastosis (EFE) did not develop, and the authors postulate that in fetal aortic stenosis, there may be an inherent myocardial microstructural abnormality [5].

Increased echogenicity of the left ventricular walls and papillary muscles of the mitral valve is often seen in critical cases. This appearance correlates well with the finding of EFE at postmortem examination and implies damage to the ventricular wall. In patients with critical AS, the presence of EFE is a risk factor for poor outcome [6]. There are also some cases that may have primary EFE but are difficult to distinguish from critical AS with EFE [7].

The aorta and aortic valve are commonly small for gestational age, although their size can be variable. The aortic valve is thickened and dysplastic, and due to the reduced left ventricular function, the Doppler velocity may be within the normal

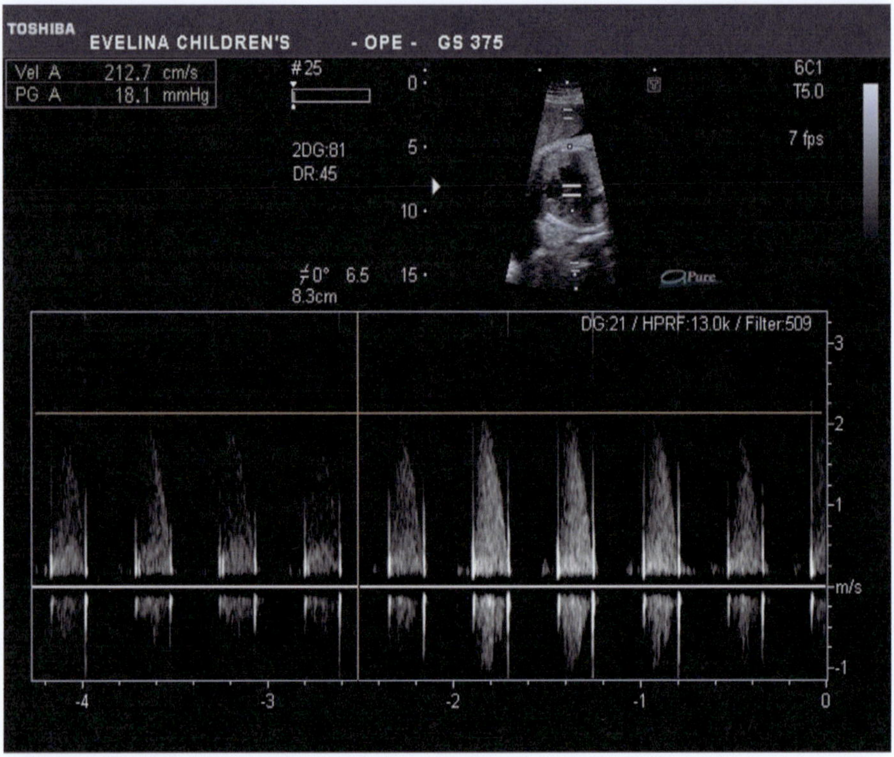

Fig. 6.2 Doppler across the left ventricular outflow tract in a patient with moderate aortic stenosis. The peak velocity of 2.1 m/s is above normal for gestational age

range. There may also be a lack of forward flow across the aortic valve with reversed flow into the transverse arch from the arterial duct. The mitral valve also appears abnormal in these cases and is restricted with reduced inflow. Mitral regurgitation is often detected with varying severity.

Critical aortic stenosis in association with an abnormal mitral valve with severe regurgitation, left ventricular dysfunction and dilatation, restrictive foramen ovale or intact atrial septum, and severe left atrium dilatation is a rare condition, frequently leading to compression of the right-sided chambers, low cardiac output, and hydrops, with a very poor prognosis (Figs. 6.4 and 6.5).

6.4 Timing

6.4.1 Obstruction in Early Gestation

In fetal aortic stenosis, a combination of hemodynamic and structural abnormalities leads to a decrease of blood flow through the left heart structures. It has been postulated that the degree of resultant hypoplasia depends on the timing of the obstruction; the earlier this occurs, the more severe the degree of hypoplasia will be [8].

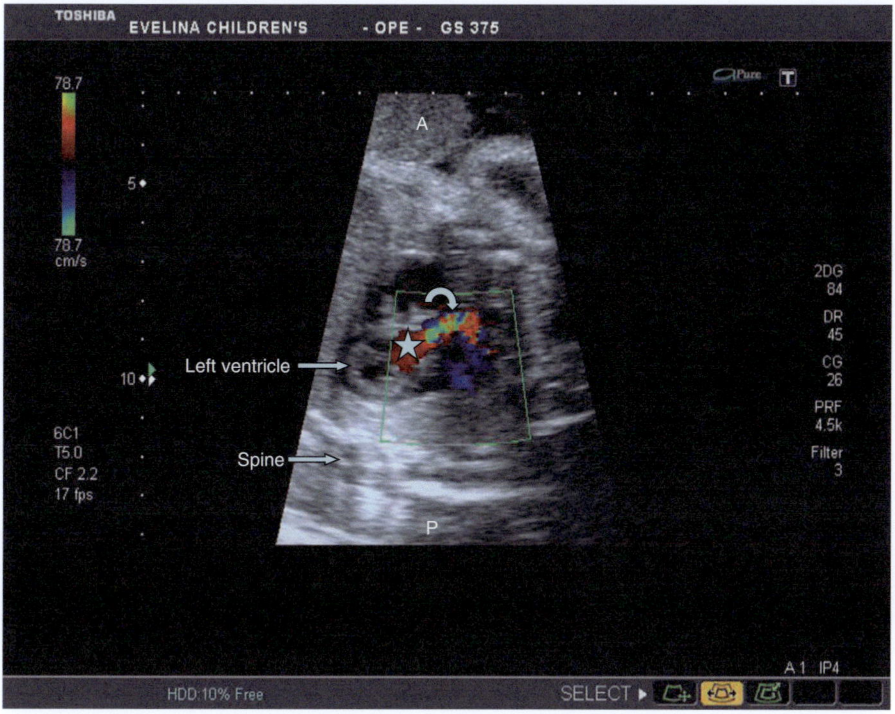

Fig. 6.3 Short axis view of left ventricle and left ventricular outflow tract in a case of moderate aortic stenosis. There is turbulent forward flow across the aortic valve into the aorta with a degree of left ventricular hypertrophy. Left ventricular outflow tract (☆) ascending aorta (↷)

With the advance of high-resolution ultrasound machines, the evaluation of the fetal heart in early gestation is possible. Aortic stenosis was detected at 11 weeks of gestation in a fetus with a normal four-chamber view, but evidence of an increased aortic Doppler velocity was subsequently shown to develop hypoplastic left heart syndrome by 17 weeks of gestation [8].

6.4.2 Obstruction in Late Gestation

For a diagnosis of aortic stenosis made in the midtrimester, the possibility of disease progression also exists. This progression may vary in severity with some fetuses ultimately developing a form of hypoplastic left heart syndrome. In these cases, the right ventricle continues to grow normally and ultimately forms the apex of the heart with the lack of growth of the left ventricle. Despite forward flow through the left heart, these ventricles would not sustain a biventricular circulation [9].

The prenatal diagnosis rate among neonates with critical aortic stenosis and ultimately a biventricular outcome is very low. This is likely due to a relatively normal four-chamber view in midgestation with the development of significant obstruction in the third trimester [10]. Not all cases of aortic stenosis will progress as some remain mild to moderate throughout the pregnancy.

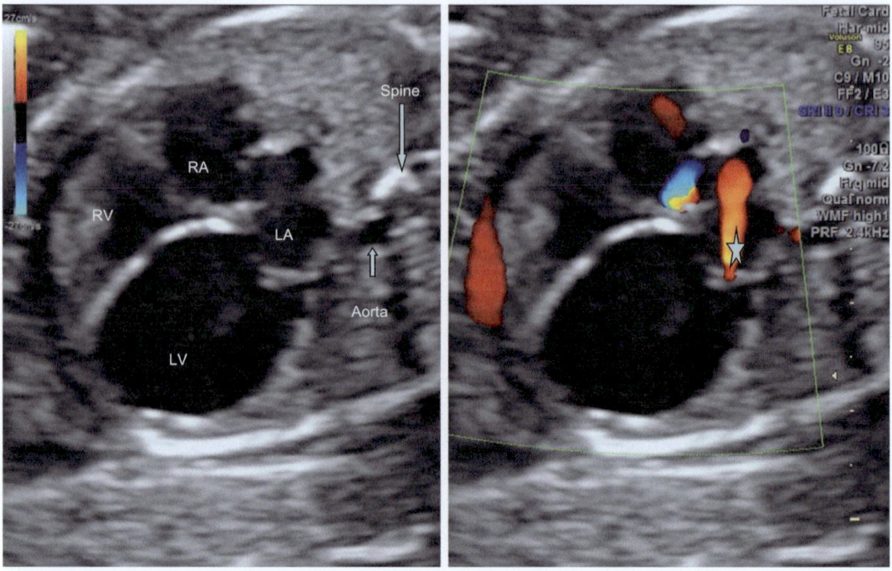

Fig. 6.4 Four-chamber view in a fetus with severe aortic stenosis. The left ventricle is dilated and globular with endocardial fibroelastosis. There is mitral regurgitation (☆). *RA* right atrium, *LA* left atrium, *RV* right ventricle, *LV* left ventricle

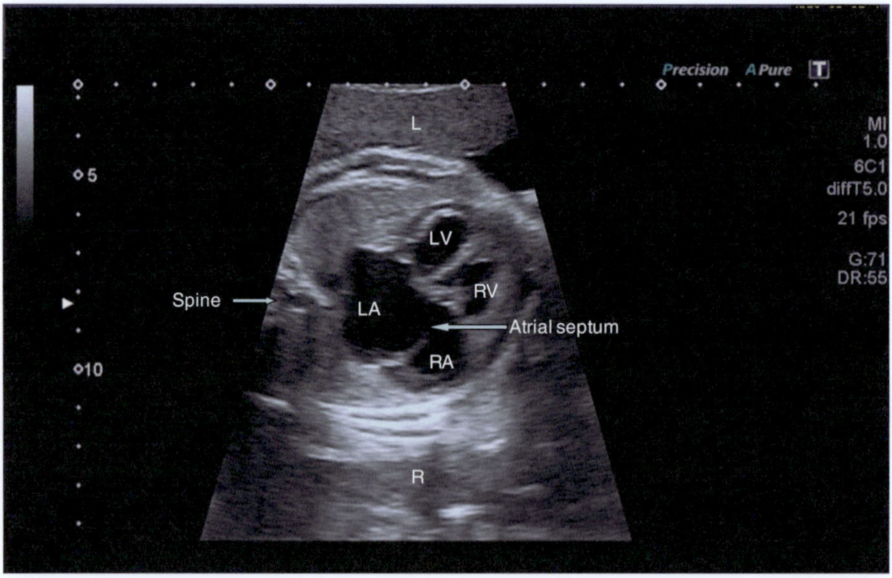

Fig. 6.5 Four-chamber view in a fetus with severe aortic stenosis and an intact atrial septum. The left ventricle is hypoplastic and is significantly dilated and bows into the right atrium. There was also significant mitral regurgitation in this fetus. *RA* right atrium, *LA* left atrium, *RV* right ventricle, *LV* left ventricle

6.5 Predictors of Progression

Sherman et al. have shown that if left ventricular growth is serially measured in fetuses with left ventricular dysfunction, the subgroup of patients who ultimately develop a hypoplastic left heart can be identified by arrested left-sided (left ventricle, aorta, and mitral valve) growth; second trimester identification of aortic obstruction in association with a dilated poorly contracting left ventricle, severe stenosis or atresia of the oval fossa, or other left heart obstructive lesions [11].

More recently, it has been shown that all of the fetuses that progressed to HLHS had retrograde flow in the transverse aortic arch, 88 % had left-to-right flow across the foramen ovale, 91 % had monophasic mitral inflow, and 94 % had significant LV dysfunction [12]. Recent data from our institution assessing progression to HLHS showed that if two or more of these criteria were present in early gestation, then a univentricular outcome occurred in 16 of 17 cases (94 %).

6.6 Outcomes

At our institution to date, there are 89 cases of aortic stenosis diagnosed prenatally. Of these, 5 % of pregnancies resulted in termination of pregnancy. If the terminations are excluded, then the outcome of the continuing pregnancies was 4 % resulting in spontaneous intrauterine death, 56 % died in the neonatal period, 4 % died in infancy, and 33 % were alive at last follow-up.

References

1. Allan LD, Sharland G, Tynan MJ. The natural history of the hypoplastic left heart syndrome. Int J Cardiol. 1989;25(3):341–3.
2. van der Linde D, et al. Birth prevalence of congenital heart disease worldwide: a systematic review and meta-analysis. J Am Coll Cardiol. 2011;58(21):2241–7.
3. Sharland G. Fetal cardiology simplified – a practical manual. Harley: tfm publishing ltd; 2013.
4. Marantz P, Grinenco S. Fetal intervention for critical aortic stenosis: advances, research and postnatal follow-up. Curr Opin Cardiol. 2015;30(1):89–94.
5. Eghtesady P, et al. Revisiting animal models of aortic stenosis in the early gestation fetus. Ann Thorac Surg. 2007;83(2):631–9.
6. McElhinney DB, et al. Assessment of left ventricular endocardial fibroelastosis in fetuses with aortic stenosis and evolving hypoplastic left heart syndrome. Am J Cardiol. 2010;106(12):1792–7.
7. Sharland GK, et al. Left ventricular dysfunction in the fetus: relation to aortic valve anomalies and endocardial fibroelastosis. Br Heart J. 1991;66(6):419–24.
8. Axt-Fliedner R, et al. Development of hypoplastic left heart syndrome after diagnosis of aortic stenosis in the first trimester by early echocardiography. Ultrasound Obstet Gynecol. 2006;28(1):106–9.
9. Simpson JM, Sharland GK. Natural history and outcome of aortic stenosis diagnosed prenatally. Heart. 1997;77(3):205–10.
10. Freud LR, et al. Low rate of prenatal diagnosis among neonates with critical aortic stenosis: insight into the natural history in utero. Ultrasound Obstet Gynecol. 2015;45(3):326–32.

11. McCaffrey FM, Sherman FS. Prenatal diagnosis of severe aortic stenosis. Pediatr Cardiol. 1997;18(4):276–81.
12. Makikallio K, et al. Fetal aortic valve stenosis and the evolution of hypoplastic left heart syndrome: patient selection for fetal intervention. Circulation. 2006;113(11):1401–5.

Fetal Aortic Valvuloplasty (FAV)

7

Carlos A.C. Pedra, Simone F. Pedra, and C. Fabio Peralta

7.1 Introduction and Historical Aspects

In the early 1990s, some renowned pediatric cardiologists such as Dr. Lindsay Allan in Europe, Dr. Norman Silverman in the USA, and Dr. Jean Claude Fouron in Canada applied evolving echocardiographic technologies to diagnose congenital heart diseases (CHD) in utero. A novel sub-specialty called fetal cardiology was born. Not only the prenatal diagnosis could be accurately made, but also serial echocardiographic examinations of fetuses with CHD allowed for a better understanding of the natural history of some diseases while still in utero. It was not long when the first fetal transcatheter aortic valvuloplasty was successfully performed in the UK under the leadership of Drs. Allan and Tynan, resulting in the advent of fetal interventional cardiology. Despite some initial resistance of the pediatric cardiology community to embrace such prenatal interventions because of legitimate concerns regarding their efficacy and ethics, the Boston group led by Dr. Tworetzky decided to push forward a strong program in this field in the early 2000s. Since then, their group have published a great deal of good data in fetal cardiac procedures, which helped to establish their role in the management of patients with fetal aortic stenosis (AS) and evolving hypoplastic left heart syndrome (HLHS), pulmonary atresia and

C.A.C. Pedra, MD, PhD, FSCAI, FACC (✉)
Catheterization Laboratory for Congenital Heart Disease, Hospital do Coração da Associação Sanatório Sírio, R Desembargador Eliseu Guilherme 147, São Paulo CEP 04004-030, Brazil
e-mail: cacpedra@uol.com.br

S.F. Pedra, MD, PhD
Echocardiography Laboratory for Congenital Heart Disease, Hospital do Coração da Associação Sanatório Sírio, R Desembargador Eliseu Guilherme 147, São Paulo CEP 04004-030, Brazil

C.F. Peralta
Hospital do Coração da Associação Sanatório Sírio, R Desembargador Eliseu Guilherme 147, São Paulo CEP 04004-030, Brazil

G. Butera et al. (eds.), *Fetal and Hybrid Procedures in Congenital Heart Diseases*, DOI 10.1007/978-3-319-40088-4_7

intact septum, and HLHS with intact interatrial septum or restrictive atrial septal defect. With evolving catheter and imaging technologies associated with favorable local scenarios, other groups also embarked on similar programs including ours in Brazil led by Dr. Fontes Pedra and the one in Vienna led by Dr. Tulzer. This chapter reviews our experience with fetal aortic valvuloplasty (FAV).

7.2 The Anatomy of the Stenotic Aortic Valve in the Fetus and Its Natural History

Aortic stenosis (AS) in the fetus can be associated with a variety of valve morphologies including tricuspid, bicuspid, unicuspid, or unicommissural. The aortic valve annulus can be normal or hypoplastic. Depending on the time period the diagnosis is made, left ventricular function can be normal or severely depressed with variable degrees of endocardial fibroelastosis (EFE). Variable degrees of mitral regurgitation (MR) and hypoplasia of the ascending aorta can be encountered as well.

Indeed, in some fetuses critical AS can evolve to HLHS while still in utero. This progression may be anticipated when some functional flow abnormalities are seen on fetal echocardiograms performed between 20 and 29 weeks of gestation. These markers were defined by the Boston group and are now used as indication criteria to dilate the valve in utero (see below) with the hope to avert this progression and achieve a biventricular (BV) circulation.

7.3 Indications of Fetal Aortic Valvuloplasty (FAV)

FAV is indicated in two scenarios: critical AS and evolving HLHS and critical AS associated with massive MR, giant left atrium (LA), and hydrops [1–3]. Critical AS is determined by the visualization of a thickened, almost immobile aortic valve with turbulent or decreased antegrade flow by color Doppler mapping on the echocardiogram. The Doppler-derived gradient across the valve can be low due to associated left ventricular (LV) dysfunction and therefore should not be used to select patients. In the former scenario, evolving HLHS is anticipated when there is moderate-to-severe LV dysfunction, reversed blood flow in the transverse aortic arch (TAA), left-to-right flow across the interatrial septum, and monophasic mitral valve (MV) inflow in mid-gestation. Dilation should be undertaken under 30 weeks' gestational age. The best candidates are those with larger LVs (LV diastolic length Z-score > −2 at the time of diagnosis), lesser degrees of EFE, and less spherical LVs. Occasionally, the procedure is performed with smaller LVs (LV diastolic length Z-score between −2 and −3) not only with the hope to avert LV hypoplasia but also to ameliorate LV function and promote antegrade flow across the aortic valve. In such patients, maternal hyperoxygenation may have a role to stimulate LV growth.

In the later scenario, although these fetuses usually have normal-sized LV, antegrade flow across the aortic valve is reduced due to valve stenosis and massive MR. Also, there is reversed flow in the TAA, heart failure, hydrops, and compression of the pulmonary veins and the right ventricle (RV). Aortic valvuloplasty and atrial septostomy (to decompress the gigantic LA and the lungs) should both be considered between 30 and 34 weeks' gestation as a "rescue" procedure to diminish the risk of fetal loss.

7.4 Center Experience and Step-by-Step Approach

From July 2007 to December 2015, we have performed 22 FAVs in 20 fetuses with critical AS with reasonable outcomes (see below). Our technique was developed based on previous publications on the subject (mainly by the Boston group) and on continuous medical education at meetings worldwide. FAV should be conducted by a multidisciplinary team, including the fetal cardiologist, the fetal medicine specialist, the anesthesiologist, and the interventionalist. Our step-by-step approach is described below.

The procedure is performed in a regular operating room (OR) under maternal conscious sedation and regional spinal blockade [1, 2]. To promote uterine relaxation, mothers are given nifedipine 20 mg TID for 48–72 h, starting 12–24 h before the procedure. If present, a large polyhydramnios is evacuated using a 15-cm-long 21-G Chiba needle (Cook Inc., Bloomington, IN, USA). After the mother has been anesthetized, an appropriate fetal position is almost always achieved by careful external version of the baby. We do not proceed if surgical uterine exposure is required. The fetus is anesthetized using a mixture of fentanyl (5–10 μg/kg), pancuronium (10–20 μg/kg), and atropine (20 μg/kg) given intramuscularly or in the umbilical cord using a 21–22-G Chiba needle [1, 2].

Under continuous two-dimensional ultrasound guidance, a 15-cm-long 17-gauge Chiba needle (with a stylet) is advanced to the LV apex across the maternal abdomen, uterine wall, and fetal chest wall. Occasionally, a transplacental and/or subcostal transhepatic needle course is required to reach the desired location. Optimal needle alignment toward the LVOT is crucial for procedural success. A pre-marked system (a rapid exchange 10-mm-long coronary balloon premounted over a cutoff 0.014″ floppy tip guidewire) is used. The needle, guidewire, and balloon shafts are premeasured and marked so that positioning within the fetal heart is known from external measurements rather than the ultrasound imaging alone. The balloon shaft is marked with sterile tapes so that no more than the full length of the balloon is extruded out of the Chiba needle tip when fully advanced. The wire is also fixed with sterile tapes so that no more than 3–4 cm of the distal flexible wire straight tip extruded out from the balloon tip. The LV is punctured at the apex, with the needle directed at the stenotic aortic valve. After stylet removal, pulsatile flow is seen coming off the needle hub. The catheter system is then introduced and advanced until the shaft mark reaches the proximal hub of the needle. Some very gentle manipulation of the catheter-wire system is required to cross the aortic valve. Seeing the wire in the ascending aorta is the unequivocal sign that the valve was properly crossed through the diminutive hole (Fig. 7.1a). Balloon positioning is primarily based on the external aforementioned measurements and ultrasound imaging. Balloons are

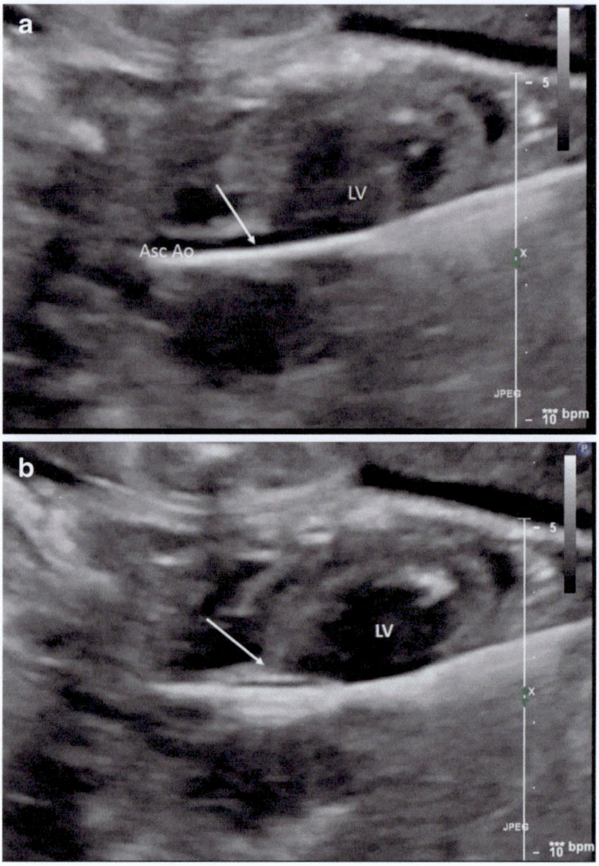

Fig. 7.1 Technical aspects of the procedure in a fetus at 25 weeks of gestational age. (**a**) The wire (marked by an *arrow*) is seen in the ascending aorta, which is an unequivocal sign that the valve was properly crossed through the diminutive hole. (**b**) The inflated balloon (marked by an *arrow*) is seen across the aortic valve annulus. *Abbreviations*: *Asc Ao* ascending aorta, *LV* left ventricle

inflated with pressure gauges to allow precise estimates of inflation diameters. Balloon diameters 10–30 % larger than the aortic valve annulus are selected for dilation. Two to four inflations are performed depending on the fetal clinical status (Fig. 7.1b). After the valve is dilated, the whole system (needle + balloon + wire) is withdrawn as a unit through the fetal cardiac wall and out of the fetal and maternal bodies to avoid shearing off the balloon from the catheter shaft. Small-volume-unit doses of epinephrine (1–10 mcg/kg) and atropine are available for immediate intracardiac injection to treat hemodynamic instability due to significant and persistent fetal bradycardia (<80–100 bpm for 3–5 min). Also a new 21–22-G Chiba needle should be readily available for pericardial drainage in case of tamponade.

After the procedure, mothers are hospitalized overnight. The fetuses are assessed the following day before planned maternal discharge. Echocardiography is performed at intervals determined by the primary fetal cardiologist. We have recommended that these mothers give birth at our own institution to customize the management strategy for each patient. In line with this policy, we believe that an elective C-section helps to better plan the next treatment step and at the same time posing less stress on such fragile patients.

7.5 Immediate Outcomes

Feasibility Success in crossing and dilating the aortic valve is observed in >90 % of patients. Reasons for failure include less than optimal fetal lie, too small fetus, poor imaging, and inadequate needle course toward the aortic valve. In our experience, we were unable to cross the valve in 2 fetuses at 22 and 23 weeks of gestation. The already small hearts in such young fetuses got even smaller after the LV apex was entered, which limited manipulations. Progressive worsening of the quality of imaging also played a role.

Complications Morbidity to the mothers is rare in the literature. We have not encountered any complications in our whole experience with fetal cardiac interventions (total of 45 procedures). On the other hand, fetal hemodynamic instability due to fetal bradycardia and hemopericardium is very common during FAV. Prompt pericardial drainage should be undertaken before the blood starts to coagulate in the pericardial space forming some sort of carapace resulting in prolonged bradycardia due to external compression. In our experience we had to drain the pericardium in 20/22 procedures. Fetal loss occurred in one of our failed cases, presumably due to excessive manipulation. This is also reported in the literature with a 10 % rate, approximately. Although fetal loss is more commonly associated with hemodynamic instability and hemopericardium, other contributing factors such as fetal and maternal anesthetic issues and mechanical stimuli may also play a role. Premature labor may ensue as in any other fetal intervention.

Efficacy A technically effective FAV is defined as one in which an unequivocal evidence of antegrade flow and/or new aortic regurgitation (AR) is seen on color Doppler echocardiography (Fig. 7.2). We have considered post-procedural AR as a marker of effective dilatation. It is well tolerated due to the low systemic vascular resistance determined by the placental circulation and the high end-diastolic left ventricular pressure and improves significantly or disappears until birth.

7.6 Follow-Up Outcomes

It is not uncommon to observe progressive improvement of LV function and size while such babies are still in utero (Fig. 7.3). Usually, satisfactory forward flow across the aortic valve is maintained until delivery. After birth, these babies are started on a prostaglandin drip for echo reassessment. The main question that rises after birth is whether the LV alone will be able to handle the whole systemic cardiac output. Many factors should be taken into account to answer this question and make the best decision for each patient including size and function of the LV, MV, and aortic valve and pattern of flow across the TAA and the ductus. We have not recommended achieving a BV circulation in the neonatal period in borderline cases. In such patients, we have employed a staged LV rehabilitation starting with a neonatal hybrid approach, which works as a bridge to a later operation in infancy

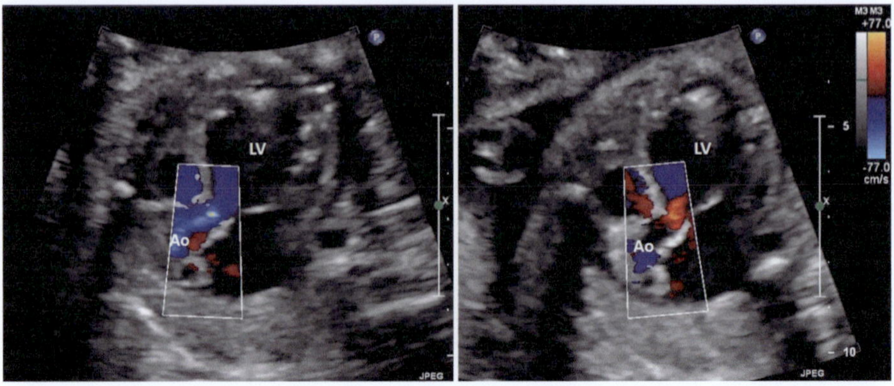

Fig. 7.2 Immediate results after successful fetal aortic valvuloplasty as assessed by echocardiography. *Left panel*: long-axis view of the left ventricular outflow tract showing unequivocal antegrade flow (*in blue*) across the aortic valve with color flow mapping. *Right panel*: same view of the left ventricular outflow tract showing aortic insufficiency (*in red*) with color flow mapping. *Abbreviations*: *LV* left ventricle, *Ao* ascending aorta

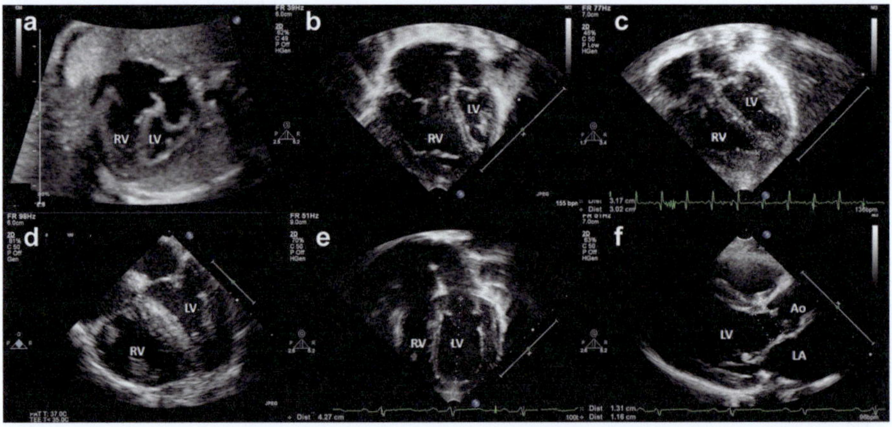

Fig. 7.3 Progressive growth over time of a small left ventricle after successful fetal aortic valvuloplasty and maternal hyperoxygenation. (**a**) Pre-procedural aspect of a smaller left ventricle that does not reach the heart apex at 27 weeks of gestational age. The *Z* value of the LV length was – 3.0. Significant and diffuse endocardial fibroelastosis is also seen. (**b**) Slight improvement of left ventricular dimensions and function in the neonatal period prior to a hybrid procedure. (**c**) Unequivocal increase in left ventricular dimensions at 5 months of age. The left and the right ventricles contribute equally to form the heart apex. The *Z* value of left ventricular length was – 1.5. (**d**) Transesophageal echocardiography immediately after surgical overhaul of the left ventricular structures at 10 months of age. A normal-sized and functioning left ventricle is appreciated. (**e**) A normal left ventricular length (*Z* value –1.0) is seen at the age of 18 months. (**f**) Normal-sized left ventricle and a widely patent aortic valve is seen on long-axis view at the age of 3 years. *Abbreviations*: *LV* left ventricle, *RV* right ventricle, *LA* left atrium

(9–12 months of age). This strategy gives more time to the LV to grow and/or improve its dimensions. The LV is overhauled later in infancy with EFE resection, aortic valve commissurotomy with leaflets thinning, MV plasty, ductal stent, and bilateral pulmonary artery band removal (Fig. 7.3).

In the literature, a neonatal BV circulation is achieved in about 30 % of fetuses who had undergone FAV. Usually these patients have a LV long-axis *Z*-score>0, a LV short-axis *Z*-score>0, an aortic annulus *Z*-score>3.5, a MV annulus *Z*-score>2, and a high-pressure LV defined by the presence of MR or AS with a maximum systolic gradient of ≥20 mmHg and milder degrees of EFE. It is our impression that even fetuses that have smaller LVs may also benefit from the procedure due to improved coronary flow and preservation of myocardial function, which may have a positive impact on neonatal outcomes, regardless of the surgical strategy (Norwood vs Hybrid) [1, 2]. In addition, promoting forward flow across the aortic valve in utero may theoretically help to minimize the neurodevelopmental abnormalities secondary to retrograde TAA perfusion. Moreover, progressive growth of the left heart structures during fetal life and over infancy resulting in an eventual BV repair has been observed our experience [1, 2] (Fig. 7.2). Out of our 18 patients who were successfully dilated in utero, only 3 had a BV circulation achieved in the neonatal period after repeat balloon aortic valvuloplasty. In five patients, a BV circulation was eventually attained after an initial hybrid operation followed by hybrid takedown and LV overhaul late in infancy. Although postnatal LV diastolic dysfunction may be an issue in these patients, we still think that this is a lesser evil than the immediate and long-term morbidity and mortality of a univentricular pathway [1]. Patients with no significant LV growth should obviously follow a univentricular pathway treatment strategy.

Fetuses with critical AS, severe MR, and gigantic LA have a somber prognosis no matter what is performed in the pre- or postnatal periods. This condition is commonly associated with either fetal loss or prematurity. In our experience, only one out of four patients with this condition survived, achieving a BV circulation after an initial hybrid procedure and LV overhaul at 9 months [2].

7.7 Future Ideas and Perspectives

Although our experience with fetal cardiac interventions in general is not huge (total of 45 cases, 22 FAV), we are comfortable at this moment to offer this treatment modality to all fetuses that need it, especially those with fetal critical AS. Proper selection is crucial to achieve better outcomes. Some might still consider ethics an issue with such interventions. However, proper multidisciplinary counseling on an individual basis generally solves any possible concerns over the procedure. Transparency is key for both the family and the hospital staff. Although we do not consider FAV an experimental procedure in our hands any more, we would agree that such intervention should only be performed by some very specific groups that can amass enough experience to analyze their own data.

Although there have been some technical refinements since its introduction, it is unlikely that we will witness a revolution with FAV in the near future. Imaging improvements will likely result in a more straightforward procedure. Miniaturization of catheters is likely to occur, which may help to minimize some complications such as tamponade.

Finally, it is unlikely that randomized trials will be ever undertaken to compare the outcomes of fetus with critical AS who underwent FAV with those who were treated conservatively. This information should be derived from large and well-designed registries. This initiative is already in motion and has provided some useful data.

References

1. Pedra SF, Peralta CF, Pedra CAC. Future directions of fetal interventions in congenital heart disease. Interv Cardiol Clin. 2013;2:1–10.
2. Pedra SR, Peralta CF, Crema L, Jatene IB, da Costa RN, Pedra CA. Fetal interventions for congenital heart disease in Brazil. Pediatr Cardiol. 2014;35:399–405.
3. McElhinney DB, Tworetzky W, Lock JE. Current status of fetal cardiac intervention. Circulation. 2010;121(10):1256–63.

8 Fetal Aortic Valvuloplasty: State of the Art

Francesca R. Pluchinotta and Wayne Tworetzky

The most commonly performed fetal cardiac intervention (FCI) is balloon aortic valvuloplasty. The primary aim of fetal aortic valvuloplasty is to modify the in utero natural history of severe aortic stenosis, characterized by left heart growth arrest, and prevent progression to hypoplastic left heart syndrome (HLHS).

Fetal aortic stenosis can be isolated or quite commonly is the dominant lesion associated with mitral valve and left ventricular myocardial disease. It includes a spectrum of severity from the mildest form, with patients requiring only a neonatal balloon aortic valvuloplasty, to the more severe form, resulting in HLHS at birth. Clinically significant aortic stenosis can occur at any gestational age. Importantly, the earlier it occurs in gestation, and in particular if it is moderate or severe in early or mid-gestation, the more likely it is to progress to HLHS.

In contrast, some fetuses have milder aortic stenosis in early and mid-gestation with it becoming more severe in late gestation. Such patients may have adequate left ventricular growth and are more commonly not detected until after birth and, if seen in late gestation, may not need fetal therapy.

At the time of diagnosis, fetuses with moderate-to-severe valvar aortic stenosis present with a normal-sized or dilated left ventricle in mid-gestation and then progress to HLHS over the course of gestation. Not all patients with HLHS have aortic stenosis as the inciting event but rather can be the result of inadequacy of a combination of left heart structures. However, the subgroup of HLHS that has captured interest for fetal therapy is those with predominant aortic stenosis and still normal-sized left heart structures. A selected group of these fetuses with aortic stenosis presents an opportunity for fetal therapy.

F.R. Pluchinotta, MD (✉)
Department of Pediatric Cardiology, Istituto Policlinico San Donato IRCCS, Via Morandi 30, San Donato Milanese 20097, Italy
e-mail: Francesca.Pluchinotta@grupposandonato.it

W. Tworetzky
Department of Cardiology, Children's Hospital, Boston, MA 02115, USA

G. Butera et al. (eds.), *Fetal and Hybrid Procedures in Congenital Heart Diseases*, DOI 10.1007/978-3-319-40088-4_8

When faced with a patient being considered for FCI, two important questions have to be considered. The first question is whether this heart defect, if left alone, will progress to HLHS at birth. The second question to be asked is whether, if a technically successful FCI is performed, the left ventricle can be salvaged resulting in a good biventricular outcome after birth. In addressing the first question, there are several papers characterizing the perinatal natural history of aortic stenosis. It is essential to understand that, unlike most other heart defects diagnosed and observed during gestation, aortic stenosis and its effects on the other heart structures is a progressive disease with a broad spectrum of severity and outcome. Predicting the natural history and likely postnatal outcome is fairly accurate at the extremes of severity, but we have to acknowledge that there is limited data predicting the natural history in those in between. Herein lies the challenge when considering patients for FCI. The consequences of making the incorrect decision for an individual patient can be as follows. On the one hand, performing a FCI on a patient whose heart disease is too far advanced may be futile in achieving the desired outcome and puts the patient at unnecessary risk. Similarly, we would not want to perform a FCI in a patient whose disease is mild enough to have an adequate result with postnatal therapy. On the other hand, not performing a FCI for a patient in whom we believe we can avert progression will result in HLHS at birth and consequently all its well-described morbidities.

Predicting progression of aortic stenosis to HLHS in fetuses with normal-sized left heart structures can be performed using color and pulse Doppler-derived physiologic aberrations that can occur alone or in combination. Most fetuses with aortic stenosis will have left ventricular dysfunction. Left to right or bidirectional flow at the foramen ovale is a consequence of elevated left atrial and left ventricular pressure that diverts flow away from the left ventricle. The elevated left ventricular diastolic pressure and dysfunction result in changes in the mitral valve inflow Doppler pattern. The normally biphasic pattern becomes either fused or monophasic with a shortened duration of diastolic filling. As the aortic stenosis progresses and/or the function deteriorates, the LV is unable to eject flow antegrade around the aortic arch. Consequently, the right ventricle (RV) takes over much of the systemic flow workload and provides flow retrograde around the aortic arch via the ductus arteriosus. Variable mitral stenosis and/or regurgitation are common although not shown to be predictive. The thought is that the higher the left ventricular pressure, the more healthy *or healthier* myocardium there is for recovery. Commonly associated anatomic features are increased endomyocardial echogenicity due to scar tissue formation and increasing left ventricular dilation or globularity. Predicting which fetuses with aortic stenosis have salvageable left ventricles has been more challenging and is the focus of ongoing research. It appears plausible that a left ventricle that still has some function, generates pressure, and has minimal scar tissue would be salvageable. Doppler estimation of the mitral regurgitation and aortic stenosis jet velocities are surrogate methods to estimate left ventricular pressure, but there is no objective technique to quantify myocardial echogenicity [1].

Surgeons have long argued that early neonatal repairs carried the promise of improved ventricular function and improved cerebral perfusion due to early removal of volume- or pressure-loading conditions on the ventricles. Logically the reverse remodeling phenomenon should be even more pronounced in fetal life where tissue is naturally prone to regeneration [2]. In selected case with aortic stenosis, opening the aortic valve in utero decreases the left ventricular afterload and promotes flow through the left heart. These may help to limit myocardial damage, prevent progressive left heart hypoplasia over the course of gestation, and may help to maintain two functioning ventricles. Moreover by improving antegrade flow through the aortic arch, brain perfusion may be improved, perhaps allowing for better neurological outcome. Indeed, brain growth, volume, and metabolism have been shown to be abnormal in the third trimester gestation in some forms of congenital heart disease with neurological morbidity recognized in up to 22 % of survivors of palliative surgery [3, 4]. However, FCI has not yet been shown to improve neurodevelopmental outcome and is the subject of ongoing research.

In 1991 Maxwell reported the first pioneering attempts at percutaneous fetal balloon aortic valvuloplasty in two human fetuses [5]. Despite the disappointing results, this work demonstrated for the first time the feasibility of the procedure in humans. From 1989 to 1997, six groups around the world attempted similar procedures and reported the result of 12 fetuses with aortic stenosis or aortic atresia who underwent ultrasound-guided balloon valvuloplasty in the third trimester of pregnancy. Technically successful balloon valvuloplasties were achieved in 7 of the 12 fetuses, but only 1 of these 7 survived beyond the newborn period. Although poor, this experience highlighted several important clinical and technical aspects, including patients' selection criteria, potential procedural complications, and equipment limitations [6].

The first reported single-center series of FCI for aortic stenosis with evolving HLHS was published by Tworetzky et al. in Boston in 2004 [7]. Of the 20 midgestation fetuses in whom the procedure was performed, aortic valvuloplasty was technically successful in 70 %. In addition, the data demonstrated improvements in fetal left heart physiology and promoted growth of the aortic and mitral valves sufficiently to achieve a biventricular circulation in almost a fourth of affected fetuses. Previously reported fetal aortic valvuloplasties were performed in the third trimester [6], which was likely too late in gestation to reverse the disease. In contrast, the encouraging data from the Boston group suggests that FCI should probably be performed as earlier as possible in gestation to have its intended effect. Interestingly, the Boston group compared the population that underwent successful fetal intervention with a control group of ten affected pregnancies wherein intervention was unsuccessful or offered but declined by the parents [7]. In the observational cohort, fetuses showed minimal growth in left heart structures during pregnancy and developed left heart hypoplasia requiring single-ventricle palliation after birth.

With growing experience in FCI and modifications of the technique, 5 years later the Boston group updated the results and published a larger series of FCI for aortic stenosis [8]. Of the 50 fetuses who underwent balloon aortic valvuloplasty, 17 (30 %) went on to have a successful biventricular outcome as neonates. Of the remaining 33 patients, 5 died and the others underwent a single-ventricle palliation. This large series of patients contributed to an enhanced understanding of the effects of fetal aortic valvuloplasty on left heart growth and function and demonstrated the importance of optimal patient selection and procedural timing.

In 2000 a group from Linz, Austria, started a FCI program [9]. In their experience, 67 % of live-born patients who had a technically successful FCI achieved a biventricular circulation after birth. The higher success rate with regard to postnatal outcomes of the biventricular group compared to the Boston data (67 vs. 24 %) might be explained by the older gestational age at the time of intervention, reflecting less severe and therefore later presentation and diagnosis of the defect and perhaps the less severe LV involvement (LV long axis *Z*-scores in Linz group 0.72 versus Boston −2.1).

In the most recent study from the Boston group that evaluated the postnatal outcome of 100 fetuses who had undergone FCI, 38 of the 88 who were live-born had a biventricular circulation, either from birth or after initial univentricular palliation [10]. Larger dimensions of left heart structures at the time of the fetal procedure and higher left ventricular pressure have been retrospectively recognized as predictors of successful fetal aortic valvuloplasty and eventual biventricular circulation [8], whereas moderate-to-severe endocardial fibroelastosis at the time of procedure is associated with lack of response despite technically successful valvuloplasty [11].

In conclusion, it is clear from present studies that in utero balloon aortic valvuloplasty can be performed successfully in selected fetuses with severe aortic stenosis and evolving HLHS with a biventricular outcome achievable in an increasing proportion of patients. Refinements in patient selection and timing of the procedure as early as possible are critical factors for success in achieving a biventricular outcome. Important in making this happen is the cooperation between specialists in maternal-fetal medicine and pediatric cardiology. Data from an international registry of cases presenting for fetal cardiac intervention [12] that includes 370 cases from 18 institutions demonstrate that overall the biventricular circulation rates for fetuses undergoing aortic valve dilation were 31 % of all procedural successes and 43 % of live-born infants with technical success.

Despite increasing procedural success and enhanced understanding of both the natural history and patient selection, in utero balloon valvuloplasty is not a standalone procedure. Almost all patients will require one or more postnatal procedures and eventually an aortic or mitral valve replacement. They remain with a variable burden of disease, the long-term outcome of which is as yet unknown. Fetal aortic valvuloplasty may improve left ventricular growth but still results in a neonatal borderline left heart requiring staged palliation or modified surgery to promote left heart growth. Centers involved in this endeavor continue to work on both improvements in technique and better understanding of this disease [9, 10, 13, 14].

References

1. Makikallio K, McElhinney DB, Levine JC, Marx GR, Colan SD, Marshall AC, Lock JE, Marcus EN, Tworetzky W. Fetal aortic valve stenosis and the evolution of hypoplastic left heart syndrome: patient selection for fetal intervention. Circulation. 2006;113:1401–5.

2. Gurtner GC, Werner S, Barrandon Y, Longaker MT. Wound repair and regeneration. Nature. 2008;453(7193):314–21.
3. Wilkins-Haug LE, Benson CB, Tworetzky W, Marshall AC, Jennings RW, Lock JE. In-utero intervention for hypoplastic left heart syndrome – a Perinatologist's perspective. Ultrasound Obstet Gynecol. 2005;26:481–6.
4. Limperopoulos C, Tworetzky W, McElhinney D, Newburger J, Brown D, Robertson Jr R, Guizard N, McGrath E, Geva J, Annese D, Dunbar-Masterson C, Trainor B, Laussen P, du Plessis A. Brain volume and metabolism in fetuses with congenital heart disease: evaluation with quantitative magnetic resonance imaging and spectroscopy. Circulation. 2010;121:26–33.
5. Maxwell D, Allan L, Tynan MJ. Balloon dilation of the aortic valve in the fetus: a report of two cases. Br Heart J. 1991;65:256–8.
6. Kohl T, Sharland G, Allan LD, Gembruch U, Chaoui R, Lopes LM, Zielinsky P, Huhta J, Silverman NH. World experience of percutaneous ultrasound-guided balloon valvuloplasty in human fetuses with severe aortic valve obstruction. Am J Cardiol. 2000;85:1230–3.
7. Tworetzky W, Wilkins-Haug L, Jennings RW, van der Velde ME, Marshall AC, Marx GR, Colan SD, Benson CB, Lock JE, Perry SB. Balloon dilation of severe aortic stenosis in the fetus: potential for prevention of hypoplastic left heart syndrome: candidate selection, technique, and results of successful intervention. Circulation. 2004;110(15):2125–31.
8. McElhinney DB, Marshall AC, Wilkins-Haug LE, Brown DW, Benson CB, Silva V. Predictors of technical success and postnatal biventricular outcome after in utero aortic valvuloplasty for aortic stenosis with evolving hypoplastic left heart syndrome. Circulation. 2009;120(15):1482–90.
9. Arzt W, Wertaschnigg D, Veit I, Klement F, Gitter R, Tulzer G. Intrauterine aortic valvuloplasty in fetuses with critical aortic stenosis: experience and results of 24 procedures. Ultrasound Obstet Gynecol. 2011;37(6):689–95.
10. Freud LR, McElhinney DB, Marshall AC, Marx GR, Friedman KG, del Nido PJ, et al. Fetal aortic valvuloplasty for evolving hypoplastic left heart syndrome: postnatal outcomes of the first 100 patients. Circulation. 2014;130(8):638–45.
11. McElhinney DB, Vogel M, Benson CB, Marshall AC, Wilkins-Haug LE, Silva V. Assessment of left ventricular endocardial fibroelastosis in fetuses with aortic stenosis and evolving hypoplastic left heart syndrome. Am J Cardiol. 2010;106(12):1792–7.
12. Moon-Grady AJ, Morris SA, Belfort M, Chmait R, Dangel J, Devlieger R, Emery S, Frommelt M, Galindo A, Gelehrter S, Gembruch U, Grinenco S, Habli M, Herberg U, Jaeggi E, Kilby M, Kontopoulos E, Marantz P, Miller O, Otaño L, Pedra C, Pedra S, Pruetz J, Quintero R, Ryan G, Sharland G, Simpson J, Vlastos E, Tworetzky W, Wilkins-Haug L, Oepkes D. International Fetal Cardiac Intervention Registry: a Worldwide Collaborative Description and Preliminary Outcomes. J Am Coll Cardiol. 2015;66(4):388–99.
13. Emani SM, Bacha EA, McElhinney DB, Marx GR, Tworetzky W, Pigula FA. Primary left ventricular rehabilitation is effective in maintaining two-ventricle physiology in the borderline left heart. J Thorac Cardiovasc Surg. 2009;138(6):1276–82.
14. Marshall AC, Levine J, Morash D, et al. Results of in utero atrial septoplasty in fetuses with hypoplastic left heart syndrome. Prenat Diagn. 2008;28(11):1023–8.

Part III

Pulmonary Valve Disease

9 Fetal Anatomy: The Pulmonary Valve in Fetal Pulmonary Valve Disease

Annalisa Angelini, Marny Fedrigo, Carla Frescura, and Gaetano Thiene

9.1 Introduction

Prenatal diagnosis has changed the understanding of the development of congenital heart defects during the gestational period. Some defects remain unchanged throughout pregnancy since the early period, while others evolve from mid to late fetal life. During gestation the pulmonary valve and trunk are slightly larger than the aortic valve and the aorta, and this difference persists until birth. The semilunar pulmonary valve is formed before the right atrioventricular valve is completed, and the cusps appear thicker early during gestation and progressively became thinner until birth. The nodules of Morgagni, identified at the line of apposition and free edge, can be identified also during fetal life. The structure of the cusp is composed by the fibrosa covered by the ventricularis and the arterialis and by the spongiosa located on the ventricular side between the fibrosa and the ventricularis.

9.2 Morphological Features

Pulmonary valve atresia and critical valve stenosis with intact ventricular septum usually develop in the setting of a hypoplastic right ventricle outflow, supporting the blood flow theory for the progressive onset of pulmonary valve stenosis and atresia and right ventricle hypoplasia during pregnancy and the development of intrauterine cardiac intervention therapeutic approach [4, 7, 8, 13, 17].

Pulmonary atresia with intact ventricular septum is a heterogeneous lesion morphologically characterized by the absence of communication between the right ventricular outflow tract and the pulmonary trunk [1, 19]. The size of the right ventricle

A. Angelini (✉) • M. Fedrigo • C. Frescura • G. Thiene
Department of Cardiac, Thoracic and Vascular Sciences, University of Padua, Padua, Italy
e-mail: annalisa.angelini@unipd.it

G. Butera et al. (eds.), *Fetal and Hybrid Procedures in Congenital Heart Diseases*, DOI 10.1007/978-3-319-40088-4_9

can vary considerably from normal size right cavity and pulmonary valve atresia at the level of the cusps with imperforate valve to severe right ventricle hypoplasia, lack of outflow tract, and pulmonary valve and abnormal right ventricle coronary artery communication. In these last settings, the hypoplasia of the right ventricle could be often ascribed to massive hypertrophy of the right wall due to the outflow tract obstruction [11, 14–16]. The associated anomalies will influence the outcome and management of these patients [3–5]. The tricuspid valve can be dysplastic or of diminutive size, and usually tricuspid valve dimension is directly proportional to the size of the right ventricular cavity [12, 18]. The presence of severe dysplastic valve cusps with severe incompetence can be a favorable parameter providing a potential right ventricle growth secondary to right ventricle overload. However massive tricuspid regurgitation can produce right ventricle negative remodeling with thinning of the parietal wall and dilatation [7]. The presence of the three components of the morphologically right ventricle, namely, the inlet, the trabecular, and the outlet portions, does not necessarily ensure an adequate size of the cavity due to the secondary hypertrophy [9]. Pulmonary arteries are usually of normal size retrogradely supplied via the ductus arteriosus. The presence of a restricted foramen ovale can reduce the right-to-left shunt and favor tricuspid and right ventricle growth. Fistulae are associated with pulmonary atresia and intact septum in one third of the fetal cases [2, 6, 8, 10, 15].

Focusing on the pulmonary valve morphology, three types of valves can be identified in pulmonary valve atresia/critical valve stenosis with intact ventricular septum:

- **Type a**: pulmonary valve atresia, due to imperforate valve, with a dome-shaped valve and two to four raphes (Fig. 9.1). Usually there is potential continuity between the right ventricle and the pulmonary trunk. Only seldom there is a muscular pulmonary atresia with no continuity between the outflow and the pulmonary trunk.
- **Type b**: critical pulmonary valve stenosis, with three dysplastic leaflets (10–20 % of patients with critical pulmonary valve stenosis) with a pinhole central jet of flow (Figs. 9.2 and 9.3).
- **Type c**: critical pulmonary valve stenosis, with the bicuspid or unicuspid valve with hypoplasia of the annulus (Fig. 9.4).

Type a is characterized by different morphologic features starting from pulmonary atresia with intact ventricular septum in the setting of imperforate valve but still with identifiable three cusps and well-formed commissures, as if the three cusps had fused after being well formed and differentiated during development. The right ventricle is variable in size but is usually small in around 50 % of the cases, moderately hypoplastic in 25 %, and normal in only 10–15 %. The right infundibulum is also hypoplastic with a hypertrophic parietal wall with an underdeveloped tricuspid dysplastic valve, small tricuspid annulus, and short chordae. The pulmonary arteries are usually normal in size and only in about 10 % of the cases can be smaller. Sinusoidal communications between the right ventricle and the coronary arteries

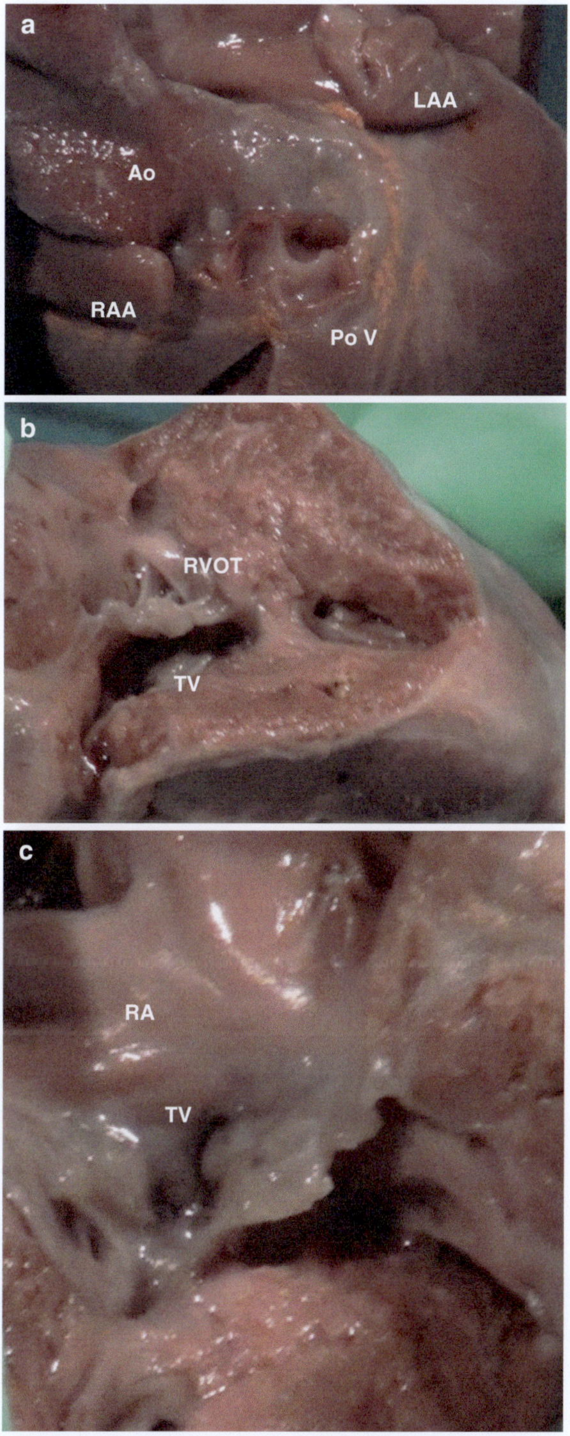

Fig. 9.1 Pulmonary valve atresia with imperforate valve. (**a**) View of the imperforate valve, after removal of the pulmonary trunk. Three cusps and well-formed commissures are still identifiable, as if the three cusps had fused after being well formed and differentiated. (**b**) The right ventricle has been opened from the apex toward the infundibulum. Note the severe hypoplasia of the right ventricle, with hypertrophic free wall. (**c**) The tricuspid valve has been opened along the acute margin of the right ventricle. Note that the tricuspid valve is also severely dysplastic. (type a). *Ao* aorta, *LAA* left atrial appendage, *PoV* pulmonary valve, *RA* right atrium, *RAA* right atrial appendage, *RVOT* right ventricular outflow tract, *TV* tricuspid valve

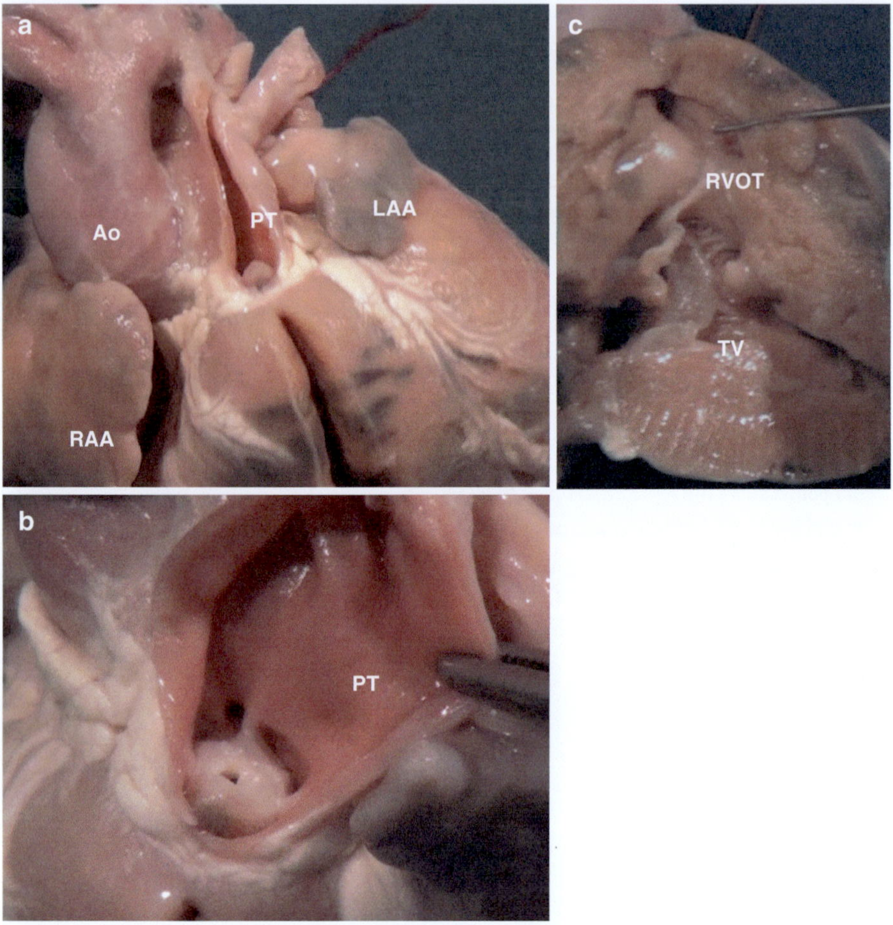

Fig. 9.2 Dome-shaped critical pulmonary stenosis. (**a**) Anterior view of the heart with hypoplasia of the pulmonary trunk and normal size aorta. (**b**) A dome-shaped pulmonary valve with a pint-point central orifice and dysplasia of the free cusps (type b). (**c**) A dysplastic and hypoplastic tricuspid valve is also present. *Ao* aorta, *LAA* left atrial appendage, *PT* pulmonary trunk, *RAA* right atrial appendage, *RVOT* right ventricular outflow tract, *TV* tricuspid valve

may develop as a mechanism of decompression of the blood from the right ventricle [6, 8, 15]. In some cases endocardial fibroelastosis can be detected in the right ventricle [8]. The right atrium is usually enlarged and hypertrophied, and the foramen ovale usually patent.

Type b is characterized by cusps with a dome-shaped pattern without clear separation in cusps, the appearance being of a thick curtain, with two to four raphes, and a pinpoint central hole allowing some blood flowing through the valve. In these cases the central hole can vary in dimension, but what seems constant is the hypoplasia of the pulmonary annulus and the dilatation of the pulmonary trunk and

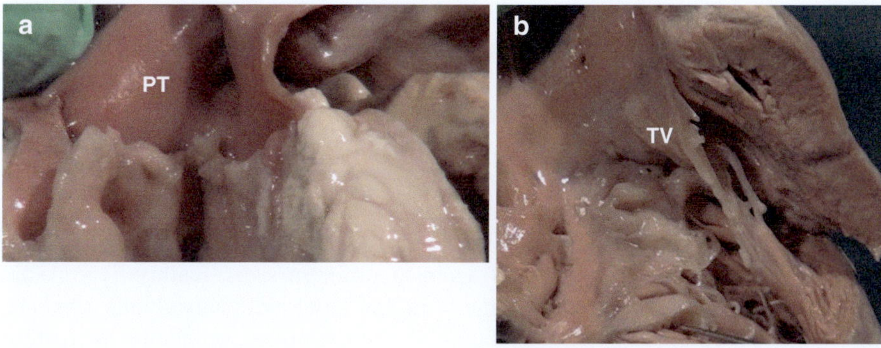

Fig. 9.3 Critical pulmonary valve stenosis and dysplastic tricuspid valve. (**a**) Note the three cusps with severe dysplastic thickening and identifiable commissures. (**b**) The tricuspid valve has been opened along the acute margin to show the severe dysplasia (type b). *PT* pulmonary trunk, *TV* tricuspid valve

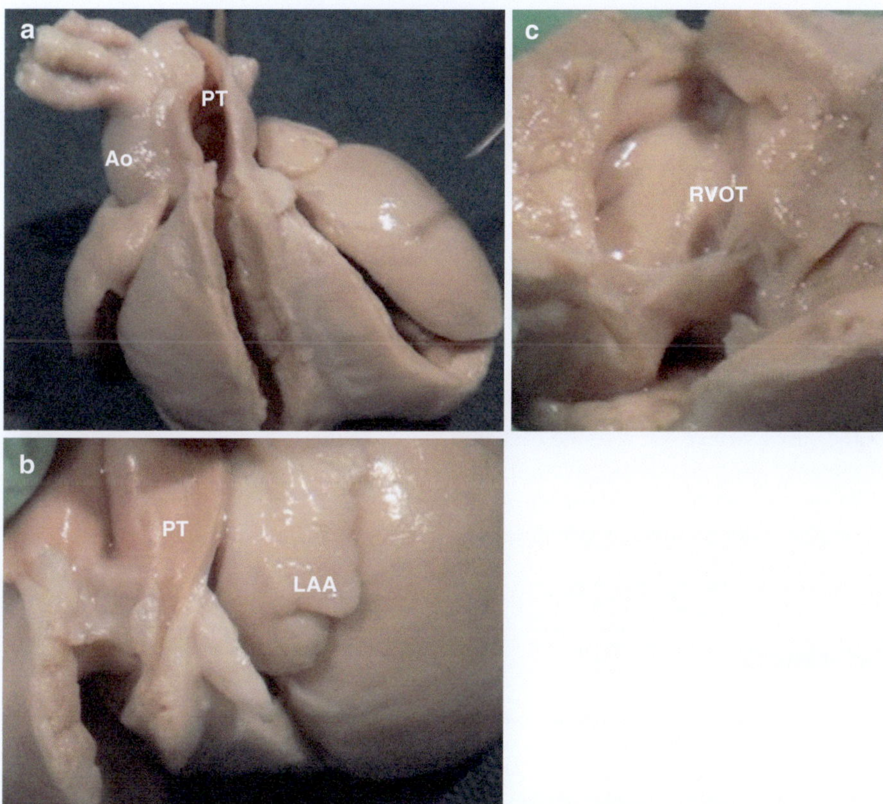

Fig. 9.4 Critical pulmonary valve stenosis with bicuspid pulmonary valve and hypoplasia of the annulus. (**a**) Anterior view of the heart with dilated pulmonary trunk. (**b**) Bicuspid and dysplastic cusps with hypoplasia of the annulus (type c). (**c**) Hypoplasia of the infundibulum and dysplasia of the tricuspid valve are present. *Ao* aorta, *LAA* left atrial appendage, *PT* pulmonary trunk, *RVOT* right ventricular outflow tract

pulmonary branches. The arterial duct is not so hypoplastic as one could expect, since it is the way through which pulmonary arterial blood flow is retrogradely guaranteed. The features of the right ventricle are similar to that of the pulmonary atresia and intact septum. In rare cases the pint-point dome-shaped valve can present with severe nodular dysplastic leaflets where it is still possible to identify three leaflets with a central hole. In other settings the three dysplastic leaflets are more developed with identifiable commissures. Histological evaluation of the leaflets showed mucoid degeneration of the fibrosa and disorganization of the leaflet structures. The right ventricular cavity is again of different sizes, mainly hypoplastic with ventricular wall hypertrophy, mainly infundibular, with subvalvular stenosis. In some cases septomarginal trabeculation can be prominent, producing the pattern of bipartitioned right ventricle.

Type c can be characterized by a bicuspid pulmonary valve with well-formed and thin bicusps, with or without a raphe but two well-formed commissures. The annulus is still smaller than in the setting of a tricuspid pulmonary valve. The right ventricle is of normal size as it is the tricuspid valve. The parietal wall is also of normal thickness. In the setting of a unicuspid valve, the morphology is that of a curtain-like cusp, with only one commissure and an eccentrically displaced hole. One or two raphes can be present as remnants of a commissure. The cusp can be dysplastic as well, and the right ventricular and atrial cavity similar to the other types previously discussed.

Conclusions

In the assessment of pulmonary atresia with intact ventricular septum/critical pulmonary valve stenosis, besides the evaluation of the valve morphology and the presence of cusp dysplasia, it is important to evaluate carefully the right ventricle dimension and hypertrophy, especially the outflow for subvalvular obstructions caused mainly by secondary hypertrophy, which is present in one third of the cases. Moreover, also the tricuspid valve desires precise assessment. Careful consideration should be given also to the left cavities since seldom aortic valve dysplasia and supravalvular aortic stenosis could be identified and could impact on fetal interventional procedure policy.

References

1. Anderson RH, Spicer D. Fistulous communications with the coronary arteries in the setting of hypoplastic ventricles. Cardiol Young. 2010;20:86–91.
2. Daubeney PE, Sharland GK, Cook AC, Keeton BR, Anderson RH, Webber SA. Pulmonary atresia with intact ventricular septum: impact of fetal echocardiography on incidence at birth and postnatal outcome. UK and Eire Collaborative Study of Pulmonary Atresia with Intact Ventricular Septum. Circulation. 1998;98:562–6.
3. Frescura C, Ho SY, Thiene G. La collezione anatomica di cardiopatie congenite dell'Università di Padova. Cleup, Padova 1996.

4. Gardiner HM, Belmar C, Tulzer G, Barlow A, Pasquini L, Carvalho JS, Daubeney PE, Rigby ML, Gordon F, Kulinskaya E, Franklin RC. Morphologic and functional predictors of eventual circulation in the fetus with pulmonary atresia or critical pulmonary stenosis with intact septum. J Am Coll Cardiol. 2008;51:1299–308.
5. Gardiner HM. Response of the fetal heart to changes in load: from hyperplasia to heart failure. Heart. 2005;91:871–3.
6. Gentles TL, Colan SD, Giglia TM, Mandell VS, Mayer Jr JE, Sanders SP. Right ventricular decompression and left ventricular function in pulmonary atresia with intact ventricular septum: the influence of less extensive coronary anomalies. Circulation. 1993;88:183–8.
7. Gómez Montes E, Herraiz I, Mendoza A, Galindo A. Fetal intervention in right outflow tract obstructive disease: selection of candidates and results. Cardiol Res Pract. 2012;2012:592403.
8. Guleserian KJ, Armsby LB, Thiagarajan RR, del Nido PJ, Mayer Jr JE. Natural history of pulmonary atresia with intact ventricular septum and right-ventricle-dependent coronary circulation managed by the single-ventricle approach. Ann Thorac Surg. 2006;81:2250–7.
9. Hawkins JA, Thorne JK, Boucek MM, Orsmond GS, Ruttenberg HD, Veasy LG, McGough EC. Early and late results in pulmonary atresia and intact ventricular septum. J Thorac Cardiovasc Surg. 1990;100:492–7.
10. Kipps AK, Powell AJ, Levine JC. Muscular infundibular atresia is associated with coronary ostial atresia in pulmonary atresia with intact ventricular septum. Congenit Heart Dis. 2011;6:444–50.
11. Lewis AB, Wells W, Lindesmith GG. Right ventricular growth potential in neonates with pulmonary atresia and intact ventricular septum. J Thorac Cardiovasc Surg. 1986;91:835–40.
12. Salvin JW, McElhinney DB, Colan SD, Gauvreau K, del Nido PJ, Jenkins KJ, Thiagarajan R, Crawford EC, Marcus EN, del Nido PJ, Tworetzky W. Fetal tricuspid valve size and growth as predictors of outcome in pulmonary atresia with intact ventricular septum. Pediatrics. 2006;118:e415–20.
13. Schidlow DN, Tworetzky W, Wilkins-Haug LE. Percutaneous fetal cardiac interventions for structural heart disease. Am J Perinatol. 2014;31:629–36.
14. Yuan S-M. Fetal cardiac interventions: an update of therapeutic options. Rev Bras Cir Cardiovasc. 2014;29:388–95.
15. Sandor GG, Cook AC, Sharland GK, Ho SY, Potts JE, Anderson RH. Coronary arterial abnormalities in pulmonary atresia with intact ventricular septum diagnosed during fetal life. Cardiol Young. 2002;12:436–44.
16. Tulzer G, Artz W, Franklin RC, Loughna PV, Mair R, Gardiner HM. Fetal pulmonary valvuloplasty for critical pulmonary stenosis/atresia with intact septum. Lancet. 2002;360:1567–8.
17. Van Aerschot I, Rosenblatt J, Boudjemline Y. Fetal cardiac interventions: myths and facts. Arch Cardiovasc Dis. 2012;105:366–72.
18. Yoshimura N, Yamaguchi M, Ohashi H, Oshima Y, Oka S, Yoshida M, Murakami H, Tei T. Pulmonary atresia with intact ventricular septum: strategy based on right ventricular morphology. J Thorac Cardiovasc Surg. 2003;126:1417–26.
19. Zuberbuhler JR, Anderson RH. Morphological variations in pulmonary atresia with intact ventricular septum. Br Heart J. 1979;41:281–8.

10 Fetal Pulmonary Valvuloplasty: Natural History and Echocardiographic Evaluation of Critical Pulmonary Stenosis/Pulmonary Atresia with Intact Ventricular Septum

Vlasta Fesslova and Savina Mannarino

Pulmonary atresia with intact ventricular septum (PAIVS) is a morphologically heterogeneous lesion characterized by variable dimensions of the right ventricle (RV) from a normal size to a variable degree of hypoplasia, often with associated anomalies of the coronary circulation. Critical pulmonary stenosis (CPS), also, is often present with an abnormal right ventricle.

Fetal diagnosis of PAIVS is relatively easy, although the differentiation between complete atresia and CPS may not be always feasible. The natural history of this complex anomaly diagnosed in utero and the predictors of neonatal outcome and of the type of postnatal correction (univentricular versus biventricular) are still objects of studies. The definition of anatomic features is fundamental for the prognosis and counseling in this anomaly.

10.1 Anatomic Features and Echocardiographic Evaluation

There is a wide anatomical spectrum involving all components of the RV.

Each echocardiographic examination should aim to:

- Achieve fetal biometry, calculation of C/T ratio, measures of the valves and ventricular chambers, and ratio of right to left heart dimensions including ventricular diameters and lengths and diameters of the atrioventricular valves and great arteries.

V. Fesslova (✉)
Center of Fetal Cardiology, Policlinico San Donato IRCCS, Milan, Italy
e-mail: vlasta.fesslova@grupposandonato.it

S. Mannarino
Pediatric Unit, Department of the Mother and Child Health,
IRCCS Policlinico San Matteo Foundation, Pavia, Italy

G. Butera et al. (eds.), *Fetal and Hybrid Procedures in Congenital Heart Diseases*, DOI 10.1007/978-3-319-40088-4_10

- Assign *z*-scores for valvular and ventricular dimensions.[1]
- Study the flow across the cardiac valves and the interatrial septum, in the fetal umbilical artery and ductus venosus (DV) in the absence of fetal breathing or movements, using the color and pulsed wave Doppler.
- Evaluate the ductus arteriosus (DA) (morphology and the direction of the flow and systolic and diastolic velocities).

10.1.1 Tricuspid Valve (TV)

TV and mitral valve (MV) dimensions are measured at the hinge points at end-diastole, immediately before the closure of the atrioventricular valves; tricuspid-to-mitral valve (TV/MV) ratio and valve *z*-score are calculated.

The TV orifice is more frequently hypoplastic, sometimes associated with dysplasia of valve leaflets. The TV appears restricted in the opening because of an increased right ventricular pressure.

More rarely the TV may seem apparently normal, or with a dilated orifice, or may present Ebstein's malformation or dysplasia.

The tricuspid regurgitant (TR) jet is visible across the valve. Continuous wave or high-pulse repetition frequency Doppler records a high-velocity jet due to the raised right ventricular pressure. To assess its severity, the visual impression, the duration of the Doppler waveform in the cardiac cycle, and the extension of the regurgitant jet into the right atrium (RA) are considered. TR is graded as absent, mild, moderate, or severe (holosystolic trace extending into diastole, TR reaching the back of the RA) [1, 2]. See Fig. 10.1.

10.1.2 Right Atrium and Atrial Septum

RA enlargement is seen in the case of a moderate/severe TR and elevated right ventricular filling pressure.

Fetal assessment of the foramen ovale includes the evaluation of the septum mobility and the recording of the interatrial Doppler flow velocities: a poor mobility of the flap and a Doppler velocity >1.5 m/s indicate a restrictive communication.

Interrogation of the DV and inferior vena cava waveforms is used as indicator of raised systemic venous pressure and is estimated as normal in the presence of a positive end-diastolic velocity or abnormal if the end-diastolic flow is absent or reversed [3, 4].

Fetal right atrial pressure (RAP) score is calculated from the combination of the severity of TR, waveform characteristics of DV, and restriction of the interatrial septum, with each parameter having a score of 0–2 [5] (Table 10.1).

---

[1] *Z*-scores representing the number of standard deviations with respect to the data of the normal population for a given gestational age, derived from echocardiographic data – Boston criteria, *Circulation*. 2009;120(15):1482–1490.

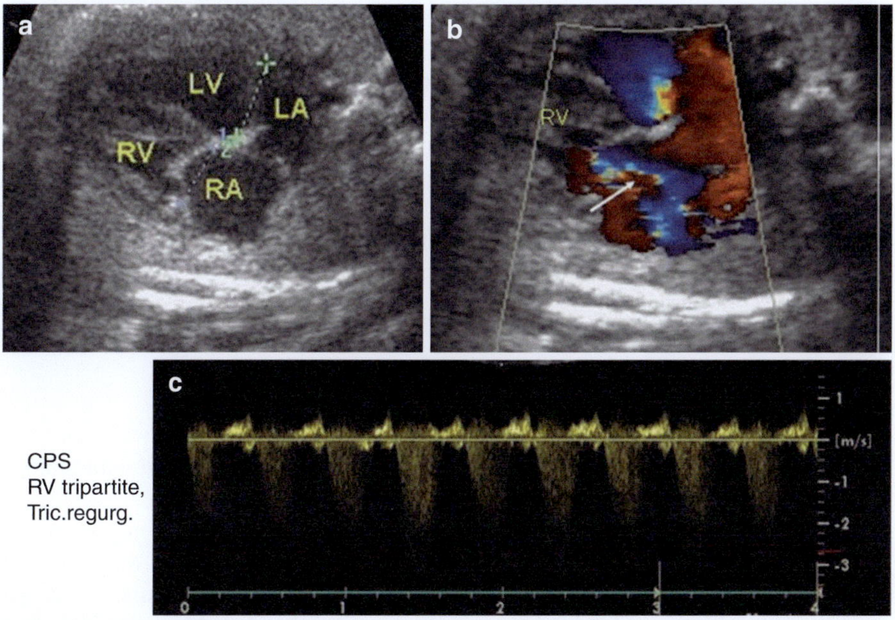

Fig. 10.1 Case with critical pulmonary stenosis with good RV (**a**), tricuspid regurgitation at color Doppler till the top of the right atrium (*RA*) in blue -arrow (**b**), and holosystolic regurgitant flow at pulsed Doppler. *LV* left ventricle, *LA* left atrium (**c**) Doppler gradient across the tricuspid valve

Table 10.1 RAP score

Points	0	1	2
Tricuspid regurgitation	None/mild	Moderate	Severe
Ductus venosus	Normal	Absent end-diastolic flow	Reversed end-diastolic flow
Foramen ovale	Normal right/left phasic flow velocities <1 m/s	Tense, bowing with moderate restriction; right/left velocities 1.0–1.5 m	Very restrictive Right/left velocities >1.5 m/s

10.1.3 Right Ventricle

The diameter of the RV is measured as the inlet length taken at closed TV from the midportion of the atrioventricular annulus to the apex of the RV at end diastole, in apical four-chamber view, to the endocardial surface [6].

The partiteness of the RV is morphologically evaluated by the number of parts of the RV not obliterated by trabecular muscular overgrowth:

- Tripartite: all three ventricular components – inlet, outlet, and trabecular – are present without intracavitary muscular overgrowth.
- Bipartite: overgrowth of the apical trabecular portion.
- Unipartite: muscular obliteration of both apical and infundibular portions.

The dimensions of the RV can worsen throughout the gestation to a pattern of a major hypoplasia with the RV progressively smaller in comparison with the left ventricle (LV). Parietal and trabecular RV hypertrophy is evident in this case and the right to left wall thickness is >1 [7]. Significant endocardial fibroelastosis is uncommon.

A septal displacement into the LV outflow tract may be present, and, when this bowing is extremely pronounced, an impairment of the left ventricular filling and function is possible.

More rarely a significant RV dilation with thin walls is observed, associated with a moderate or severe TR.

10.1.4 Pulmonary Valve (PV)

Differential diagnosis between pulmonary atresia and critical pulmonary stenosis (CPS) is difficult. In some cases severe pulmonary stenosis can progress to pulmonary atresia during the prenatal period [8–10].

Among different types of atresia, valvular atresia is more commonly *membranous* (in about 75 %), due to a complete fusion of the valve leaflets with a patent infundibulum existing in the latter setting up to the level of the valvular tissue. At echocardiography this valve is visible also during the systole with a potential for a continuity between the RV and pulmonary trunk.

In a minority of cases, a *muscular* atresia with infundibular obliteration is present, without echocardiographic continuity between the RV and the pulmonary trunk.

In the cross-sectional view of the great vessels, a retrograde flow through the ductus confirms the diagnosis.

In the CPS the valvular orifice is reduced by the fusion of the commissures of the valve, thickened and doming. An accelerated forward pulmonary blood flow can be detectable, in addition to the reversed flow from the DA at color Doppler, in severe cases. See Fig. 10.2.

All vessel measurements are estimated at their maximum dimensions, at the end of systole, and z-score is calculated. Pulmonary/aorta ratio is obtained at the level of the annulus of both vessels. The PV and pulmonary trunk are usually smaller than normal for gestational age and of aortic annulus.

The pulmonary arteries are confluent ranging from slightly smaller dimensions in comparison with the normal values to a severe hypoplasia and are usually supplied in the fetal life in a retrograde way from the DA.

10.1.5 Ductus Arteriosus

An acute angled ductus tends to arise more proximally from the aortic arch than usual. The flow at color Doppler is interrogated – showing a total retrograde flow toward the valvular plane in the case of PAIVS (see Fig. 10.3) and a partial component of an anterograde flow in the case of CPS.

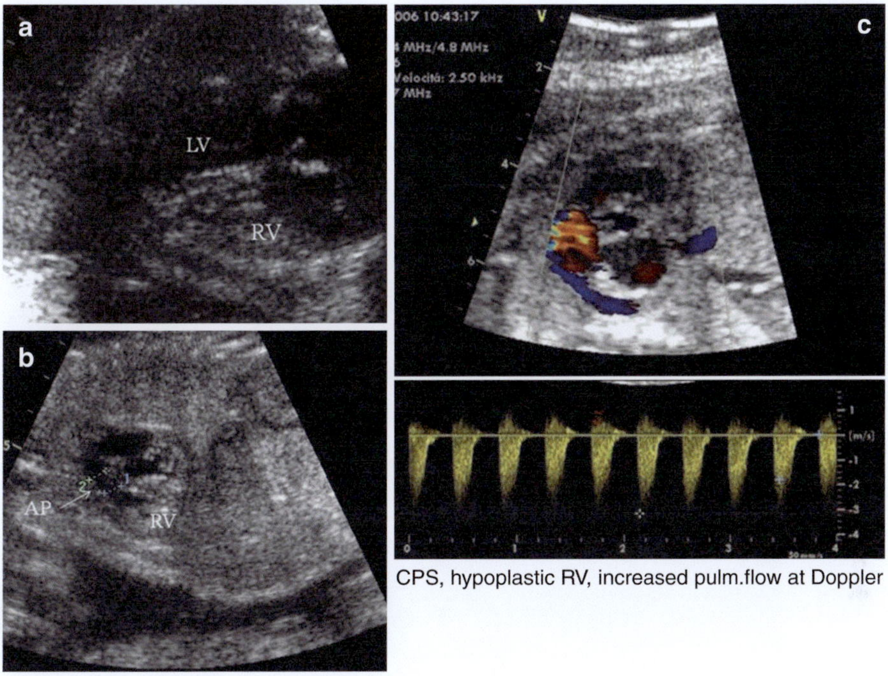

Fig. 10.2 Case with critical pulmonary stenosis with hypoplastic RV (**a**), small pulmonary valve annulus (**b**), and increased pulmonary flow at Doppler (**c**)

10.1.6 Ventriculocoronary Connections (VCCs)

Coronary artery anomalies in PAIVS include RV-to-coronary artery fistulae and/or coronary artery stenosis and occlusions.

VCCs occur as a persistence of the primitive connections in the condition of a high pressure, from the RV to the aorta in systole and from the aorta to the RV in diastole. They are reported both in cases of PAIVS and CPS [11].

VCCs are more frequent in cases with RV hypoplasia (z-score < −3) and major hypoplasia of the main pulmonary artery and the sigmoid shape of the DA [11, 12].

RV-to-coronary artery fistulae have been reported to occur in 31–68 % of patients with PAIVS [13–15].

RV-dependent coronary circulation (RVDCC) is defined by:

1. The presence of ventriculocoronary fistulae with severe obstruction of at least two major coronary arteries
2. Complete aortocoronary atresia
3. Situations in which a significant portion of the LV myocardium is supplied by the RV

PAIVS,
reversed
flow from
the duct

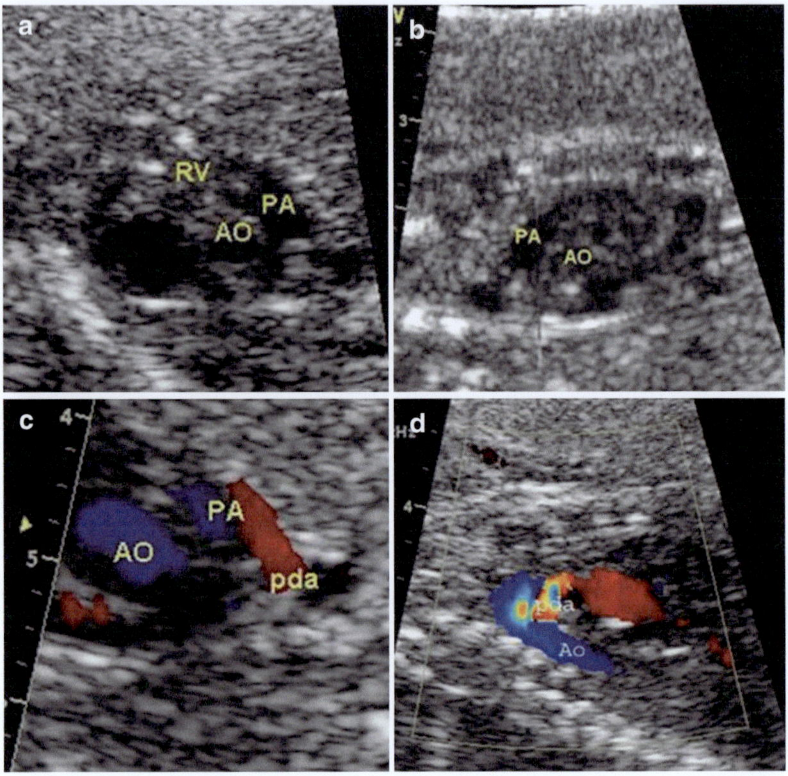

Fig. 10.3 Two-D echocardiographic images (**a** and **b**). Case with pulmonary atresia and intact septum (PAIVS) and reversed pulmonary flow from the duct at color Doppler – in *red* (**c**, **d**). *PA* pulmonary artery, *Ao* aorta, *pda* ductus arteriosus

RVDCC may cause RV "steal" in the presence of fistulae alone and ischemia, coronary isolation, or myocardial infarction in the presence of coronary stenosis [13, 16].

The coronary stenosis is usually not detectable prenatally by echocardiography, while a more precise evaluation of the VCCs is possible by a postnatal angiography.

Echocardiographic Evaluation The evaluation of the fetal coronary circulation is now possible with high-resolution 2-D imaging and with new color Doppler techniques.

The coronary arteries in normal heart are difficult to detect by fetal echocardiography. In PAIVS or CPS, the systematic evaluation to assess VCCs involves scanning the aortic root and the right ventricular myocardium using color Doppler mapping with a low-velocity setting.

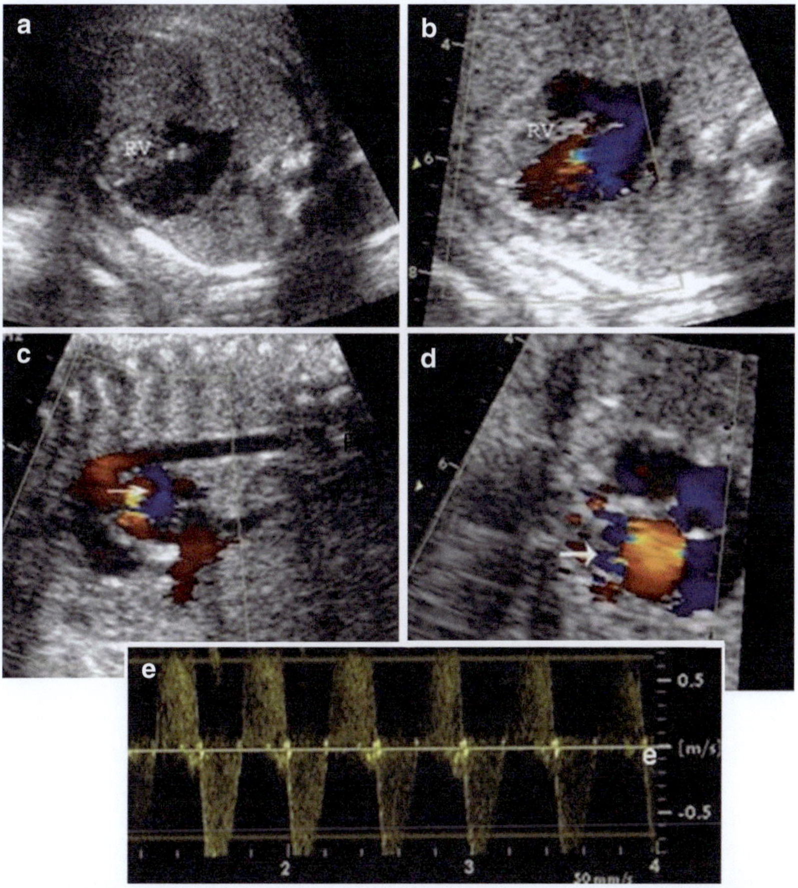

PAIVS,
+
sinusoids

Fig. 10.4 Case of PAIVS and hypoplastic RV (**a**, **b**), reversed flow from the duct (**c**), and turbulent flow at color Doppler due to sinusoids (**d**), with systodiastolic flow at pulsed Doppler (**e**)

When turbulent color signal is identified only on the epicardial surface of the myocardium and within trabeculations of the RV, *minor fistulae or sinusoids* may be suspected (see Fig. 10.4). In this case there is a connection between trabeculations of the RV and coronary capillaries with a slight filling of nondilated coronary arteries. In the presence of intracavitary right ventricular connections, the coronary turbulent diastolic flow pattern is best seen at the transverse section of the fetal heart, immediately over the five-chamber view, but sometimes this flow is difficult to record.

The existence of a VCC between the right ventricle and right coronary artery (*mayor fistulae*) is suspected when a dilated vessel along the right ventricular wall is observed, and color flow imaging reveals that this blood flow arises from the aortic root and faces the right ventricular chamber. The pulsed Doppler interrogation shows a forward diastolic and reversed systolic flow.

Multiple VCCs with the possibility of RVDCC are suspected when other abnormal blood flows are found between the right ventricular wall and the left coronary artery [13, 17–19].

10.1.7 Other Abnormalities

LV: very rarely, it is possible to observe spongiform noncompactile interventricular septum, dysplastic MV, or concentric LV hypertrophy [20].

Also left superior caval vein, right aortic arch, and aberrant subclavian artery are rarely described.

Associated extracardiac or chromosomal anomalies are reported: chromosome 22 deletion and, rarely, chromosome 4p deletion and Dandy-Walker syndrome [20, 21].

10.2 Natural History

When the right heart is small in the second and third trimester, its dimensions can worsen during the remaining gestation to a pattern of a major degree hypoplasia. Equally, severe pulmonary valvular stenosis can progress to a complete atresia [22].

The possibility of the development of a hypoplastic RV led to the idea of performing an early valvuloplasty already in utero with the aim of making possible a postnatal biventricular repair: the selection criteria of cases and the results obtained until now will be treated in a specific chapter.

Severe anomalies of the tricuspid valve as Ebstein or non-Ebstein anomaly with important valvular regurgitation may predispose to the hydrops fetalis and intrauterine death [23].

Fetal growth may be restricted in some cases of PAIVS and CPS.

Failed differentiation between CPS and PAIVS in fetal life will not in any case affect the prenatal and postnatal management of the case, because of a similar strategy.

10.2.1 Postnatal Treatment

Postnatally, a ductus-dependent circulation with desaturation and cyanosis is present, often with a need of a respiratory assistance. The first procedure after birth is the prostaglandin treatment. Then, after a reevaluation of the cardiac features, the decision is taken with regard to the possibility of the RV decompression in suitable cases (without VCCs), by means of pulmonary valvuloplasty, usually with the need of radiofrequency opening of the valve, establishing so the RV-PA continuity with a potential for the subsequent RV and TV growth. Otherwise, systemic pulmonary shunt is performed, in alternative to the ductal stenting. This approach may be needed also after the valvuloplasty, if the arterial saturation does not improve, due to inadequacy of the RV to provide a valid pulmonary flow [24].

A disproportional growth of the tricuspid valve with respect to the somatic growth can occur, especially in patients with small tricuspid valves and lower right ventricular pressures after decompression [25].

The size of the TV and RV will determine the type of the final repair – the possibility of a Fontan operation. Long-term outcome after Fontan is comparable to other complex cardiac anomalies treated this way.

Management of Cases with VCCs A main surgical option is the creation of a systemic-to-pulmonary shunt. However, there is a rather relevant postnatal mortality due to ischemia/coronary events, in these cases. Subsequently, a single-ventricle palliation provides a good long-term clinical outcome even in this category of patients [26]. In some cases, however, there may be a progression of the size and numbers of coronary fistulae at the long term, with clinical symptomatology of ischemia at exercise, and this should be kept in mind.

More rarely, an option of the tricuspid valve closure is chosen [27].

10.2.2 Predictors for the Postnatal Outcomes and Treatment

Different studies have used tricuspid and pulmonary valve fetal *z*-scores to predict a postnatal biventricular or univentricular repair.

For Gardiner et al. [5], the TV *z*-score was a good predictor in all cases studied, but the best predictive scores for a postnatal biventricular repair were the PV *z*-score > −1 and the median TV *z*-score > −3.4 before 23 weeks, the median TV score > −3.95 before 26 weeks, the combination of median PV *z*-score and the median TV/MV ratio (at 26–31 weeks), and the combination of median TV *z*-score and median TV/MV ratio (>31 weeks). The RAP score and the evidence of coronary fistulae were good independent predictors: RAP score > 3 predicted biventricular repair, and the detection of fistulae usually predicted a univentricular route.

In the study of Salvin et al. [11] on 13 fetuses with a midgestation fetal TV *z*-score < −3, only 1 achieved biventricular repair, compared with 5 of 5 with a TV *z*-score > −3. Of 13 fetuses with a midgestation fetal TV *z*-score < −3, 8 were diagnosed postnatally with a right ventricular-dependent coronary circulation, compared with none who had a TV *z*-score > −3.

The average rate of TV growth between mid- and late fetal echocardiograms was significantly lower in patients who did not achieve biventricular repair.

The presence of TR was found to be a good predictor of a better outcome with a biventricular repair, having these fetuses larger RV dimensions, without VCCs [28]. This is in agreement with the study of Peterson et al. [29], who suggest that TR can facilitate the growth of the RV and TV despite the pulmonary atresia. Also, in this study, both a fetal TV *z*-score of −4 or less beyond 23 weeks of gestation and a fetal

TV annulus of 5 mm or less beyond 30 weeks of gestation were predictive of poor postnatal outcomes. In addition, right/left ventricular length or width less than 0.5 and/or the absence of TR were predictive of poor outcome.

Roman et al. [30] suggested a four-criteria scoring system to predict the postnatal outcome of PAIVS/CPS. They found the best sensitivity and specificity for a non-biventricular outcome as follows: TV/MV ratio <0.7, RV/LV length ratio <0.6, TV inflow duration <31.5 % of cardiac cycle length, and the presence of RV sinusoids. If three of these four criteria were fulfilled, this predicted a non-biventricular outcome with sensitivity of 100 % and specificity of 75 %.

In conclusion, the echocardiographic diagnosis of PAIVS/CPS is feasible. However, as reported above, both outcomes and management are still under evaluation.

References

1. Bolger AF, Eigler NL, Maurer G. Quantifying valvular regurgitation. Limitations and inherent assumptions of Doppler techniques. Circulation. 1988;78:1316–8.
2. Rivera JM, Vandervoort PM, Vazquez de Prada JA, et al. Which physical factors determine tricuspid regurgitation jet area in the clinical setting? Am J Cardiol. 1993;72:1305–9.
3. Kiserud T, Eik-Nes. SH, Blaas HG, Hellevik LR. Ultrasonographic velocimetry of the fetal ductus venosus. Ultrasound Obstet Gynecol. 1991;338:1412–4.
4. DeVore GR, Horenstein J. Ductus venosus index: a method for evaluating right ventricular preload in the second-trimester fetus. Ultrasound Obstet Gynecol. 1993;3:338–42.
5. Gardiner HM, Belmar C, Tulzer G, Barlow A, Pasquini L, Carvalho JS, Daubeney PE, Rigby ML, Gordon F, Kulinskaya E, Franklin RC. Morphologic and functional predictors of eventual circulation in the fetus with pulmonary atresia or critical pulmonary stenosis with intact septum. J Am Coll Cardiol. 2008;51(13):1299–308.
6. Tan J, Silverman NH, Hoffman JIE, Villegas M, Schmidt KG. Cardiac dimensions determined by cross-sectional echocardiography in the normal human fetus from 18 weeks to term. Am J Cardiol. 1992;70:1459–67.
7. Hornberger LK, Benacerraf BR, Bromley BS, Spevak PJ, Sanders SP. Prenatal detection of severe right ventricular outflow tract obstruction: pulmonary stenosis and pulmonary atresia. J Ultrasound Med. 1994;13:743–50.
8. Gardiner HM. Progression of fetal heart disease and rationale for fetal intracardiac interventions. Semin Fetal Neonatal Med. 2005;10:578–85.
9. Shinebourne EA, Rigby ML, Carvalho JS. Pulmonary atresia with intact ventricular septum: from fetus to adult. Heart. 2008;94:1350–7.
10. Sharland GK, Tynan M, Qureshi SA. Prenatal detection and progression of right coronary artery to right ventricle fistula. Heart. 1996;76:79–81.
11. Salvin JW, McElhinney DB, Colan SD, Gauvreau K, del Nido PJ, Jenkins KJ, Lock JE, Tworetzky W. Fetal tricuspid valve size and growth as predictors of outcome in pulmonary atresia with intact ventricular septum. Pediatrics. 2006;118:e415–20.
12. Maeno YV, Boutin C, Hornberger LK, McCrindle BW, Cavallé-Garrido T, Gladman G, Smallhorn JF. Prenatal diagnosis of right ventricular outflow tract obstruction with intact ventricular septum, and detection of ventriculocoronary connections. Heart. 1999;81:661–8.
13. Giglia TM, Mandell VS, Connor AR, Mayer JE, Lock JE. Diagnosis and management of right ventricle-dependent coronary circulation in pulmonary atresia with intact ventricular septum. Circulation. 1992;86:1516–28.
14. Calder AL, Co EE, Sage MD. Coronary arterial abnormalities in pulmonary atresia with intact ventricular septum. Am J Cardiol. 1987;59:436–42.

15. Powell AJ, Mayer JE, Lang P, Lock JE. Outcome in infants with pulmonary atresia, intact ventricular septum, and right ventricle-dependent coronary circulation. Am J Cardiol. 2000;86:1272–4.
16. Guleserian KJ, Armsby LB, Thiagarajan RR, del Nido PJ, Mayer Jr JE. History of pulmonary atresia with intact ventricular septum and right-ventricle-dependent coronary circulation managed by the single-ventricle approach. Ann Thorac Surg. 2006;81:2250–8.
17. Cha HH, Choo YS, Seong WJ. Prenatal diagnosis of multiple ventriculocoronary connections in pulmonary atresia with an intact ventricular septum: a case report. J Obstet Gynaecol Res. 2015;41:1278–81.
18. Chaoui R, Tennstedt C, Goldner B, Bollmann R. Prenatal diagnosis of ventriculo-coronary communications in second-trimester fetus using transvaginal and transabdominal color Doppler sonography. Ultrasound Obstet Gynecol. 1997;9:194–7.
19. Sandor GG, Cook AC, Sharland GK, Ho SY, Potts JE, Anderson RH. Coronary arterial abnormalities in pulmonary atresia with intact ventricular septum diagnosed during fetal life. Cardiol Young. 2002;12:436–44.
20. Daubeney PEF, Delany DJ, Anderson RH, et al. Pulmonary atresia with intact ventricular septum: range of morphology in a population-based study. J Am Coll Cardiol. 2002;39:1670–9.
21. Vesel S, Rollings S, Jones A, Callaghan N, Simpson J, Sharland GK. Prenatally diagnosed pulmonary atresia with ventricular septal defect: echocardiography, genetics, associated anomalies and outcome. Heart. 2006;92:1501–5.
22. Todros T, Presbitero P, Gagliotti P, Demarie D. Pulmonary stenosis with intact ventricular septum: documentation of development of the lesion echocardiographically during fetal life. Int J Cardiol. 1988;19:355–60.
23. Song TB, Lee JY, Kim YH, Oh BS, Kim EK. Prenatal diagnosis of severe tricuspid insufficiency in Ebstein's anomaly with pulmonary atresia and intact ventricular septum: a case report. J Obstet Gynaecol Res. 2000;26:223–6.
24. Mallula K, Vaughn G, El-Said H, Lamberti JJ, Moore JW. Comparison of ductal stenting versus surgical shunts for palliation of patients with pulmonary atresia and intact ventricular septum. Catheter Cardiovasc Interv. 2015;85:1196–202.
25. Huang SC, Ishino K, Kasahara S, Yoshizumi K, Kotani Y, Sano S. The potential of disproportionate growth of tricuspid valve after decompression of the right ventricle in patients with pulmonary atresia and intact ventricular septa. J Thorac Cardiovasc Surg. 2009;138:1160–6.
26. Yoshimura N, Yamaguchi M. Surgical strategy for pulmonary atresia with intact ventricular septum: initial management and definitive surgery. Gen Thorac Cardiovasc Surg. 2009;57:338–46.
27. Waldman JD, Karp RB, Lamberti JJ, Sand ME, Ruschhaupt DG, Agarwala B. Tricuspid valve closure in pulmonary atresia with important RV-to-coronary artery connections. Ann Thorac Surg. 1995;59:933–41.
28. Iacobelli R, Pasquini L, Toscano A, Raimondi F, Michielon G, Tozzi AE, Sanders SP. Role of tricuspid regurgitation in fetal echocardiographic diagnosis of pulmonary atresia with intact ventricular septum. Ultrasound Obstet Gynecol. 2008;32:31–5.
29. Peterson RE, Levi DS, Williams RJ, Lai WW, Sklansky MS, Drant S. Echocardiographic predictors of outcome in fetuses with pulmonary atresia with intact ventricular septum. J Am Soc Echocardiogr. 2006;19:1393–400.
30. Roman KS, Fouron JC, Nii M, Smallhorn JF, Chaturvedi R, Jaeggi ET. Determinants of outcome in fetal pulmonary valve stenosis or atresia with intact ventricular septum. Am J Cardiol. 2007;99:699–703.

Indications for Fetal Pulmonary Valvuloplasty

11

Roland Gitter, Wolfgang Arzt, and Gerald Tulzer

In parallel to the interventions on the aortic valve, pulmonary valvuloplasty in utero may follow two different indications. The first is to simply ensure fetal survival by reversing fetal hydrops caused by severe right-ventricular decompensation. The second and more ambitious goal is reducing fetal morbidity, by promoting intrauterine growth on ventricular, valvular, and vascular level so as to avoid the development of a functionally univentricular heart. The achievements of these goals depend on an evidence-based selection of suitable candidates, on the level of expertise and cooperation of the team performing the intervention, and on the availability of adequate technical equipment. In light of improving results of postnatal treatment ranging from postnatal dilatation, radio-frequency perforation of atretic valves, and surgical strategies of one-and-a-half heart or univentricular course, only limited types of lesions have the potential to benefit from prenatal interventions.

The selection of suitable candidates remains difficult and is still based on the center's experience, the level of expertise and ability of cooperation of the team performing the intervention, and at last the adequate technical equipment.

Contraindications for fetal pulmonary valvuloplasty result from valvular, right-ventricular, and other cardiac malformations as well as extracardiac lesions, chromosomal aberrations, and twin pregnancies. An atretic or subatretic right-ventricular outflow tract cannot be perforated by the needle and is thus not feasible for intervention. Large coronary sinusoids, which indicate a right-ventricular-dependent coronary perfusion, represent another contraindication for intrauterine treatment. Severe extracardiac malformations have to be taken into account as well as twin

R. Gitter (✉) • G. Tulzer
Department of Pediatric Cardiology, Children's Heart Center Linz,
Kepler University Hospital Linz, Linz, Austria
e-mail: Roland.gitter@gespag.at

W. Arzt
Institute of Prenatal Medicine, Kepler University Hospital Linz, Linz, Austria

G. Butera et al. (eds.), *Fetal and Hybrid Procedures in Congenital Heart Diseases*, DOI 10.1007/978-3-319-40088-4_11

pregnancies as both conditions raise the important ethical issue of exposing the mother or the sibling to the risks of the intervention. The ethical question is even more ostensible in the case of weighing up the indication against the experience of the team. A fetus with critical pulmonary valve stenosis in good circulatory status judged to be suitable for in utero treatment should not be treated by an inexperienced team doing the intervention every now and then, but referred to a center with sufficient expertise which is able to deal with unfavorable fetal positions and periprocedural complications.

The ideal patient for intrauterine intervention on the pulmonary valve comes with an obstruction solely on the valvular level. The RVOT is developed; the size of the right ventricle is not too small to be determined as clearly hypoplastic but on the other hand not of normal size which would favor postponing treatment to the postnatal period (Fig. 11.1). Roman et al. in 2007 tried to identify cutoff values of measurements regarding the size of the tricuspid valve in comparison to the mitral valve and the right-ventricular to the left-ventricular length, respectively, to predict a uni- or biventricular course [1] (Fig. 11.2). Gomez Montes et al. in 2012 published a scoring system to predict the most likely course of circulation in PA/IVS by means of combining cardiac dimensions and functional parameters [2].

The ideal patient therefore should match the criteria for a non-biventricular outcome as close as possible to justify fetal treatment. Furthermore and again under ideal auspices, close monitoring of the fetal heart's status, especially the size of the right ventricle to depict growth arrest, allows setting of the indication and the proper timing for in utero valvuloplasty. If the right ventricle does not show any increase in size over a period of 3–4 weeks in the midterm gestation, a spontaneous reversal of this process is unlikely and can be achieved only by decompressing the right ventricle by opening the pulmonary valve.

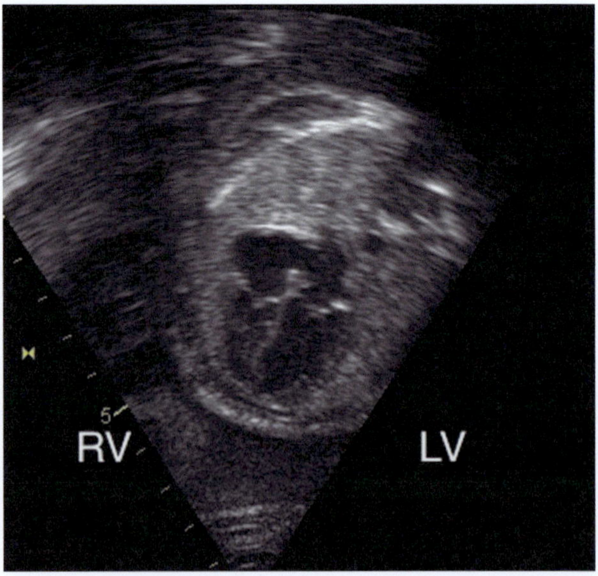

Fig. 11.1 This 2D echo picture shows a typical borderline right ventricle due to pulmonary atresia with equivocative prediction concerning biventricular outcome and therefore basically a potential candidate for intrauterine treatment

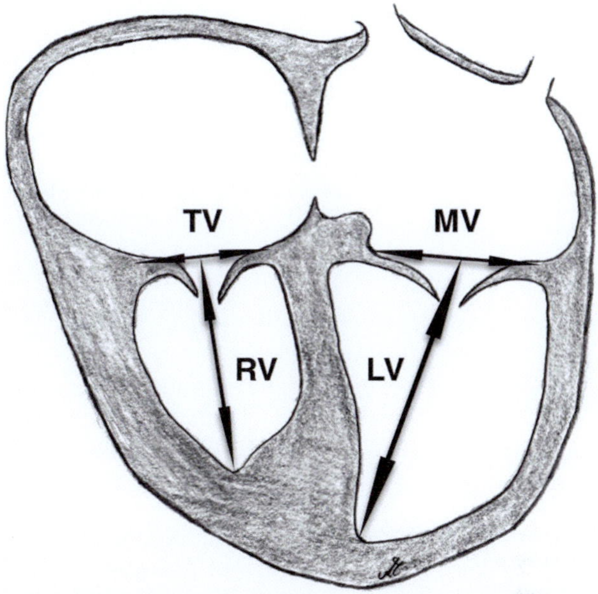

Fig. 11.2 This illustration of a heart with hypoplastic right ventricle shows how to measure RV and LV parameters which are used for the estimation of the further intrauterine course

So in summary the indication for intrauterine treatment of the pulmonary valve is by far more difficult to determine when compared to postnatal dilatation and covers more or less the field between a clear-cut hypoplastic right ventricle which is lost for biventricular circulation and a well-sized right heart without additive structural abnormalities which may be preserved for intervention after birth. Further studies, especially dealing with the comparison in the outcome of treated fetuses and fetuses with the intention to treat and abandoned procedure, will modify and adjust the indication for intrauterine valvuloplasty in the future (Table 11.1).

Besides these two traditional indications mentioned above, another issue may be stressed when pondering about future perspectives of in utero therapy. If the strategy of treatment as soon as possible to avoid damages for the myocardium or the heart rhythm – as it is well established in the treatment of atrial septal defects or tetralogy of Fallot – is transferred and applied to the treatment of critical pulmonary valve stenosis, the indications for intrauterine treatment will include another subgroup of patients. Currently the intervention itself bears still an immanent risk for the babies' heart function and survival and a not negligible risk for the pregnancy and mother's health. On the other hand, it is obvious that systemic or suprasystemic pressures in the right ventricle do have negative effects on both right-ventricular architecture and function. Unloading the suffering subpulmonary ventricle in utero remains therefore a more or less technical question. The more experience in performing the intervention is present, better equipment is available, and image quality is improved, the less risk emanates from the intervention. This therapeutic principle – bringing the right ventricle into optimal shape and function by intervening early even in cases of expected biventricular course – may turn out to be an important third indication for pulmonary valvuloplasty in the fetus (Table 11.2).

Table 11.1 Indications for intrauterine pulmonary valvuloplasty

Severe stenosis or membranous atresia on the level of the pulmonary valve with
Retrograde flow in the duct
Intact or highly restrictive ventricular septum
Identifiable but small right ventricle
Prediction of most likely univentricular course with
RV/LV ratio < 0.6
TV/MV < 0.7
TV *Z*-score ≤ −3
Tricuspid inflow time < 31,5 % of cardiac cycle
Growth arrest of the RV over 3–4 weeks
Fetal hydrops in pulmonary valve stenosis or atresia due to
Severe right heart failure
Restrictive foramen ovale
Severe tricuspid regurgitation

Table 11.2 Contraindications for intrauterine pulmonary valvuloplasty

Atresia of the RVOT
Unipartite right ventricle
Ventricular septal defect
Large coronary sinusoids
Unexperienced team
Severe extracardiac malformations and chromosomal abnormalities
Twin pregnancy

References

1. Roman K, Fouron JC, Nii N, Smallhorn J, Chaturvedi R, Jaeggi E. Determinants of outcome in fetal pulmonary valve stenosis or atresia with intact ventricular septum. Am J Cardiol. 2007;99:699–703.
2. Gomez Montes E, Herraiz I, Mendoza A, Galindo A. Fetal intervention in right outflow tract obstructive disease: selection of candidates and results. Cardiol Res Pract. 2012;2012:592403.

Center Experience and Step-by-Step Approach for Fetal Pulmonary Valvuloplasty

12

Gerald Tulzer and Wolfgang Arzt

12.1 Center Experience

In our center (the Children's Heart Center Linz), the fetal cardiac intervention program was started in the year 2000. In fact, the very first procedure, which we performed, was in a fetus with pulmonary atresia with intact ventricular septum (PAIVS) at 28 weeks [1]. Since then a total of 91 interventions have been here conducted, the majority in fetuses with critical aortic stenosis, few in fetuses with hypoplastic left heart syndrome and restrictive foramen ovale, and altogether 20 procedures in 14 fetuses with PAIVS or critical pulmonary stenosis with intact ventricular septum. We reported our first case together with a case that was done in the UK in a publication in the year 2002. This fetus was thought to develop restriction at the atrial level with increased central venous pressures and imminent hydrops as indicated by severely abnormal venous Doppler waveforms – a complication that may result in fetal hydrops and intrauterine death. The fetus had a hypoplastic RV with growth arrest and suprasystemic right ventricular pressures, a significant tricuspid regurgitation (TR), and a favorable anatomy with a membranous atresia of the pulmonary valve and well-developed confluent pulmonary arteries. For this first procedure, we used a 16-gauge needle and managed to perforate the membrane between the RV and main pulmonary artery. Clear antegrade as well as retrograde flow across the pulmonary valve annulus was observed immediately after the procedure by color-flow and CW Doppler. This fetus was followed longitudinally in our center, and over the following weeks, significant changes in hemodynamics were documented: growth of RV long axis, growth of

G. Tulzer (✉)
Department of Pediatric Cardiology, Children's Heart Center Linz,
Kepler University Hospital Linz, Linz, Austria
e-mail: Gerald.Tulzer@gespag.at

W. Arzt
Institute of Prenatal Medicine, Kepler University Hospital Linz, Linz, Austria

G. Butera et al. (eds.), *Fetal and Hybrid Procedures in Congenital Heart Diseases*, DOI 10.1007/978-3-319-40088-4_12

tricuspid valve annulus, change from a short monophasic to a longer biphasic RV inflow, as well as complete disappearance of the TR jet. Six weeks after the procedure, TR reappeared again with high velocities due to an increasing restenosis of the perforated pulmonary valve. This baby was delivered at 38 + 2 weeks; postnatally it received a pulmonary valvuloplasty, and because of a still borderline RV output, a 3.5 mm modified right BT shunt was placed. This shunt was successfully removed at the age of 8 months. Now 15 years later, this girl still has had no other interventions; she has mild to moderate pulmonary stenosis and mild pulmonary regurgitation with some dilation of the main pulmonary artery. She is on no medication, is very sportive, and has no exercise intolerance at all.

This encouraging preliminary experience motivated us to continue and to further develop in utero treatment of PAIVS. Our experience with the first series of five and six cases, respectively, was published in 2006 and 2011 [2, 3]. At that time we had a technical success rate – which means that we were able to perforate and to dilate the pulmonary valve – in four out of six cases. Of the successful cases, three became biventricular and one ended up with a one-and-a-half ventricle circulation. In 2015 we presented our experience of 12 procedures in ten fetuses. We were able to perforate and to dilate the valve in 80 % of these fetuses. Again we saw RV and TV growth and longer RV inflow durations but with remaining high PV gradients in most of them. Six of them became biventricular, one with a one-and-a-half ventricle and one with a univentricular circulation. Currently our experience consists of 20 procedures in 14 fetuses; three of them are still in utero.

12.2 Step-by-Step Approach

12.2.1 Assessing Fetal Position

The single most important factor for a successful procedure is the fetal position. Once the fetus is in a dorso-posterior position with the RV facing toward the maternal abdomen and the fetal spine is positioned between 5 and 7 o'clock, the procedure has a very high chance of being successful. There are "borderline" positions, where an intervention theoretically is still possible but certainly more difficult and a challenge for the whole team: amount of amniotic fluid, position of the placenta, distance between maternal skin and fetal heart, maternal obesity, and obvious obstacles in the way of the intended needle insertion (umbilical cord, fetal extremities, etc.). Additionally there are fetal positions, where a successful intervention is impossible (e.g., spine anterior), and the procedure has to be postponed until a better position is present. This initial evaluation is usually done by both perinatologist and cardiologist together and certainly needs a lot of experience.

12.2.2 Setting Up the OR

All procedures were performed in the operating theater with enough space for the anesthesia team (we performed all procedures under general anesthesia); on one side of the table, there is the ultrasound machine positioned and on the other side the catheter table with the necessary equipment. Our interventional team consists of an anesthetist with one or two nurses, one perinatologist for the needling, two fetal cardiologists for scanning and handling of the catheter, and one physician or nurse handling the balloon inflation.

12.2.3 Preparing the Procedure

Mother: After having given informed consent on the day before the procedure, an ultrasonic assessment of the fetal position is done. If the fetus is found to be in a favorable position, the mother is brought into the theater and scanned again, and if the fetus has not changed position, anesthesia is started instantly. Only after effective anesthesia of the mother and fetus has been confirmed, all other necessary preparations continue: positioning of the mother, skin sterilization, and preparing the operation field.

Fetus Fetal weight is estimated by ultrasound and emergency medication is prepared (epinephrine, atropine).

Catheter and needling equipment (Fig. 12.1): The following items were prepared: 18G or 19G needles (Cook Medical®) depending on gestational age and distance to the fetal heart, floppy 0.0014 in. guidewires, and 2.5–4 mm semi-compliant, monorail coronary artery balloon catheters (Maverick®, Boston Scientific) with a manometer-equipped syringe and sterile strips to mark catheters and wires. The guidewire is inserted into the catheter and then both together through the needle after the trocar was removed. Markers on the catheter and the wires are placed to make sure the depth of insertion can be controlled. Then catheter and wire are removed from the needle; the trocar is inserted back again and handed over to the perinatologist to perform the puncture. The wire remains in the catheter and both will be inserted together, once the needle will be in place.

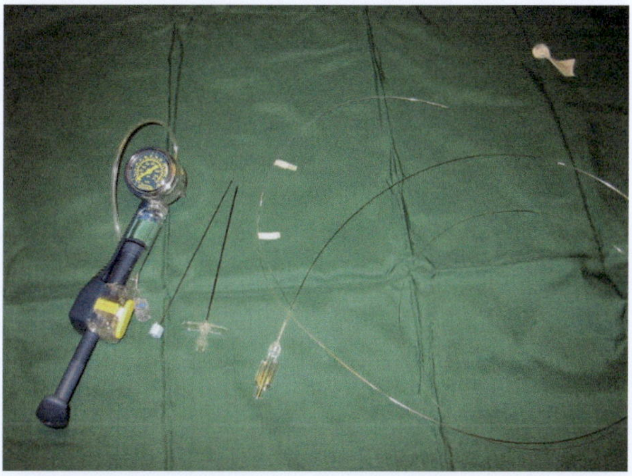

Fig. 12.1 Equipment used for fetal valvuloplasty: *left*, syringe with manometer for balloon inflation; *middle*, 18G needle with the trocar removed; and *right*, monorail balloon catheter with a 0.0014 in. floppy wire inside. Note the two markers on the catheter and on the guidewire, respectively

Ultrasound We use a Voluson E8 (GE Healthcare) ultrasound machine for imaging with standard curve array scanners equipped with Doppler and color Doppler. Keyboard and probe get a sterile cover. All procedures are recorded continuously on DVD.

12.2.4 Procedure

Puncture + imaging: This is the most critical part. The direction of the needle has to be perfect from the beginning, because larger manipulations or angle corrections are not possible once inside the fetal heart. So the synchronization between the scanning and needling person is crucial; sometimes both have to be done simultaneously by the same person. This procedure is significantly more challenging than aortic valve dilation, because the target, the hypoplastic RV, is usually very small. It has to be entered in the region of the RVOT about 1 cm proximal to the atretic valve and almost perpendicular to the fetal chest.

Testing the right needle position: Before perforating the atretic pulmonary valve or advancing a guidewire across a critical pulmonary stenosis, one has to be sure to be inside the cavity of the RV, which by ultrasound alone is very difficult to judge. So at this time, the trocar is slowly removed, and if blood is coming out through the needle (usually with quiet a high pressure), one can be sure to have an intracardiac position.

Perforation of the atretic valve: In the case of pulmonary atresia, the trocar has to be inserted again – be careful to do it very slowly; otherwise, one will push air bubbles into the RV and imaging will be a dramatic worse afterward. Under ultrasound guidance the needle is then advanced through the valve into the main PA. If there is critical pulmonary stenosis with still a tiny opening, the trocar should stay outside, and the whole ensemble (catheter with guidewire) will be slowly inserted. The ultrasound picture as well as the markers on the catheter will show you when the catheter tip has reached the tip of the needle. Then only the guidewire is advanced forward to cross the tiny opening, which is successful in most of the cases after a few attempts. Once the guidewire is clearly seen in the main PA or in the ductus arteriosus, the catheter is manipulated over the wire into an optimal position across the valve annulus (Fig. 12.2).

Performing the dilatation: Now the balloon is inflated with the respective diameter. Balloon size should be at least 10–20 % larger than the valve diameter. With the current available equipment, a 4 mm balloon will be the largest size that would fit through an 18G needle. Using larger needles will allow larger balloons, but will increase the likelihood for complications.

Withdrawal of all equipment: A deflated balloon sometimes cannot be retracted back into the needle again. Instead of applying increased force, we prefer to withdraw the needle together with the deflated balloon, which is still outside. After a successful dilatation, one should see good antegrade flow as well as some pulmonary regurgitation (Fig. 12.3a, b).

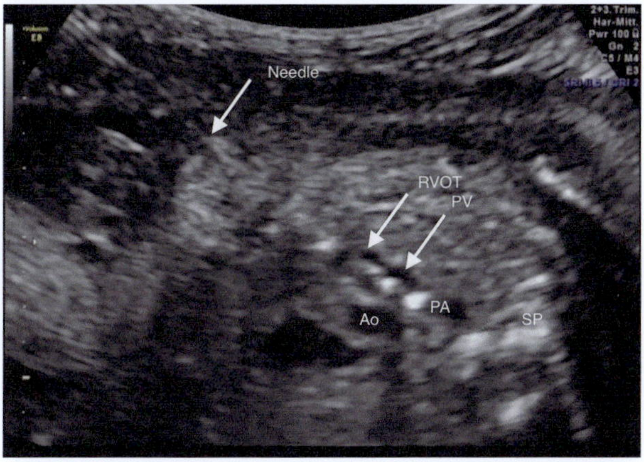

Fig. 12.2 Fetal pulmonary valvulotomy procedure: the needle is already passed from the right ventricular outflow tract through the perforated pulmonary valve in the main pulmonary artery. *Ao* aorta, *PA* pulmonary artery, *PV* pulmonary valve, *RVOT* right ventricular outflow tract

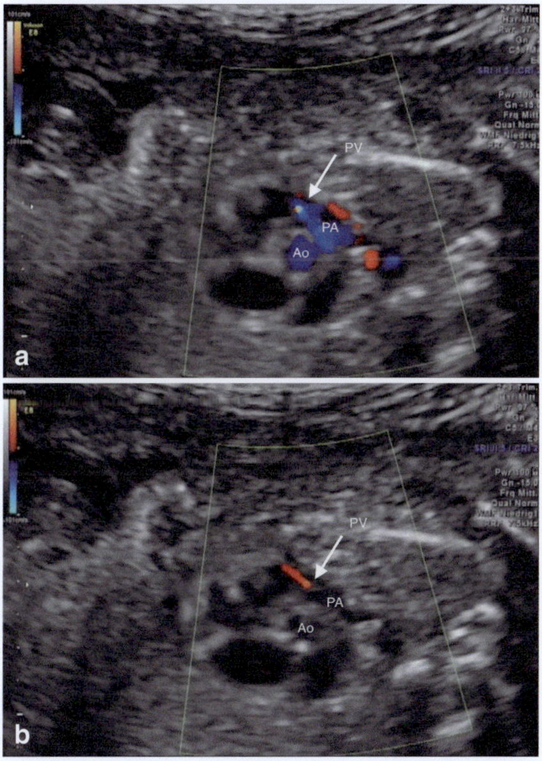

Fig. 12.3 Color Doppler after a successful pulmonary valvuloplasty: (**a**) picture in systole (note the blue color across the pulmonary valve indicating now antegrade flow from the right ventricle into the pulmonary artery) and (**b**) picture in diastole (note the red pulmonary regurgitation jet back into the right ventricle indicating some damage of the pulmonary valve after valvuloplasty). *Ao* aorta, *PA* pulmonary artery, *PV* pulmonary valve

12.2.5 Post-procedural Assessment

Immediate: Watch for pericardial effusion and drain instantly if it gets too large with signs of hemodynamic compromise. If persistent bradycardia develops, epinephrine is administered (according to estimated fetal weight) into the left ventricle (now using a 22G needle).

First 24–48 h: Nonstress test to watch for premature labor or fetal arrhythmias; observe if there are signs of premature rupture of the membranes or amnioinfection.

Long term: The patients were discharged 2 days after the procedure is stable, and follow-up visits were recommended every 2 or 4 weeks to assess hemodynamic changes.

So far we did not see any major maternal complication from this procedure [4].

References

1. Tulzer G, Arzt W, Franklin RC, Loughna PV, Mair R, Gardiner HM. Fetal pulmonary valvuloplasty for critical pulmonary stenosis or atresia with intact septum. Lancet. 2002;360(9345):1567–8.
2. Tulzer G, Gardiner H. Cardiac Interventions in the fetus: potential for right-sided lesions. Prog Pediatr Cardiol. 2006;22(1):79–83.
3. Arzt W, Tulzer G. Fetal surgery for cardiac lesions. Prenat Diagn. 2011;31(7):695–8.
4. Wohlmuth C, Tulzer G, Arzt W, Gitter R, Wertaschnigg D. Maternal aspects of fetal cardiac intervention. Ultrasound Obstet Gynecol. 2014;44(5):532–7.

Pulmonary Valvuloplasty: Fetal, Neonatal, and Follow-Up Outcomes

13

Eva Grohmann, Andreas Tulzer, Wolfgang Arzt, and Gerald Tulzer

The primary management and outcome of unborn children with atresia (PA/IVS) or critical stenosis of the pulmonary valve (CPS) and intact ventricular septum are still under discussion. The degree of the morphological and clinical picture of this disease can vary from a hypoplastic right heart syndrome with a univentricular physiology to a biventricular heart only with the need for valvuloplasty after delivery. Neonates with CPS or PA/IVS show considerable variation of abnormalities of the right ventricle, tricuspid valve (TV), and coronary arteries. Therefore, there is a wide range in the reported 5-year survival rate from 50 to 86% [1]. This cardiac malformation is rarely associated with chromosomal defects or extra-cardiac malformations. Therefore, the cardiologist's prediction of a univentricular or biventricular circulation could have even more influence on the parents' choice regarding the future of the pregnancy [2]. The focus of this chapter lies especially on the fetal and neonatal outcome of fetuses, who underwent pulmonary valvuloplasty in utero.

A fetal pulmonary valve dilatation is a technically highly challenging procedure, thus making the outcome of fetuses undergoing intervention dependent on an experienced team that knows how to deal with the accompanying difficulties and complications, both fetal and maternal, respectively. The most common complications are pericardial effusions or episodes of severe bradycardia. Without adequate therapy intrauterine death may occur. Complications from the maternal side with the potential of endangering the fetus are premature rupture of membranes and preterm labor resulting in premature delivery with its known problems.

E. Grohmann • A. Tulzer • G. Tulzer (✉)
Department of Pediatric Cardiology, Children's Heart Center Linz, Kepler University Hospital Linz, Linz, Austria
e-mail: Gerald.Tulzer@gespag.at

W. Arzt
Institute of Prenatal Medicine, Kepler University Hospital Linz, Linz, Austria

G. Butera et al. (eds.), *Fetal and Hybrid Procedures in Congenital Heart Diseases*, DOI 10.1007/978-3-319-40088-4_13

Fetuses undergoing intrauterine pulmonary valvuloplasty in our institution experienced bradycardias and pericardial effusions to the same extent (approximately 35–40 %). Due to prompt intracardiac administration of epinephrine, so far no intrauterine deaths occurred because of bradycardia. In the case of pericardial effusions, the fluid was drained immediately as soon as hemodynamic impairment was seen. Another rare complication was the formation of a clot inside the right ventricle with the potential of filling even the whole cavity of the right ventricle, thus impairing the visibility by ultrasound and making the continuation of the procedure impossible. In these cases the procedure had to be aborted and repeated later.

There are several predictors and scores to predict the outcome and eventual circulation of fetuses with PA/IVS or CPS. Gardiner and colleagues [2] published specific criteria depending on gestational age to predict an eventual postnatal outcome. The variables included the ratio of tricuspid valve and mitral valve annular diameter, pulmonary valve *z*-scores, a right atrial pressure score (combination of tricuspid valve Doppler, foramen ovale, and ductus venosus flow patterns), and the presence of coronary fistulae. Another scoring system established by a Canadian group [1] used four criteria to discriminate between fetuses, who would undergo univentricular or biventricular management after delivery. This scoring system included a ratio of tricuspid valve and mitral valve annular diameter with a ratio of less than 0.7 predicting a univentricular circulation; a ratio of the right ventricular over left ventricular length of less than 0.6 predicted a univentricular circulation; furthermore biventricular repair was unlikely if the tricuspid valve inflow duration was less than 32 % of the cardiac cycle or if there were sinusoids to the right ventricle. If three of these factors were fulfilled, univentricular physiology was detected with 100 % sensitivity and 75 % specificity in fetuses below 31 weeks of gestation. Currently there are no studies that prove an improvement of one of these scores after successful fetal pulmonary valvuloplasty [1].

To optimize the overall outcome, delivery should be planned in a specialized center with an experienced team and the possibility to perform cardiac catheterization in newborns. After delivery all newborns with CPS or PA/IVS, who underwent valvuloplasty in utero, should receive prostaglandins for initial hemodynamic stabilization; as in many cases, a residual gradient can impair pulmonary arterial perfusion.

Up to now there is only little experience on the overall outcome of children with CPS or PA/IVS, who underwent in utero valvuloplasty. The biggest series reported so far by Tworetzky et al. in 2009 reported ten cases, who underwent fetal pulmonary intervention since 2002 [3]. In this study fetuses with membranous pulmonary atresia and identifiable pulmonary valve (PV) leaflets or membrane, an intact or highly restrictive ventricular septum, with a tricuspid valve annulus *z*-score of −2 or below, and an identifiable but small right ventricle underwent fetal intervention. Cardiac puncture was performed under ultrasound guidance percutaneously or through a limited laparotomy, and a coronary angioplasty balloon was used for valvuloplasty. Here six of ten procedures were technically successful and lead to significant growth of right heart structures compared to control fetuses, which did not undergo prenatal intervention [3].

We recently reported our experience with 12 pulmonary valve procedures in ten fetuses, all with hypoplastic RVs and suprasystemic RV pressures. The median TV z-score was −3.13. The procedures were performed at a median gestational age of 27 + 4 weeks. Technical success was achieved in 8 out of 12 interventions or in eight out of ten fetuses. No maternal side effects from the procedure or anesthesia were observed. In all successful cases, some improvements of right-sided structures or RV filling were observed, but high pulmonary valve gradient remained in most cases, and these gradients increased again toward the term indicating restenosis. After a median follow-up of 38 years, all successful dilated patients are alive, six have a good biventricular circulation (three of them had transient BT shunts), one patient had a one-and-a-half ventricle repair, and one patient remained univentricular.

13.1 Case Reports from Our Institution

In the year 2000, our very first fetus with PA/IVS and signs of heart failure with imminent fetal hydrops underwent intrauterine intervention at 27 + 6 weeks of gestation [4]. The procedure was successful; growth of RV structures as well as disappearance of the TR and a change from monophasic to biphasic filling of the RV was observed. After elective delivery at 38 weeks of gestation, the patient underwent a successful balloon valvuloplasty on her second day of life. Suprasystemic right ventricular pressures could be reduced to nearly normal values. Due to the hypertrophic and still somewhat hypoplastic right ventricle, we decided to put in a modified BT shunt to ensure adequate pulmonary perfusion.

At the age of 8 months, the BT shunt was removed, and a repair of a double orifice tricuspid valve was performed. Right ventricular growth and function were close to normal at that time. Up to today the child was doing well with mild to moderate pulmonary regurgitation. She was always asymptomatic and is now a very sportive young lady without any medication. A cardiac MRI at the age of 14 years showed excellent right ventricular function and a mildly dilated RV (97 ml RVEDV/m2 BSA).

Another case was a fetus with a severe pulmonary stenosis, a subpulmonary stenosis, a hypoplastic right ventricle with nearly no trabecular part, a borderline tricuspid valve, and a coronary fistula. In the year 2007, we performed an unsuccessful intervention at 31 + 1 and a partially successful one at 32 + 1 weeks of gestation in this fetus. After elective delivery at 37 + 2 weeks of gestation, the patient underwent a successful balloon valvuloplasty on his second day of life. Due to the borderline right ventricle, the patient received a modified Blalock-Taussig shunt on his tenth day of life. The BT shunt was removed at the age of 7 months, and a one-and-a-half ventricle repair with a bidirectional Glenn shunt, valvulotomy of the pulmonary valve with muscle bundle resection in the RVOT, and closure of the ASD was done. A previously performed catheterization showed a good development of the pulmonary vascular bed, a moderately elevated right atrial pressure of 12 mmHg, and a reduced growth of the right ventricle. At the age of 7 years, the boy is still doing fine with no exercise intolerance and no medication.

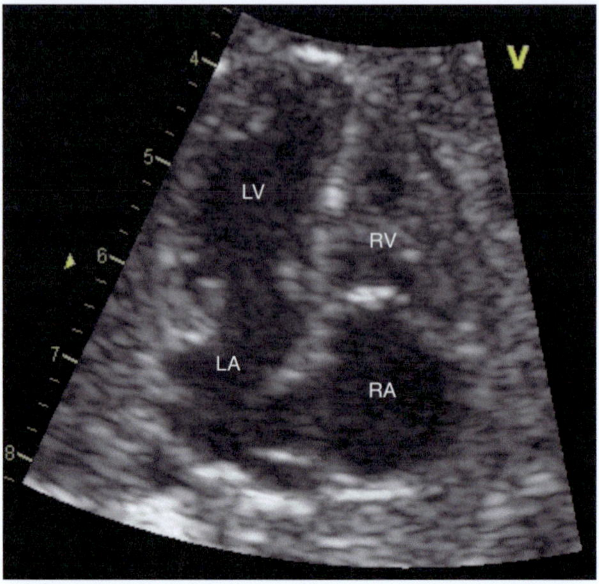

Fig. 13.1 Four-chamber view of a fetus with a small hypertrophic right ventricle (case 3)

Another fetus with diagnosis of PA/IVS and a small but tripartite right ventricle underwent a successful intrauterine intervention at 25+0 weeks of gestation (Fig. 13.1). This intervention resulted in severe pulmonary regurgitation. Right ventricular filling was primarily retrograde during the rest of pregnancy. The baby was delivered spontaneously at 37+1 weeks of gestation, and a modified BT shunt with repair of the pulmonary valve was performed at the 20th day of life. Follow-up echocardiograms showed a good growth of the right ventricle, a normal tricuspid valve inflow, and a moderate pulmonary regurgitation. Due to the satisfactory growth and function of the right ventricle, the BT shunt could be closed by intervention at the age of 8 months. Three years later the girl is doing fine with excellent exercise tolerance and no medication.

References

1. Roman KS, Fouron J-C, Nii M, Smallhorn JF, Chaturvedi R, Jaeggi ET. Determinants of outcome in fetal pulmonary valve stenosis or atresia with intact ventricular septum. Am J Cardiol. 2007;99(5):699–703.
2. Gardiner HM, Belmar C, Tulzer G, Barlow A, Pasquini L, Carvalho JS, et al. Morphologic and functional predictors of eventual circulation in the fetus with pulmonary atresia or critical pulmonary stenosis with intact septum. J Am Coll Cardiol. 2008;51(13):1299–308.
3. Tulzer G, Arzt W, Franklin RCG, Loughna PV, Mair R, Gardiner HM. Fetal pulmonary valvuloplasty for critical pulmonary stenosis or atresia with intact septum. Lancet. 2002;360(9345):1567–8.
4. Tworetzky W, McElhinney DB, Marx GR, Benson CB, Brusseau R, Morash D, et al. In utero valvuloplasty for pulmonary atresia with hypoplastic right ventricle: techniques and outcomes. Pediatrics. 2009;124(3):e510–8.

14 Literature on Fetal Therapy After Pulmonary Valvuloplasty

Roland Gitter and Gerald Tulzer

Due to the relative rarity of the lesion and the complexity of patient selection and the intervention itself, current numbers of reported cases are limited to approximately two dozens. The first publication worldwide was issued in 2002 by Tulzer et al. [1] from Children's Heart Center Linz, describing a successful valvulotomy of the pulmonary valve, performed in a fetus with heart failure at 28 weeks of gestation. Following the procedure significant growth of the tricuspid valve and the right ventricle was observed. The neonate was delivered at 38 weeks with a RV suitable for biventricular repair leading the authors to the conclusion that in utero pulmonary valvulotomy is feasible and may change the natural history of the condition in affected fetuses with PA/IVS [1]. In 2006 another successful intervention was reported by Galindo et al. [2] performed in a fetus with critical PS-IVS and heart failure at 25 weeks of gestation. After the procedure a significant improvement in fetal hemodynamics was seen up to 34 weeks, when a significant restenosis with signs of circulatory failure leads to premature delivery of the baby and an immediate postnatal valvuloplasty provided a biventricular repair for the baby [2].

Another 3 years later in 2009, the first consecutive series was published by Tworetzky W. et al. from the Boston group [3]. During a 6-year period, ten fetuses at a median gestational age of 24 weeks (range from 21–28 weeks) underwent the attempt of balloon dilation of the PV in utero. Whereas the first four procedures were technically unsuccessful, the most recent six were technically successful. Success was defined by the inflation of a balloon within the pulmonary valve followed by unequivocal antegrade blood flow across the valve detected by color Doppler imaging. Compared to 15 control fetuses with PA/IVS who did not undergo prenatal intervention and out of whom nine had univentricular outcomes after birth, the tricuspid

R. Gitter (✉) • G. Tulzer
Department of Pediatric Cardiology, Children's Heart Center Linz,
Kepler University Hospital Linz, Linz, Austria
e-mail: Roland.gitter@gespag.at

G. Butera et al. (eds.), *Fetal and Hybrid Procedures in Congenital Heart Diseases*, DOI 10.1007/978-3-319-40088-4_14

valve annulus, right ventricle length, and PV annulus grew significantly more from mid- to late gestation in the six fetuses who underwent successful interventions. Five of these successfully treated patients had maintained antegrade pulmonary blood flow postnatally and underwent neonatal augmentation of the right ventricular outflow tract combined with a systemic to pulmonary shunt, which could be closed later on in four patients – the fifth patient in the intermediate period at the time of the paper's publication. Biventricular circulation – in which per definition the right ventricle is the only source of pulmonary blood flow, with systemic arterial saturation of more than 90 % in room air, with or without interatrial communication – was the primary goal of the intervention and could be achieved in five out of six successfully treated valves. The authors conclude that the initial results are promising, but fetal intervention for PA/IVS remains an experimental therapy, and it is necessary to compare the outcomes of this approach with those of postnatal transcatheter and surgical interventions that are currently the standard of care. The risk/benefit balance must be clear before prenatal intervention becomes an accepted therapy.

In 2012 Polat et al. [4] yielded a case of PA/IVS which they followed during midgestation from 24–28 weeks, observing increased tricuspid regurgitation and a lack of growth of the right ventricle ending up with a tricuspid valve annulus Z-score of −2.8. Intervention was successfully performed at 28 weeks. Immediately after the procedure, there was an improvement in fetal hemodynamics, but no further follow-up is described in this case report. Another small series of four interventions was published by Gomez-Montes et al. [5] in 2012. Fetal valvuloplasty was offered to three fetuses with signs of heart failure and one fetus with a predicted univentricular course. All interventions were considered successful; two babies died postnatally, but the other two were fine with a biventricular course at follow-up period of 8 years and one-and-a-half ventricle repair after 21 months, respectively [5].

In 2014 the group of Children's Heart Center Linz reported their experience of 12 attempted fetal valvuloplasties performed in 10 fetuses with suprasystemic RV pressures. Eight cases were considered successful and the intervention resulted in better RV filling and continuous, but slower than normal growth of the tricuspid valve and RV. Out of the first five newborns, four were biventricular at the end of the first year; one child received a Glenn shunt. One 6-month-old patient still has a Blalock-Taussig shunt; two fetuses were still in utero at the time of publication. Currently there is no literature available concerning the definitive treatment of fetuses, who underwent intrauterine pulmonary valvuloplasty. This field is predominantly still unexplored resulting in a lack of publications.

References

1. Tulzer G, Arzt W, Franklin RCG, Loughna PV, Mair R, Gar- diner HM. Fetal pulmonary valvuloplasty for critical pulmonary stenosis/atresia with intact septum. Lancet. 2002;360(9345):1567–8.
2. Galindo A, Gutierrez-Larraya F, Velasco JM, de la Fuente P. Pulmonary balloon valvuloplasty in a fetus with critical pulmonary stenosis/atresia with intact ventricular septum and heart failure. Fetal Diagn Ther. 2006;21:100–4.

3. Tworetzky W, McElhinney DB, Marx GR, et al. In utero valvuloplasty for pulmonary atresia with hypoplastic right ventricle: techniques and outcomes. Pediatrics. 2009;124(3):e510–8.
4. Polat T, Danısman N. Pulmonary valvulotomy in a fetus with pulmonary atresia with intact ventricular septum: first experience in Turkey. Images Paediatr Cardiol. 2012;14(3):6–11.
5. Gómez Montes E, Herraiz I, Mendoza A, Galindo A. Fetal intervention in right outflow tract obstructive disease: selection of candidates and results. Cardiol Res Pract. 2012;2012:592403.

15 Future Perspectives on Fetal Pulmonary Valvuloplasty

Gerald Tulzer

Prenatal intracardiac interventions for PA/IVS or CPS are still in its early stages. So far it has been shown that pulmonary valve perforations and dilations are technically feasible and have the potential to change fetal hemodynamics. The first case series and our experience have been promising, but a lot of issues have to be clarified and improved before it will become clinical routine.

15.1 Patient Selection

The proper patient selection is still unclear: the current selection criteria have been described already earlier in this chapter, and it is clear that these criteria are not really satisfactory. If there is severe congestive heart failure and hydrops, the rational for a fetal intervention is, as mentioned above, fetal survival. If the goal is a biventricular instead of a univentricular circulation, it becomes complicated. We are still lacking exact predictors of univentricular vs biventricular outcomes, and a lot of work is still ahead of us to better understand and predict the natural history of this cardiac lesion. However, the goal could be even more ambitious: not only biventricular instead of univentricular but to optimize RV size and function already prenatally to prepare the RV for a lifelong excellent performance. It is evident that suprasystemic RV pressures have deleterious effects on RV size, growth, and function and that these RVs should be decompressed as early as possible to avoid more secondary damage (in the absence of large ventricular to coronary communications). The only reason to wait until after birth is that prenatal interventions (1) are very difficult and (2) expose fetuses (who are not in heart failure and would survive

G. Tulzer
Department of Pediatric Cardiology, Children's Heart Center Linz, Kepler University Hospital Linz, Linz, Austria
e-mail: Gerald.Tulzer@gespag.at

G. Butera et al. (eds.), *Fetal and Hybrid Procedures in Congenital Heart Diseases*, DOI 10.1007/978-3-319-40088-4_15

to term without major problems) and healthy mothers to the risks of anesthesia and intervention. If theoretically there would be no risk at all to the mother and child, everyone would agree to decompress the RV as soon as possible. Therefore one of the future perspectives would be to minimize the risks for mother and fetus and to optimize the procedure for a technical success.

15.2 Equipment

In order to minimize risks and optimize technical success, currently used equipment has to be improved significantly. Future directions could be better needles, better balloons, and better imaging.

Eighteen or 19 gauge needles are still too large for small fetal hearts. They result in increased trauma to amniotic membranes (risk for premature rupture of membranes) and to the fetal heart (risk for bradycardia, thrombus, and pericardial effusions). The use of significant smaller needles is necessary to minimize these risks. Another important point is the ability to maneuver the needle tip, once inside the fetal heart. The RV cavity is small, the angulation toward the RV outflow tract very difficult. Angulated needles of even better needles with variable angulations would improve safety and technical success rates.

There are no dedicated balloon catheters for fetal intervention: the currently used standard coronary balloon catheters from the adult cath lab are too long, their profile is too high, and the balloon is too small. A fetal cardiac catheter has to be short for easy manipulation with according guide wires; it needs to have a very low profile in order to fit through small needles, and the balloon on the tip has to be short (max 10 mm) but with a large inflated diameter.

Clear imaging is the clue to a successful intervention: 2D resolution has already improved but still could be better. Three-dimensional (3D) orientation can be extremely difficult, so a real-time 3D imaging system with excellent image quality and high-frame rate would be optimal.

Proof of efficacy: important questions to be answered are as follows: Does a fetal pulmonary valvuloplasty in this condition always lead to improved growth of RV and tricuspid valve or is it dependent on certain conditions? What are the mechanisms of prenatal RV growth: proliferation versus hypertrophy? What would be the best time for intervention, what is the earliest possible or the latest date in pregnancy that makes sense? What are the mechanisms of early fetal pulmonary restenosis or atresia and how to avoid or treat it? All these questions and many more are unclear at this moment and need a scientific evaluation. However, the main problems are low numbers, lack of standardization, and too many centers performing valvuloplasties in different ways and settings. The best way at this stage would be to define few centers and to conduct RCT trials.

15.3 Training

As mentioned above, currently too many centers are starting with fetal cardiac interventions. Patient selection is unclear, the equipment is far from optimal, different teams in different settings are performing interventions in a non-standardized way, and assessment of success and hemodynamic changes are poor as well as postnatal assessment and decision-making. If fetal intracardiac interventions and fetal pulmonary valvuloplasties for fetuses with PA/IVS or CPS in particular will have a chance to evolve into a useful clinical routine, treatment in the future is largely dependent on the clarification of most of these abovementioned issues. In my opinion, centralization and concentration to few dedicated centers are absolutely necessary to advance the skills and our knowledge about this exiting new promising treatment option.

Part IV

Procedures on the Interatrial Septum

The Embryology of the Interatrial Septum

16

Paolo Versacci, Walter Vignaroli, Gioia Mastromoro, Flavia Ventriglia, and Bruno Marino

The interatrial septum develops from the 27th to the 37th days of gestation, when the human embryo goes from 5 mm to 16–17 mm in length [23].

To better understand the complex structure of the interatrial septum and its embryological development, it is first useful to describe the embryological constitution of the atria.

16.1 Right Atrium

In human beings, the anatomical right atrium is constituted embryologically by the primitive right atrium and by sinus venosus. The primitive left atrium and the sinus of the pulmonary veins form the anatomical left atrium [6, 26]. In the mature heart, the parts that are derived from sinus venosus are easily distinguished by their smooth internal wall, in contrast to the wall of the atrial components, which carries pectinate muscles. The atria acquire their septal wall by means of the septation process.

According to the bilateral right and left symmetry of organisms, the primitive atria are the only primitive cardiac segments that are situated one to the right and the other to the left from the time of their initial appearance [19]. All other primitive cardiac segments develop in series. As a result of this process, the atria and the atrial appendages are the only cardiac structures that can be used for the diagnosis of the type of situs [17]. The primordial right and left atria appear before the sinus venosus, which is progressively incorporated into the right atrium during its development. At the beginning, the sinus venosus is a vascular sac in a dorsocranial position with respect to the dorsal wall of both atria, and it receives the venous blood from the right and left side of the embryo. It is made of a central portion and two lateral

P. Versacci • W. Vignaroli • G. Mastromoro • F. Ventriglia • B. Marino (✉)
Department of Pediatrics, "Sapienza" – University of Rome, Rome, Italy
e-mail: bruno.marino@uniroma1.it

G. Butera et al. (eds.), *Fetal and Hybrid Procedures in Congenital Heart Diseases*, DOI 10.1007/978-3-319-40088-4_16

horns: the right and the left horns of the sinus venosus [5]. They are connected to the rest of the heart tube through the sinoatrial foramen and collect blood from the common cardinal, vitelline, and umbilical veins, which are all the venous blood returning to the heart. The junction of the sinus venosus with the common atrium is called the sinoatrial junction [14]. Contrary to what occurs in most vertebrate embryos, asymmetry of the venous pole in human embryos appears to be present from the beginning onward [6]. In fact, the sinoatrial connection gradually shifts to the right side of the common primitive atrial chamber so that all the systemic venous drainage is limited to what will become the right atrium [14, 15].

At the beginning of the process that leads to the incorporation of the sinus venosus into the right atrium, the sinoatrial foramen has no valves, but it has muscular wall and cardiac jelly, which seem to prevent the retrograde blood flow during atrial contraction. Afterward, the right sinus valve (right sinoatrial valve) and the left sinus valve (left sinoatrial valve) appear, which grow from their onset into the right primitive atrium cavity [25]. The sinus valves are oriented craniocaudally, and where they meet cranially, they form a structure called the septum spurium [14]. This septum flanks the inlet of the future superior caval vein and will finally be incorporated into the terminal crest, which separates the right auricle from the rest of the right atrium [22, 30]. The left venous valve is no longer apparent in the mature heart, because it fuses with the atrial septum by the end of the embryonic period. The right venous valve, however, remains present as the valve of the inferior vena cava, called the Eustachian valve, and the valve of the coronary sinus, called the Thebesian valve [16, 25]. The Eustachian valve continues into the terminal crest, which courses along the posterior atrial wall surrounding the access of the superior vena cava. In the mature heart, the anatomical limits of the sinus region of the right atrium are cephalically, the orifice of the superior vena cava; caudally, the orifices of the inferior vena cava and of the coronary sinus; to the right, the crista terminalis; to the left, the septal wall of the right atrium [16]. In summary, the anatomical right atrium has a sinus region, which originates from the right horn of the sinus venosus, and a fan-shaped pectinate muscles region, which originates from the primitive right atrial myocardium. The boundary between these two regions is the crista terminalis, which takes origin from the right sinus valve [6].

16.2 Left Atrium

The definitive left atrium is constituted by the primitive left atrium and the pulmonary sinus venosus. Completion of the development of the left atrium requires the formation of the lungs and the pulmonary vasculature. The lungs themselves develop as outpouchings from the trachea [23]. As the lung buds form, a plexus of vessels develops around them [19]. This pulmonary plexus drains through a short vessel, which anastomoses to form common pulmonary veins that open into the dorsal wall of the left atrium. Afterward, the common pulmonary vein divides into two branches, each one of which in turn branches into a pair of pulmonary veins [21]. As a result of the incorporation of the common pulmonary vein and its two branches into the wall of the left atrium, the four pulmonary veins will each have an individual opening into this chamber [26]. The incorporated venous tissue also constitutes a major portion of the smooth-walled surface of this atrium. In the mature heart there is no morphological structure that can suggest the limit between the pulmonary sinus venosus and the primitive left atrium [11].

16.3 Atrial Septation

In human beings, the interatrial septum consists of several embryological components including the septum primum, the anterosuperior and the posteroinferior cushions of the atrioventricular canal, the septum secundum, the left sinus valve, and the extracardiac mesenchyme called "spina vestibuli" [4, 13, 27]. Atrial septation starts with formation of the septum primum that grows out from the roof of the common atrium as a thin muscular structure with an endocardial cushion like mesenchymal cap lining the free under-rim (Fig. 16.1). The direction of the growth of the septum primum is from cranioposterior toward the atrioventricular canal, thereby reducing the size of the space between the free edge of the septum primum and fusing atrioventricular cushions [3]. This space is called ostium primum. Despite the fact that the anterosuperior and the posteroinferior endocardial cushions of the atrioventricular canal are a part of the perimeter of the ostium primum, only the posteroinferior endocardial cushion contributes to the closure of this foramen, as confirmed by *in vivo*-labelling experiments in chick embryo hearts [10]. Before the closure of the ostium primum, multiple perforations appear in the septum in the region adjacent to the future drainage of the superior vena cava and the right superior pulmonary vein, most likely by a process of apoptosis. These perforations coalesce to form the so-called ostium secundum (Fig. 16.1) [20].

Another important component of the interatrial septal complex is the "spina vestibuli," which in human beings is constituted by extracardiac mesenchyme, which is involved in the incorporation of the different components to form the definitive interatrial septal complex [6]. The origin of this structure is a matter of some controversy, but its importance in atrial septation now appears to be well established. The "spina vestibuli" was initially described by His in 1880, as a triangular mesenchymal wedge, which protruded into the lumen of the atrium from a nonmuscular area, which he called the "area interposita" in the dorsal wall of the common atrium [12, 18, 27]. It originates in the splanchnic mesoderm ventral to the foregut as a mesenchymal protrusion that contributes to the final formation of the basal part of the developing atrial septum [29]. This structure, in direct continuity with the mediastinal mesenchyme, protrudes into the atrial cavity at the caudal end of commissure between the valves of the sinus venosus. Normal growth of the "spina vestibuli" is important for separate formation of the right and left atrioventricular junction [1, 2]. When development proceeds in a normal way, the "spina vestibuli" grows to reinforce the right side of the area over which the mesenchymal cap on the septum primum fuses with the atrial surface of atrioventricular endocardial cushions [18]. The fusion of the mesenchymal tissues with the atrioventricular endocardial cushions leads to the closure of the ostium primum [6]. Failure of the mesenchymal cap to fuse with atrioventricular cushions results in atrial septal defects [8, 24, 30]. The

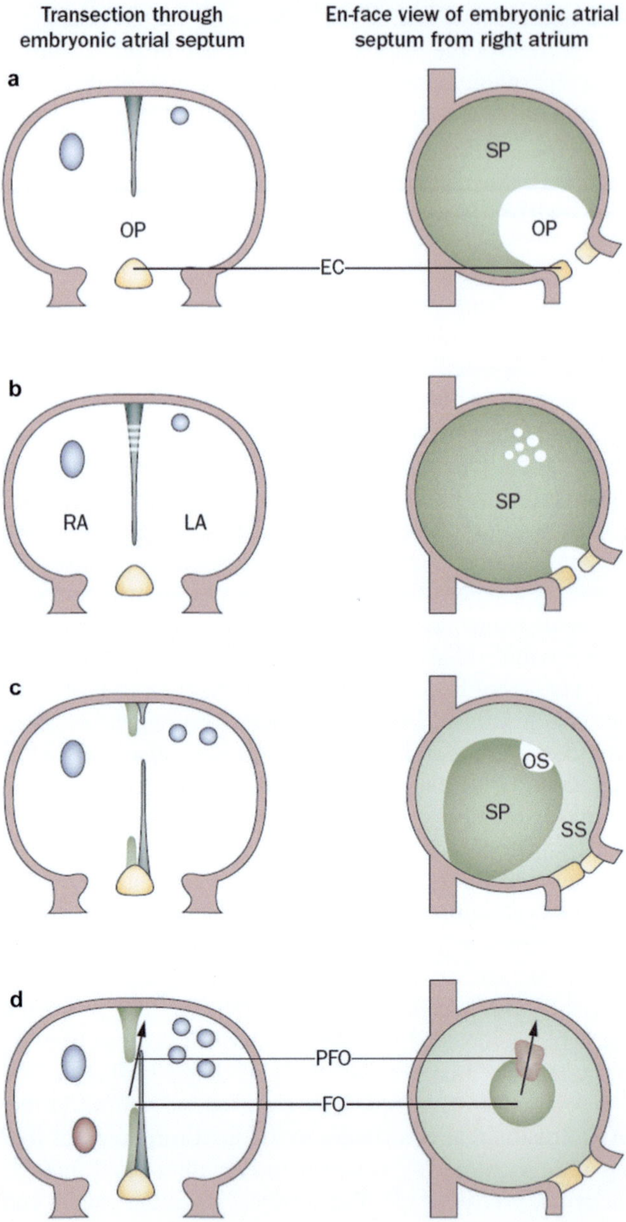

Fig. 16.1 Development of the atrial septum in utero. (**a**) The septum primum grows from the roof of the atria. (**b**) Fenestrations develop within the septum primum. (**c**) The septum secundum develops by an infolding of the atrial walls. The ostium secundum acts as a conduit for right-to-left shunting of oxygenated blood. (**d**) At the anterosuperior edge of the fossa ovalis, the primum and secundum septum remain unfused, which constitutes a PFO. *Arrow* denotes blood flowing through the PFO from the embryonic right atrium to the left atrium. Abbreviations: *EC* endocardial cushion, *FO* fossa ovalis, *LA* left atrium, *OP* ostium primum, *OS* ostium secundum, *PFO* patent foramen ovale, *SP* septum primum, *RA* right atrium, *SS* septum secundum (Adapted by permission from Macmillan Publishers Ltd.: (Patrick et al. [9]), copyright (2011))

derivation and position of the "spina vestibuli" are fundamental, because alterations in the connection of the atrial chamber to the body of the embryo, through the dorsal mesocardium and "spina vestibuli," influence the atrial relationship to the extracardiac midline mesenchyme. The connection with the midline is critical, as this area of attachment encloses the pulmonary pit, which represents the entrance of the pulmonary vein [22, 28]. Variation in the connection gives the potential for abnormal positioning of the pulmonary vein, which would allow the possibility of abnormal pulmonary venous return.

The septum secundum grows later in the development out of the roof of the primitive common atrium, to the right of the septum primum, to form a crescent-shaped structure. The complex of the lower rim of the septum secundum and the ostium secundum is called foramen ovale (Fig. 16.1). One limb of the septum secundum extends ventrally and the other cephalodorsally, thus forming the limbus of the foramen ovale [14, 29]. Moreover, the left sinus valve fuses with the right side of the septum secundum. During the embryologic and fetal period, due to a higher pressure in the right atrium, the limbus of the foramen ovale allows the passage of blood from the right atrium to the left atrium through the ostium secundum (Fig. 16.1). After birth, when lung circulation begins its function, the pressure in the left atrium rises, and the foramen ovale is functionally closed by the septum primum or valve of the foramen ovale, which is pressed against the free border of the septum secundum. The right atrium receives the systemic blood through the superior vena cava, inferior vena cava, and coronary sinus. The left atrium receives the pulmonary venous blood through the pulmonary veins. Functional closure is followed by anatomical closure during the neonatal period due to a process of laminar thrombosis. When anatomical closure takes place, this area is nominated the fossa ovale: the floor is the septum primum, and the limbus is the free border of the septum secundum [7].

References

1. Anderson RH, Brown NA, Webb S. Development and structure of the atrial septum. Heart. 2002;88:104–10.
2. Anderson RH, Ho SY, Becker AE. Anatomy of the human atrioventricular junctions revisited. Anat Rec. 2000;260:81–91.
3. Anderson RH, Spicer DE, Brown NA, Mohun TJ. The development of septation in the four-chambered heart. Anat Rec. 2014;297:1414–29. doi:10.1002/ar.22949.
4. Anderson RH, Webb S, Brown NA. Clinical anatomy of the atrial septum with reference to its developmental components. Clin Anat. 1999;12:362–74. doi:10.1002/(SICI)1098-2353(1999)12:5<362::AID-CA6>3.0.CO;2-F.
5. Anderson RH, Webb S, Brown NA, et al. Development of the heart: (2) septation of the atriums and ventricles. Heart. 2003;89:949–58. doi:10.1136/heart.89.8.949.
6. Anselmi G, de la Cruz MV. Embryological development of the atria. Septation and viscero-atrial situs. In: Living morphogenesis of the heart. Birkhäuser: Soft cover reprint of the original 1st ed. 1998 edition; 2012. pp. 169–86.
7. Asami I, Koizumi K. Development of the atrial septal complex in the human heart: contribution of the spina vestibuli. In: Clark E, Markwald R, Takao A, editors. Developmental mechanism of the heart disease. Armonk: Futura Publishing Co.; 1995. p. 255–60.
8. Briggs LE, Kakarla J, Wessels A. The pathogenesis of atrial and atrioventricular septal defects with special emphasis on the role of the dorsal mesenchymal protrusion. Differentiation. 2012;84:117–30. doi:10.1016/j.diff.2012.05.006.

9. Calvert PA, Rana BS, Kydd AC, Shapiro LM. Patent foramen ovale: anatomy, outcomes, and closure. Nat Rev Cardiol. 2011;8:148–60.
10. De la Cruz MV, Giménez-Ribotta M, Saravalli O, Cayré R. The contribution of the inferior endocardial cushion of the atrioventricular canal to cardiac septation and to the development of the atrioventricular valves: study in the chick embryo. Am J Anat. 1983;166:63–72. doi:10.1002/aja.1001660105.
11. DeRuiter MC, Gittenberger-De Groot AC, Wenink AC, et al. In normal development pulmonary veins are connected to the sinus venosus segment in the left atrium. Anat Rec. 1995;243:84–92. doi:10.1002/ar.1092430110.
12. His W. Anatomie menschlicher Embryonen. Leipzig: Vogel; 1880.
13. Kim JS, Virágh S, Moorman AF. Development of the myocardium of the atrioventricular canal and the vestibular spine in the human heart. Circ Res. 2001;88:395–402. doi:10.1161/01.RES.88.4.395.
14. Kirby ML, Waldo K. Cardiac development. Oxford/New York: Oxford University Press; 2007.
15. Knauth A, McCarthy KP, Webb S, et al. Interatrial communication through the mouth of the coronary sinus. Cardiol Young. 2002;12:364–72. doi:10.1017/CBO9781107415324.004.
16. Licata RH. The human embryonic heart in the ninth week. Am J Anat. 1954;94:73–125. doi:10.1002/aja.1000940104.
17. Macartney FJ, Zuberbuhler JR, Anderson RH. Morphological considerations pertaining to recognition of atrial isomerism. Consequences for sequential chamber localisation. Br Heart J. 1980;44:657–67.
18. Mommersteeg M, Soufan A, de Lange F. Two distinct pools of mesenchyme contribute to the development of the atrial septum. Circ Res. 2006;99:351–3. doi:10.1161/01.RES.0000238360.33284.a0.
19. Moorman A, Webb S, Brown NA, et al. Development of the heart : (1) formation of the cardiac chambers and arterial trunks. Heart. 2003;89:806–14.
20. Moss & Adams' Heart Disease in Infants, Children, and Adolescents, Including the Fetus and Young Adults, vol. 1. Philadelphia: Lippincott Williams & Wilkins; 2008.
21. O'Rahilly R, Muller F. Developmental stages in human embryos. Washington: Carnegie Institution of Washington; 1987.
22. Oostra RJ, Steding G, Lamers WH, Moorman AFM. Development and septation of the atria and venous pole. In: Steding's and Virágh's scanning electron microscopy atlas of the developing human heart. New York: Springer; 2007. p. 48–88.
23. Sadler TW. Cardiovascular system. In: Langman's medical embryology. 12th ed. Philadelphia: Lippincott Williams & Wilkins/a Wolters Kluwer business; 2012. p. 162–200.
24. Snarr BS, Wirrig EE, Phelps AL, et al. A spatiotemporal evaluation of the contribution of the dorsal mesenchymal protrusion to cardiac development. Dev Dyn. 2007;236:1287–94. doi:10.1002/dvdy.21074.
25. Steding G, Xu JW, Seidl W, et al. Developmental aspects of the sinus valves and the sinus venosus septum of the right atrium in human embryos. Anat Embryol (Berl). 1990;181:469–75.
26. Streeter GL. Contribution to embryology. Washington: Carnegie institution of Washington; 1945.
27. Tasaka H, Krug EL, Markwald RR. Origin of the pulmonary venous orifice in the mouse and its relation to the morphogenesis of the sinus venosus, extracardiac mesenchyme (spina vestibuli), and atrium. Anat Rec. 1996;246:107–13. doi:10.1002/(SICI)1097-0185(199609)246:1<107::AID-AR12>3.0.CO;2-T.
28. Webb S, Anderson RH, Lamers WH, Brown NA. Mechanisms of deficient cardiac septation in the mouse with trisomy 16. Circ Res. 1999;84:897–905. doi:10.1161/01.RES.84.8.897.
29. Webb S, Brown NA, Anderson RH. Formation of the atrioventricular septal structures in the normal mouse. Circ Res. 1998;82:645–56. doi:10.1161/01.RES.82.6.645.
30. Wessels A, Anderson RH, Markwald RR, et al. Atrial development in the human heart: an immunohistochemical study with emphasis on the role of mesenchymal tissues. Anat Rec. 2000;259:288–300. doi:10.1002/1097-0185(20000701)259:3<288::AID-AR60>3.0.CO;2-D.

Fetal Anatomy: The Interatrial Septum in the Fetus with Congenital Heart Disease

17

Annalisa Angelini, Marny Fedrigo, Carla Frescura, and Gaetano Thiene

Hypoplastic left heart syndrome (HLHS) [12] represents a complex congenital defect which is characterized by different entities as:

- Mitral stenosis or atresia
- Aortic stenosis or atresia
- Hypoplastic left ventricle

In the setting of HLHS, a restrictive foramen ovale (FO) is reported in 25 % of the cases [10, 13], while complete closed interatrial septum is reported in only 1 % of pathological series [2, 5] and 6 % in clinical series [10, 13]. The closed or restricted foramen ovale produces nonimmune fetal hydrops, left atrial hypertension. As a consequence abnormal lung development occurs characterized by congenital pulmonary cystic lymphangiectasias and pulmonary vein muscularization, which will be irreversible as long as the condition persists in the fetus, impacting on survival at birth or even later after delivery when bidirectional shunt is attempted [3, 6, 9]. The lack of communication between the two atria hinders the systemic oxygenated blood from the placenta to reach the left cavities and ultimately the ascending aorta and systemic circulation resulting in structural heart abnormalities known as hypoplastic left heart syndrome [7].

Atrial septation is a complex process which produces separation of the right and left atrial component of the primitive common atrium and starts early during fetal life. By 33 days the septum primum is formed as an outward expansion of the posterior-superior atrial wall [1]. Later the reabsorption of the septum primum produces a communication in the septum known as ostium secundum. At day 43 the septum secundum develops, again as an eversion from the posterior wall, on the

A. Angelini (✉) • M. Fedrigo • C. Frescura • G. Thiene
Department of Cardiac, Thoracic and Vascular Sciences, University of Padua, Padua, Italy
e-mail: annalisa.angelini@unipd.it

G. Butera et al. (eds.), *Fetal and Hybrid Procedures in Congenital Heart Diseases*, DOI 10.1007/978-3-319-40088-4_17

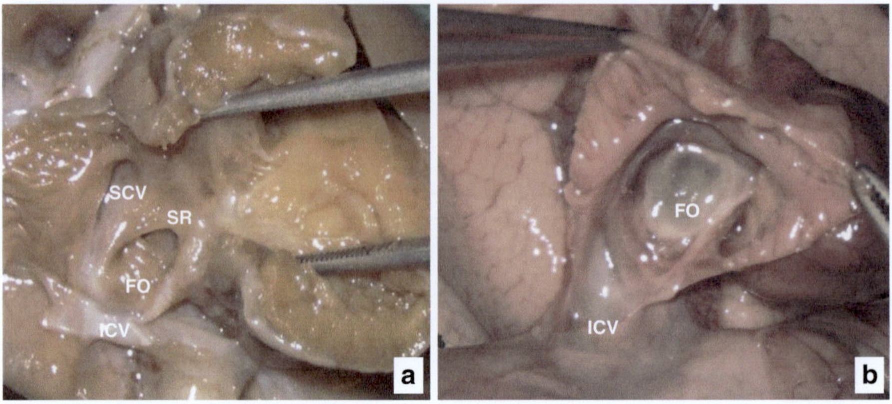

Fig. 17.1 (**a**) Female fetus 21 gestational weeks, spontaneous abortion. The heart was structurally normal. The right atrium has been opened to show the interatrial septum with a well-formed rim of the fossa ovalis, flap valve, and patent foramen ovale. (**b**) Female fetus 22 gestational weeks, voluntary abortion for congenital heart disease (HLHS). The right atrium has been open from the inferior vena cava toward the apex of the right atrial appendage. The foramen ovale is closed by the flap valve which is plastered against the muscular rim of the foramen and appeared aneurismatic with bulging toward the left atrium

right end side of the septum primum, forming what becomes the rim of the fossa ovalis, which remains muscular even after birth. By the third month of gestation the atrial septation is completed. The floor of the fossa ovalis is then represented by septum primum; it acts as a valve in which remnants patent in the anterior part (Fig. 17.1). This fossa ovalis is one of the essential pathways during fetal life, ensuring the blood flow from the right atrium to the left atrium, left ventricle, and ascending aorta. The fossa is oval in shape and has the same size as the inferior caval vein orifice. With atrial growth the dimension of the fossa ovalis will decrease, and at term of gestation, the size is reduced to 60 % of the caval orifice. The valve of the fossa ovalis exceeds the area demarked by the rim. It can then balloon into the left atrium if the pressure in the right atrium is high. At birth, with increasing pulmonary venous return, the flap valve is pushed against the rims of the fossa and progressively fused with it. Originally the valve is a muscular structure which progressively becomes fibrous.

Three different patterns of atrial cavity and atrial septum can be recognized in HLHS with intact or restrictive foramen ovalis [4, 10]:

- Type A: A relatively large left atrium with a thick septum secundum and a thin septum primum adherent to each other, often associated with leftward and posteriorly deviated septum primum and massively dilated pulmonary veins. Decompression pathway from the left atrium can be to the innominate vein, right superior vena cava, and right atrium. This pathway is unobstructed.
- Type B: A small, muscular left atrium with circumferential thickening of the atrial walls and a thick "spongy" muscular atrial septum without ostensible

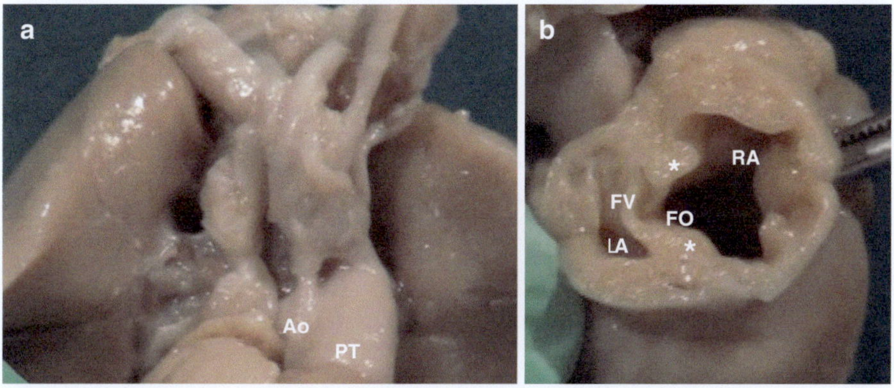

Fig. 17.2 Female fetus 23 gestational week, voluntary abortion for hypoplastic left heart syndrome. (**a**) Anterior view of the heart and the lungs. Note the pulmonary trunk (*PT*) and the severe hypoplastic ascending aorta (*Ao*) in the setting of the aortic atresia. (**b**) Transverse cut at the level of the left and right atrial cavity showing the restricted foramen ovale with well-formed muscular rims (*asterisk*) and the thick flap valve

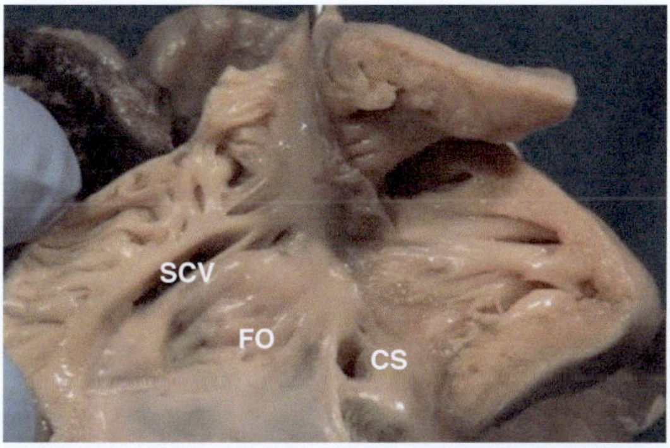

Fig. 17.3 Hypoplastic left heart syndrome. The right atrium is opened from the inferior vena cava toward the apex of the right atrial appendage and the right ventricle along the acute margin of the heart. The foramen ovale is completely closed by a thick valve. *SCV* superior caval vein, *FO* foramen ovale, *CS* coronary sinus orifice

distinction between septum primum and septum secundum. The atrial septum is thickened without distinction between septum primum and secundum. The left atrium appears muscular. The pulmonary veins are usually small (Fig. 17.2b).

- Type C: A giant left atrium with a thin, rightward bulging septum with identifiable septum primum and secundum, this in the setting of severe mitral regurgitation. The pulmonary veins are usually large [14].

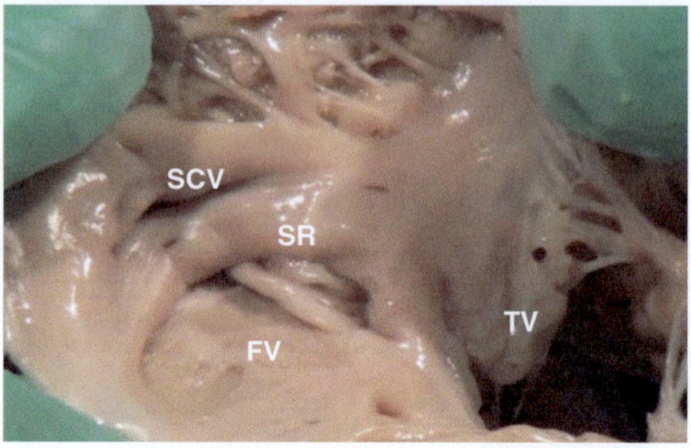

Fig. 17.4 Hypoplastic left heart syndrome. The right atrium is opened from the inferior vena cava toward the apex of the right atrial appendage and the right ventricle along the acute margin of the heart. The foramen ovale is restricted by an aneurismatic and redundant flap thick valve. *SCV* superior caval vein, *FO* foramen ovale, *SR* superior rim of the fossa ovalis

Even during the fetal life, a thin atrial septum (type C) will favor septostomy/septoplasty (Fig. 17.1b), whereas a thick atrial septum (type A and B) will favor interatrial stenting (Fig. 17.2b).

The premature closure of the foramen ovalis (Figs. 17.1b and 17.3) or its severe restriction (Figs. 17.2b and 17.4) results in diversion of blood flow from the left atrium and cardiac chamber remodeling (Fig. 17.2a). The right ventricle with the tricuspid valve is well developed since they are handling the entire systemic blood flow, which reaches the right atrium. The tricuspid valve can present with some degree of dysplasia of the leaflet and abnormalities of the subvalvular apparatus [11]. The pulmonary trunk (PT) is dilated, and the arterial duct is prominent such it carries all systemic circulation (Fig. 17.2a). The left ventricle is usually small with hypoplasia and dysplasia of the mitral valve apparatus, often associated with endocardial fibroelastosis. The aorta is hypoplastic with normal origin of the coronary arteries [8]. The aortic valve is hypoplastic as well, with all the leaflet spectrum, from imperforate to unicuspid, bicuspid, or tricuspid cups. Dysplasia is a constant feature of unicuspid, bicuspid, or tricuspid leaflets, with myxoid nodular degeneration. In the setting of atresia and imperforate valve, the aortic orifice is guarded by a thin, curtain-like membrane in the absence of clearly identifiable cups and raphes. The commissures can be identified as tiny raphe at the sinotubular junction.

Key Points

- Dimension of the left atrium and left ventricle
- Morphological substrate of interatrial septum
  - Type A: discrete identifiable FO, thicker border of FO, aneurism of FO
  - Type B: muscular, more disadvantageous
  - Type C: large atrium with interatrial septum of type B or type A.

References

1. Anderson RH, Webb S, Brown NA, Lamers W, Moorman A. Development of the heart: (2) Septation of the atriums and ventricles. Heart. 2003;89:949–58.
2. Bharati S, Lev M. The surgical anatomy of hypoplasia of aortic tract complex. J Thorac Cardiovasc Surg. 1984;88:97–101.
3. Canter CE, Moorehead S, Huddleston CB, Spray TL. Restrictive atrial septal communication as a determinant of outcome of cardiac transplantation for hypoplastic left heart syndrome. Circulation. 1993;88:II456–60.
4. Chaturvedi RR, Ryan G, Seed M, van Arsdell G, Jaeggi ET. Fetal stenting of the atrial septum: technique and initial results in cardiac lesions with left atrial hypertension. Int J Cardiol. 2013;168:2029–36.
5. Frescura C, Ho SY, Thiene G. La collezione anatomica di cardiopatie congenite dell'. Padova: Università di Padova. Cleup; 1996.
6. Graziano JN, Heidelberger KP, Ensing GJ, Gomez CA, Ludomirsky A. The influence of a restrictive atrial septal defect on pulmonary vascular morphology in patients with hypoplastic left heart syndrome. Pediatr Cardiol. 2002;23:146–51.
7. Hove JR, Köster RW, Forouhar AS, Acevedo-Bolton G, Fraser SE, Gharib M. Intracardiac fluid forces are an essential epigenetic factor for embryonic cardiogenesis. Nature. 2003;421:172–7.
8. Ilbawi AM, Spicer DE, Bharati S, Cook A, Anderson RH. Morphologic study of the ascending aorta and aortic arch in hypoplastic left hearts: surgical implications. J Thorac Cardiovasc Surg. 2007;134:99–105.
9. Maeda K, Yamaki S, Kado H, Asou T, Murakami A, Takamoto S. Hypoplasia of the small pulmonary arteries in hypoplastic left heart syndrome with restrictive atrial septal defect. Circulation. 2004;110(11 Suppl1):II139–46.
10. Rychik J, Rome JJ, Collins MH, DeCampli WM, Spray TL. The hypoplastic left heart syndrome with intact atrial septum: atrial morphology, pulmonary vascular histopathology and outcome. J Am Coll Cardiol. 1999;34:554–60.
11. Stamm C, Anderson RH, Ho SY. The morphologically tricuspid valve in hypoplastic left heart syndrome. Eur J Cardiothorac Surg. 1997;12:587–92.
12. Tchervenkov CI, Jacobs JP, Weinberg PM, Aiello VD, Béland MJ, Colan SD, Elliott MJ, Franklin RC, Gaynor JW, Krogmann ON, Kurosawa H, Maruszewski B, Stellin G. The nomenclature, definition and classification of hypoplastic left heart syndrome. Cardiol Young. 2006;16:339–68.
13. Vida VL, Bacha EA, Larrazabal A, Gauvreau K, Dorfman AL, Marx G, Geva T, Marshall AC, Pigula FA, Mayer JE, del Nido PJ, Fynn-Thompson F. Surgical outcome for patients with the mitral stenosis-aortic atresia variant of hypoplastic left heart syndrome. J Thorac Cardiovasc Surg. 2008;135:339–46.
14. Vogel M, McElhinney DB, Wilkins-Haug LE, Marshall AC, Benson CB, Juraszek AL, Silva V, Lock JE, Marx GR, Tworetzky W. Aortic stenosis and severe mitral regurgitation in the fetus resulting in giant left atrium and hydrops: pathophysiology, outcomes, and preliminary experience with pre-natal cardiac intervention. J Am Coll Cardiol. 2011;57:348–55.

Literature on Fetal Therapy on Interatrial Septum

18

Simona Anna Marcora

Atrial septal restriction during fetal age is widely recognized as a lethal defect mostly in patients with hypoplastic left heart syndrome (HLHS) and intact atrial septum (IAS) or highly restrictive atrial septum (HRAS). The poor outcome has been attributed to structural abnormalities of the pulmonary venous vasculature with arterialization of pulmonary veins and dilatation of lymphatics due to prenatal left atrial hypertension [1]. This hypothesis has been recently supported by an interesting histopathologic study on changes in alveoloseptal lung parenchyma in fetuses with atrial septal restriction; these authors observed that severe lung disease is already evident in the second trimester, precisely in week 23 [2]. Efforts to decompress the hypertensive left atrium in utero have been made since 2000 to treat neonatal hypoxia and hemodynamic instability, to improve anatomic lung abnormalities and outcome. This chapter is a review of the most significant experiences reported in literature on procedural and clinical results of fetal atrial septostomy procedures in HLHS and IAS/HRAS.

Table 18.1 reports procedural outcome after fetal atrial septostomy for IAS/HRAS in HLHS [3–7]. Key points are:

- Feasibility and high rate of technical success with low procedural-related death.
- Different techniques (ballooning, septostomy, stenting) have been introduced during years to obtain a permanent larger atrial defect; stenting should be preferred to balloon dilatation to avoid recoil in thick atrial septum; however, risks of infection, thrombosis, or late embolization of stents are still unknown.
- Best timing for the procedure not yet known; risks of fetal demise and early delivery have to be balanced against lung disease due to prolonged left atrium hypertension.

S.A. Marcora
ASST Papa Giovanni XXIII, Bergamo, Italy
e-mail: smarcora@asst-pg23.it

G. Butera et al. (eds.), *Fetal and Hybrid Procedures in Congenital Heart Diseases*, DOI 10.1007/978-3-319-40088-4_18

Table 18.1 Procedural outcomes after fetal atrial septostomy for IAS/HRAS in HLHS

Group (ref); period	No. patients (pts); EGA (weeks)	Stent	Outcome of fetal atrial septostomy	Complications of fetal procedures	Fetal procedure-related death	Postnatal atrial septostomy	Postnatal outcomes
Boston (Ref. [3]); 2000–2003	7 pts; 26–34 weeks	None	Technical success: 6/7 (86 %)	Fetus: hemothorax 1/7 (14 %) Mother: none	1/7 (14 %)	3/6 (50 %)	Mortality: 66 % (1/6 at birth, 3 after Norwood) Survival: 34 % (1/6 Norwood, 1/6 Glenn)
Boston (Ref. [4]); 2001–2007	21 pts; 23–34 weeks	1/21	Technical success: 19/21 (90 %)	Fetus: arrhythmias, pericardial and pleural effusion 8/21 (40 %) Mother: none	2/21 (9.5 %)	12/19 (63 %)	Mortality: no death at birth; 58 % (7/12 with postnatal decompression) died after Norwood versus 14 % (2/7 who had a routine Stage I procedure)
Boston (Ref. [5]); 2002–2009	14 pts aortic stenosis, mitral regurgitation in giant left atrium 5/14 fetal procedures 22–33 weeks	1/5	Technical success: 5/5		None	3/14 (21 %)	Mortality 85 % (2/14 alive)
Toronto (Ref. [6]); 2000–2012	10 pts 4/10 fetal procedures 20–36 weeks	4/4	Technical success: 4/4 (2/4 stent stenosis)	Fetus: pericardial effusion and stent embolization 2/4 (50 %) Mother: none	None	4/4 (100 %, in two cases associated to pulmonary bibanding)	Mortality: 50 % (2/4 death in pts with prenatal septostomy), 100 % (2/6 fetal demise, 4/6 pre-Norwood in pts without prenatal septostomy)
Boston (Ref. [7]); 2005–2012	9 pts; 24–31 weeks	9/9	Technical success 5/9 (55 %)	Fetus: hemopericardium, arrhythmias 5/9 (88 %) Mother: none	1/9 (11 %)	1/8 (12.5 %)	Mortality: 43 % (3/7 at birth) Survival: 1 discharge, 2 Glenn, 1 biventricular

- Successful fetal atrial septostomy is associated with less frequent need for emergent postnatal intervention, but clinical efficacy, mostly in reverse lung pathology, cannot be demonstrated by these small series.

Table 18.2 reports clinical outcomes after fetal atrial septostomy for IAS/HRAS in HLHS. Table 18.3 compares clinical outcomes in patients with postnatal septostomy or without fetal atrial restriction in the same years [8–13]. Key points are:

- Patients born with HLHS and IAS have high morbidity and mortality at birth and first stage palliation comparing with HRAS but patent a or no restriction.
- Trends toward improved survival after birth improved in recent years compared with early experience; this is due to the introduction of fetal atrial procedures, the progress in catheter postnatal techniques as an alternative to surgical septostomy, and the advance in pre-Norwood strategies as left atrial decompression plus pulmonary bibanding to minimize pulmonary injury and promote healing of the lung.
- Data about outcomes after stage 2, Fontan and their interstages are contrary; some studies show that patients with restriction have the same survival as patients without; other studies show a worse survival.
- Higher mortality after Glenn and Fontan can be explained by vascular pulmonary reactivity due to lung disease, late pulmonary vein stenosis.
- Fetal atrial septostomy can be considered a savage procedure for high-risk candidate, however has not yet been associated to improve in late outcome and reversal of lung disease due to fetal left atrial hypertension.

In the last part of bibliography, review articles [14–23], written after the introduction of fetal atrial septostomy procedures, are reported to suggest more general readings on this topic. Among these, it is mandatory to reflect on this citation, "Rather than await a proliferation of such procedures at centers that are unlikely to amass a critical volume of experience to ensure clinical competence, a prospective multicenter trial should be considered to address the nuances of technical performance of the procedures, to evaluate the short and mid term result and to compare these results with those of children undergoing various form of palliation for HLHS. Only then can we determine whether this is a rationale strategy for the management of these patients or merely the application of a technique in search of an indication" [23].

Table 18.2 Clinical outcomes after fetal atrial septostomy for IAS/HRAS in HLHS

Group (ref); period	No. patients (pts); fetal procedures (type)	Neonatal outcome	Norwood mortality	Interstage 1 mortality/ transplant (OHT)	Glenn mortality	Interstage 2 mortality/OHT	Fontan mortality	Pulmonary veins stenosis
Boston (Ref. [8]); 2001–2006	32 pts; 14/32 fetal procedures (5 atrial septostomy)	Postnatal atrial septostomy: 29/32 (91 %) Neonatal death 0	10/32 (30 %)	4/22 (18 %)	1/18 (5.5 %)	2/17 (12 %)	2/3 (12 waiting Fontan)	11/32 (34 %)
Philadelphia (Ref. [9]); 1997–2006	16 pts HLHS/IAS (severe form) No fetal procedures	Postnatal atrial septostomy: 16/16 Neonatal death: 8/16 (50 %)	3/5 (60 %)	Not available (n.a.)	1/3 (33 %)	75 % at 3 years ($^{\S}p<0.001$)	0/3	2/16 (12.5 %)
	22 pts HLHS/ HRAS (less severe form); 2/2 fetal procedures	Postnatal atrial septostomy: 20/22 (90 %) Neonatal death: 0/22	*1/19 (5 %)*	n.a.	*5/21 (23 %)*	30 % at 3 years§	3/12 (25 %)	
Texas (Ref. [10]); 2010–2013	6 pts HLHS IAS/RAS 2/6 fetal procedure	Postnatal atrial septostomy: 6/6 Neonatal death: 2/6 (33 %) Pulmonary bibanding (0–7 days): 4/6	0/4	None	0/4			

$^{\S}(p<0.001)$

Table 18.3 Clinical results of patients with HLHS/IAS without fetal atrial septostomy or patients with HLHS without IAS

Group (ref); period	No. and type of patients (pts)	Neonatal outcome	Norwood mortality	Interstage 1 Mortality/transplant (OHT)	Glenn mortality	Interstage 2 mortality/OHT	Fontan mortality	Pulmonary veins stenosis
Boston (Ref. [11]); 1990–2002	33 pts HLHS/IAS (55 % prenatal diagnosis) 66 pts HLHS no IAS	Postnatal atrial Septostomy: 33/33 Neonatal death: 7/33 (21 %) Postnatal atrial Septostomy: 0/66 Neonatal death: 0	16/26 (38 %) 20/66 (30 %)	At 1,6 months 48 %, 58 % At 1,6 months 9 %, 21 %	Early 3/16 (19 %) n.a.	At 12 months 66 % At 12 months 28 %	0/10 n.a.	n.a n.a.
San Francisco (Ref. [12]); 1999–2009	14 pts HLHS/IAS 35 pts HLHS no IAS	Postnatal atrial septostomy: 5/14 (36 %) Neonatal death: 4/14 (28.5 %) Postnatal atrial septostomy and death: 0/3	0/10 3/35 (8.5 %)	4/10 (12.5 %) 3/32 (6 %)	n.a. n.a.	At 2 years 40 % At 2 years 17 %	n.a. n.a.	n.a. n.a.
New York (Ref. [13]); 2003–2011	20 pts HLHS/HRAS (75 % prenatal diagnosis) 121 pts HLAS no HRAS	Postnatal atrial septostomy: 20/20 No neonatal death No postnatal atrial septostomy and death	4/20 (20 %) 7/121 (6 %)	1 lost follow-up (LFU) 5/114 (4.5 %) 10 LFU	3/15 (20 %) 6/99 (6 %)	2 LFU 6/93 (6.4 %) 7 LFU 1 BIV	0/6 4 waiting Fontan 2/52 Fontan (3.8 %) 27 waiting Fontan	4/20 (20 %) n.a.

References

1. Rychik J, et al. The hypoplastic left heart syndrome with intact atrial septum: atrial morphology, pulmonary vascular histopathology and outcome. J Am Coll Cardiol. 1999;34:554–60.
2. Goltz D, et al. Left ventricular obstruction with restrictive inter-atrial communication leads to retardation in fetal lung maturation. Prenat Diagn. 2015;35:1–8.
3. Marshall AC, et al. Creation of an atrial septal defect in utero for fetuses with hypoplastic left heart syndrome and intact or highly restrictive atrial septum. Circulation. 2004;110:253–8.
4. Marshall A, et al. Results of in utero atrial septoplasty in fetuses with hypoplastic left heart syndrome. Prenat Diagn. 2008;28:1023–8.
5. Vogel M, et al. Aortic stenosis and severe mitral regurgitation in fetus resulting in giant left atrium and hydrops. J Am Coll Cardiol. 2011;57:348–55.
6. Chaturvedi RR, et al. Fetal stenting of the atrial septum: technique and initial results in cardiac lesions with left atrial hypertension. Int J Cardiol. 2013;168:2029–36.
7. Kalish BT, et al. Technical challenges of atrial septal stent placement in fetuses with hypoplastic left heart syndrome and intact atrial septum. Catheter Cardiovasc Interv. 2014;84:77–85.
8. Vida VL, et al. Hypoplastic left heart syndrome with intact or highly restrictive atrial septum: surgical experience from a single center. Ann Thorac Surg. 2007;84:581–5.
9. Glatz JA, et al. Hypoplastic left heart syndrome with atrial level restriction in the era of prenatal diagnosis. Ann Thorac Surg. 2007;84:1633–9.
10. Barker GM, et al. Optimization of preoperative status in hypoplastic left heart syndrome with intact atrial septum by left atrial decompression and bilateral pulmonary artery bands. Pediatr Cardiol. 2014;35:479–84.
11. Vlahos P, et al. HLHS with IAS. Outcome after neonatal transcatheter atrial septostomy. Circulation. 2004;109:2326–30.
12. Lowenthal A, et al. Prenatal diagnosis of atrial restriction in hypoplastic left heart syndrome is associated with decreased 2-year survival. Prenat Diagn. 2012;32:485–90.
13. Hoque T, et al. Current outcomes of hypoplastic left heart syndrome with restrictive atrial septum: a single center experience. Pediatr Cardiol. 2013;34:1181–9.
14. Tworetzky W, et al. Fetal interventions for cardiac defects. Pediatr Clin North Am. 2004;51:1503–31.
15. Sekar P, et al. The role of fetal echocardiography in fetal intervention: a symbiotic relationship. Clin Perinatol. 2009;36:301–27.
16. McElhinney DB, et al. Current status of fetal cardiac intervention. Circulation. 2010;121:1256–63.
17. Bacha EA. Impact of fetal cardiac intervention on Congenital Heart Surgery. Semin Thorac Cardiovasc Surg Pediatr Card Surg Annu. 2011;14:35–7.
18. Van Aerschot I, et al. Fetal cardiac interventions: myths and facts. Arch Cardiovasc Dis. 2012;105:366–72.
19. Allan LD. Rationale for and current status of prenatal cardiac intervention. Early Hum Dev. 2012;88:287–90.
20. Tulzer G, et al. Fetal cardiac interventions: rationale, risk and benefit. Semin Fetal Neonatal Med. 2013;18:298–3011.
21. Herberg U, et al. Foetal therapy: what works? Closed interatrial septum. Cardiol Young. 2014;24:47–54.
22. Schidlow DN, et al. Percutaneous fetal cardiac interventions for structural heart disease. Am J Perinatol. 2014;31:629–36.
23. Kleinman CS. Fetal cardiac intervention. Innovative therapy or a technique in search of an indication? Circulation. 2006;113:1378–81.

19 Procedures on the Atrial Septum: Approach, Outcomes and Future Perspective

Edgar Jaeggi, Rajiv Chaturvedi, and Greg Ryan

This chapter provides an overview of the normal atrial septum and the main lesions that are associated with prenatal septal restriction, proposes selection criteria of patients and procedures for possible in utero interventions, and illustrates the fetal and postnatal outcome after intrauterine intervention.

19.1 Natural History and Pathophysiology

19.1.1 The Foramen Ovale in the Normal Fetal Circulation

In the normal fetal circulation with two parallel functioning ventricles, the foramen ovale (FO) is an important provider of oxygenated umbilical blood from the placenta to the left heart, the ascending aorta, and the upper body. The crescent-shaped FO is typically located in the central portion of the secundum atrial septum and progressively increases in width from about 3 mm at 18 weeks to 6 mm at term [1]. The thin and mobile septum primum is positioned on the left side of the atrial septum and functions as a flap valve of the FO. During most of the cardiac cycle, it is

E. Jaeggi, MD, FRCP(C) (✉)
Department of Pediatrics, Labatt Family Heart Centre, The Hospital for Sick Children, University of Toronto, 555 University Avenue, Toronto, ON M5G 1X8, Canada

Fetal Cardiac Program, Labatt Family Heart Centre, Toronto, ON, Canada
e-mail: edgar.jaeggi@sickkids.ca

R. Chaturvedi, MB BChir, MD, PhD
Department of Pediatrics, Labatt Family Heart Centre, The Hospital for Sick Children, University of Toronto, 555 University Avenue, Toronto, ON M5G 1X8, Canada

G. Ryan, MB, FRCSC, FRCOG
Department of Obstetrics and Gynecology, Faculty of Medicine, Mount Sinai Hospital, University of Toronto, 700 University Avenue, Toronto, ON M5G 1X5, Canada

G. Butera et al. (eds.), *Fetal and Hybrid Procedures in Congenital Heart Diseases*, DOI 10.1007/978-3-319-40088-4_19

pushed into the left atrium (LA) by the steady stream of blood that enters the FO. After birth, as the arterial duct closes, the pulmonary blood flow increases, and the LA pressure exceeds that of the right; the septum primum flap is forced against the septum secundum, functionally closing the foramen ovale. In time the septae fuse, leaving the fossa ovalis as a remnant of the FO.

19.1.2 Premature Restriction of the Atrial Septum (RAS)

The prenatal development of RAS is associated with either a primary developmental abnormality of the atrial septum that leads to a small or absent FO orifice or, secondary to fetal LA hypertension, the premature adhesion of the primum septal flap to the atrial septum causing partial or total FO occlusion. Premature RAS may occur as an isolated anomaly or in combination with other pathologies and may have life-threatening lesion-specific clinical consequences. The rationale for prenatal therapy is to improve the survival for conditions with a high risk for perinatal death or at least to modify the outcome sufficiently to justify the risk of the prenatal intervention. These principles most obviously but not exclusively apply to two forms of obstructive left heart disease that may present with severe atrial septal restriction: hypoplastic left heart syndrome (HLHS) and critical aortic stenosis (AS) with severe mitral regurgitation (MR).

HLHS with an intact atrial septum (*IAS*) represents a particularly lethal combination of serious anomalies. If left untreated before birth, HLHS/IAS has been associated with overall mortality of 50% or more [2–7]. Atrial septal restriction severe enough to require early postnatal catheter septostomy affects about 10% of newborns with a fetal diagnosis of HLHS [2, 8], but in about half of these cases, the septum is intact or nearly intact [2, 9]. As there is no relevant egress of blood entering the LA via the pulmonary veins (PVs), this causes marked elevation in left atrial and pulmonary venous pressure with concomitant reduction in lung perfusion and remodeling of the pulmonary vasculature. The lung pathology commonly observed in HLHS/IAS includes severely dilated lymphatics and thickened "muscularized" pulmonary veins and arteries [2, 10]. At birth, the newborn with severe impediment to left-right atrial shunting in the setting of HLHS or critical aortic stenosis becomes profoundly hypoxemic and acidotic and thus will require the urgent creation of an atrial communication for immediate survival. Some centers therefore perform caesarean sections in pediatric operating rooms or hybrid catheterization laboratories to shorten the interval between delivery and the neonatal atrioseptostomy. Nonetheless, recent studies have shown that even with a prenatal diagnosis and optimized perinatal management, the prognosis of HLHS/IAS remains dismal due to persistent pulmonary vascular abnormalities and high pulmonary vascular resistance that may preclude the option of a successful surgical palliation to a bicavopulmonary anastomosis [4, 5, 9–12]. The grim outlook of HLHS/IAS has prompted efforts to develop criteria and techniques to intervene for this condition before birth [13, 14], in the hope that the prenatal creation of a sufficiently large left atrial communication to lower the LA pressure may also improve the pulmonary vascular development and the likelihood of survival.

Fetal AS with severe MR typically leads to severe dilation of the left ventricle and atrium. The severe aortic stenosis results in left ventricular failure and mitral regurgitation secondary to annular dilation. The combination of an elevated left ventricular end-diastolic pressure and mitral regurgitation leads to left atrial hypertension which is further increased by the secondary atrial septal restriction or closure. This combination of progressive aortic stenosis and atrial restriction blocks all routes of blood egress from the left heart. Progressive dilation of the left heart cavities can cause mechanical compression of the right atrium and ventricle, impede the filling and emptying of the right heart, increase the systemic venous pressure, and lead to low cardiac output and fetal hydrops. Similar echocardiographic findings can occur with a primary left ventricular cardiomyopathy. The prognosis of this constellation of findings is very poor with survival rates beyond the neonatal period of <20 % [7]. To prevent in utero demise from progressive heart failure, options for salvage rescue therapy may include fetal aortic valve dilation to reduce the amount of MR by improving the left ventricular function and aortic forward flow, fetal atrial septoplasty to decompress the LA and improve the right ventricular preload and output, or the two procedures in combination.

Other cardiac lesions may be affected by severe atrial septal restriction than HLHS, which makes them potential indications for a prenatal intervention. This includes the subset of patients with transposition of the great arteries (TGA) that has IAS and ductus arteriosus constriction and is likely to present with profound hypoxemia at birth due to the poor mixing of blood between the pulmonary and systemic circulations [15–18]. While the prenatal assessment of the FO and the arterial duct is crucial to identify TGA patients at risk of severe neonatal complications, demise immediately following delivery has occurred despite the prenatal diagnosis of IAS, suggesting that adequate mixing may not always be obtained in time with the usual postnatal emergency measures. RAS resulting in fetal hydrops and death has been reported in association with Ebstein's anomaly of the tricuspid valve, severe tricuspid regurgitation, and obligatory right-left atrial shunting [19]. Finally, in the offspring with an otherwise structurally normal heart, RAS has been associated with neonatal pulmonary hypertension and death [20].

19.2 Echocardiographic Evaluation and Selection Criteria

19.2.1 Obstructive Left Heart Lesions

Careful fetal echocardiographic assessment of the left atrium, the atrial septum, and the pulmonary veins (PV) provides important information on atrial septal patency in obstructive left heart lesions [8, 10, 21]. By two-dimensional echocardiography, three patterns of atrial morphology may be distinguished in left heart lesions with IAS according to Rychik and colleagues (Fig. 19.1a–c): [9] Two thirds of cases in their study had a thick atrial septum, large LA, and massively dilated pulmonary veins (*type A*). The remaining third either had the *type B* morphology with a thick atrial septum with small LA and pulmonary veins or a *type C* pattern with a thin

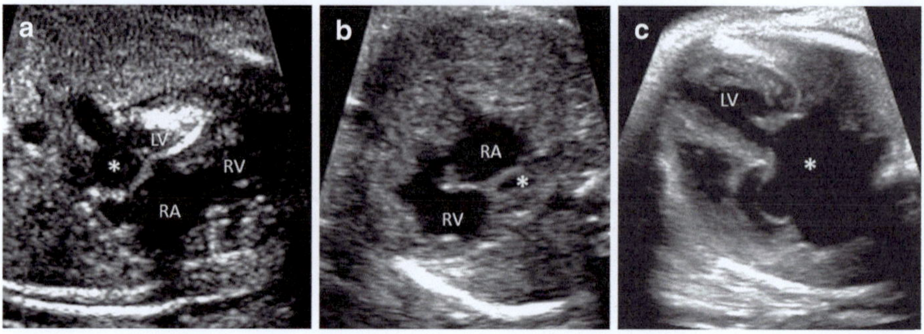

Fig. 19.1 (**a–c**) Types of left atrial (*) and atrial septal morphology that occur in association with obstructive left heart with a severely restricted atrial septum. Type A: thick septum, dilated left atrium, dilated pulmonary veins; type B: thick septum, tiny left atrium, and pulmonary veins; type C: thin septum, massively dilated left atrium

atrial septum, giant LA, severe mitral regurgitation, and dilated pulmonary veins. In our experience, the type A morphology was mainly observed in conjunction with fetal aortic atresia and severe mitral valve obstruction with a small, hypertensive left ventricle [3]. The type B was seen in a case with mitral and aortic atresia and tiny left heart structures which, because of the small LA size precludes any option of a prenatal intervention on the atrial septum [22]. Alternate vascular pathways of LA decompression, such as levoatrial cardinal veins, can be detected in some patients with HLHS/IAS, which may also be obstructed. In contrast, the thin type C atrial septum was predominantly seen with severe MR secondary to critical AS rather than in HLHS/IAS [7]. Several authors have shown that in HLHS and other severe obstructive left heart lesions, the severity of fetal FO restriction and LA hypertension is best predicted by pulse wave Doppler interrogation of the PV flow (Fig. 19.2) [3, 8, 23]. In the absence of left heart pathology, the pulmonary veins appear non-distended and display a pulse wave Doppler flow pattern with low peak velocities in ventricular systole (s-wave) and early diastole (d-wave) of similar magnitude and cessation of flow during atrial systole (a-wave). In HLHS with unrestricted left-right atrial shunting, there is also normal continuous PV forward flow in systole and early diastole, but this is followed by brief a-wave flow reversal as the left atrium pumps blood against the FO and the simultaneously contracting right atrium (Fig. 19.2a). The ratio of the velocity-time integrals (VTI) of PV forward/reverse flow is high (>10:1) as the combined VTI of the forward s- and d-waves is much larger than the VTI of the small and brief reversed a-wave. Where there is more atrial septal restriction, there is a rise in pressure and volume within the PVs, owing to restricted flow during diastole. This is reflected by a decrease in the early diastolic forward flow to the LA, an increase in the duration and peak velocity of a-wave flow reversal, and thus a lower PV forward/reverse VTI ratio (Fig. 19.2b). Where the atrial septum is closed, the PV Doppler flow pattern is to and fro, showing only a forward s-wave during ventricular systole and a similarly large and broad a-wave in the opposite direction during atrial systole and thus a forward/reverse VTI ratio of 1. There is no

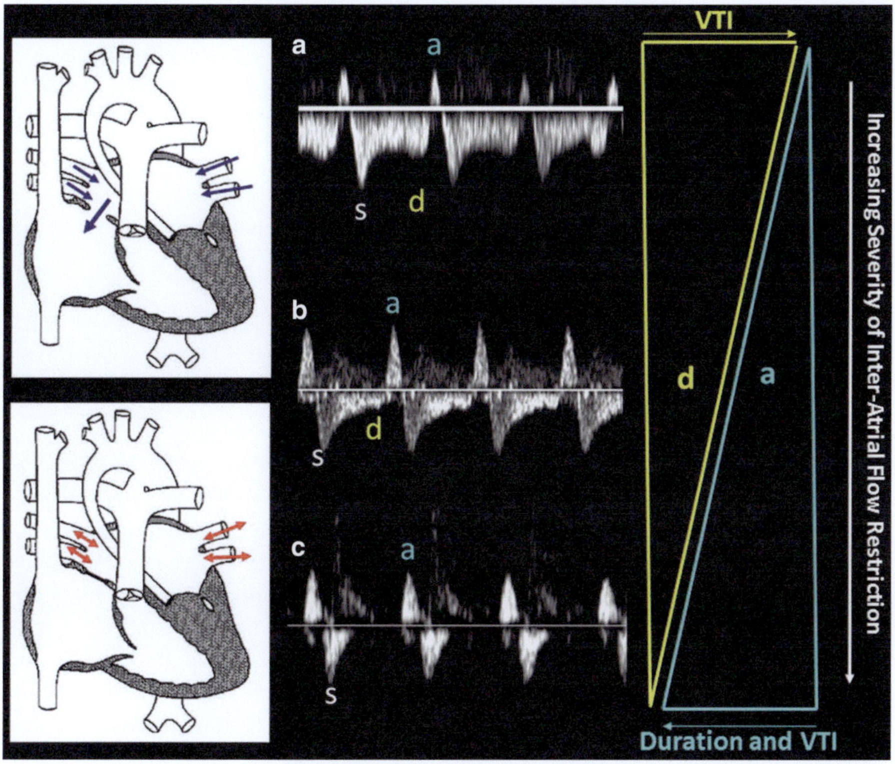

Fig. 19.2 (**a**–**c**) Pulmonary venous (PV) Doppler findings in hypoplastic left heart syndrome with various degrees of atrial septal restriction. (**a**) Without obstruction, there is only minimal a-wave flow reversal. (**b**) With some restriction, there is decreased PV forward flow in early diastole (*d*-wave) and increased flow reversal in atrial systole (*a*-wave) due to the increase in left atrial pressure. (**c**) Intact atrial septum with to-and-fro pulmonary vein Doppler flow. VTI, velocity-time interval of the d-wave (*yellow*) and a-wave (*blue*), respectively

or only a tiny discernable d-wave during early diastole (Fig. 19.2c). Where the atrial septum is closed due to severe MR, however, the d-wave flow may still be present due to the additional volume load of the LA and PV although the duration of the a-wave flow reversal is significantly prolonged reflecting the increase in LA pressure. Thus, if there is severe MR, the PV VTI ratio should therefore not be used to quantify the RAS unlike the a-wave flow duration.

Patient selection criteria for in utero fetal atrial decompression in HLHS or AS with IAS are based on a small number of patients. In cases with *HLHS/IAS*, Michelfelder and colleagues found a PV forward-reverse velocity-time integral (VTI) ratio of 5 or less to be the strongest predictor of the need for neonatal balloon atrial septostomy (BAS) within the first 48 h of life [8, 23]. Nonetheless, we and others have used more stringent criteria that more than fulfill the above Michelfelder criteria (Table 19.1) [3, 24, 25]. In a Hospital for Sick Children, Toronto, review of prenatally untreated cases with severe left heart obstruction and RAS, there were no

Table 19.1 Echocardiographic criteria for fetal atrial septal intervention and type of procedure

Hypoplastic left heart syndrome
Toronto:
a-wave duration ≥ 90 ms by pulmonary vein Doppler
Type A or C atrial morphology
Pulmonary lymphangiectasia by fetal MRI
Boston:
Atrial septal defect ≤1 mm or closed
Prominent flow reversal in pulmonary veins
Sao Paolo:
Atrial septal defect ≤1 mm or closed
Type A or C atrial morphology
Bidirectional to-and-fro pulmonary vein flow

fetal and neonatal survivors if the duration of a-wave flow reversal in the PV was ≥90 ms while fetal cases with a PV duration <90 ms had typical HLHS outcomes [3]. In addition, in HLHS cases with an a-wave duration of 95–115 ms, invasive pressure measurements prior to in utero LA decompression demonstrated high LA pressures of 15–30 mmHg [3]. There was a strong association between a PV a-wave duration ≥ 90 ms and pulmonary lymphangiectasia as demonstrated by histology and/or fetal magnetic resonance imaging in all our cases, independent of whether they were prenatally treated or not [3, 22]. We have used the same findings to consider in utero atrial septal interventions for fetuses with HLHS and variants with the type A or C morphology. Fetal MRI is routinely used in Toronto to screen for pulmonary lymphangiectasia and to measure pulmonary blood flow [26]. Indications published by others (Table 19.1) to perform prenatal atrial septoplasties for HLHS included an intact atrial septum or a tiny atrial communication ≤1 mm, either with "prominent flow reversal" in the PVs [27] or bidirectional to-and-fro PV Doppler tracing [25].

There are no well-established indications for intervention on the atrial septum of *AS/IAS with severe MR*. On the one hand, successful aortic valve dilation may be sufficient as the only in utero procedure to decrease the amount of MR, reopen the atrial communication, resolve fetal hydrops, and prevent in utero demise [7, 25, 28, 29]. On the other hand, while the creation of an interatrial septal defect may have theoretical benefits [27], atrial septoplasty alone for AS/MR was considered ineffective and, when attempted in combination with aortic valvuloplasty, was rarely technically successful [7]. Still, survival has been reported in a few fetal cases that underwent in utero atrial septoplasty alone or in combination with aortic valve dilation [7, 25, 30].

Indications and results for prenatal atrial septal procedures for other cardiac conditions than HLHS and AS have not been reported. Nonetheless, reasons to attempt an in utero intervention on the atrial septum may include fetal cardiac conditions that are expected to result in perinatal demise but can be improved with a fetal intervention. *Obstructive right heart lesions with an obligatory right-left atrial shunt* such as pulmonary atresia with an intact ventricular septum or tricuspid atresia carry a high risk of in utero demise if the atrial septum becomes restrictive. In this situation, the obstructed egress from the right to the left atrium causes systemic venous congestion and reduced lymphatic drainage from the thoracic duct, followed by the appearance of ascites, skin edema, and hydrops. At our center, in utero stenting across the atrial secundum septum has been successfully attempted in a midtrimester fetus with progressive ascites related to tricuspid atresia and a severely restrictive, redundant septum primum aneurysm. The procedure allowed for the pregnancy continuation and the postnatal survival with single ventricle surgery.

Despite planned caesarean section and cardiac catheterization to shorten the interval between delivery and the neonatal atrial septostomy, newborns with *TGA with severe RAS and arterial duct constriction* are at a high risk of neonatal death due to low systemic arterial oxygenation and persistent pulmonary hypertension [18, 31]. FO restriction in fetal TGA has been associated either with a thin, hypermobile septum primum or with a thickened, immobile atrial septum [31, 32]. The constricted arterial duct appeared narrowed at the pulmonary artery end, with a diameter that was significantly below the published normal data [29]. Whether these criteria are sensitive enough to offer prenatal atrial, septostomy is uncertain. As of late 2015, there are no publications on in utero therapy for TGA/IAS [18].

19.3 Technical Approach

19.3.1 BAS Versus Stenting

Techniques that have been used to create atrial septal defects (ASD) in the human fetus include balloon dilation, stenting, and radiofrequency or laser perforation of the atrial septum [3, 7, 13, 24, 25, 27, 29, 33, 34]. Atrial septal radiofrequency or laser procedures resulted in only small defects that almost immediately closed [3, 34, 35]. Balloon atrial septoplasty (BAS) or septal stenting of the fetal interatrial septum are therefore the only currently recommended options to achieve persistent atrial septal patency at birth. Our approach in Toronto has been to perform fetal BAS for the thin type C atrial septum and to use atrial septal stenting for those patients with the rigid thick muscular type A septum (see under results).

19.3.2 Step-By-Step Approach

We have used our previously reported ultrasound-guided percutaneous approach for all types of fetal atrial septal procedures [3]. This includes maternal premedication with local anesthesia with 2 % lidocaine, prophylactic antibiotics, and mild intravenous (IV) sedation with midazolam and fentanyl. We wait until the fetal position is optimal, either lying supine or with the right atrium upward, and then the fetus is rapidly paralyzed and sedated using intrahepatic vein rocuronium 1.2 mg/kg, fentanyl 2 mcg/kg, and atropine 0.02 mg/kg. A 20 cm non-beveled 18G needle (Cook Medical, Bloomington, IN, USA) is used as a delivery sheath for a coronary balloon (3.5 mm diameter, 10 or 15 mm long Pantera, Biotronik

AG, Bülach, Switzerland) or a coronary stent (3.0 mm diameter, 13 or 15 mm long, PRO-Kinetic, Biotronik AG, Bülach, Switzerland). The balloon/stent is premounted on a short 0.014″ wire (Hi-Torque Floppy II, 50 cm long, Abbott Vascular, Santa Clara, CA). The shaft of the balloon is marked (Steri-Strip, 3 M Health Care, St. Paul, MN) to indicate that the shoulder of the advancing balloon is completely beyond the needle tip. This physical marker of the relationship of the needle tip to the balloon/stent is an important supplement to the ultrasound images. An additional marker is placed on the 0.014″ wire to indicate the position when it is 2 cm beyond the tip of the balloon. Particularly in the case of stent delivery, the needle's trajectory must be chosen with the eventual stent deployment in mind. Too acute an angle of engagement with the atrial septum will result in an oblique course of the stent across the atrial septum. This leaves little space to retract the 18G needle so that the stent and the shoulder of its balloon are fully beyond the needle tip which must remain within the RA. A trajectory resulting in the stent being deployed approximately parallel to the plane of the atrioventricular ring often gives the most space. Under continuous ultrasound guidance, the 18G needle is advanced into the RA, through the interatrial septum and then positioned within the LA close to the mouth of a left pulmonary vein (PV) (Fig. 19.3a). To confirm the needle tip is within a cardiac chamber, blood is aspirated upon entry into the RA and then LA. The ensemble of a 0.014″ wire with premounted balloon/stent is advanced through the lumen of the 18G needle, so that the 0.014″ wire is deployed deep in the left pulmonary vein. The needle is retracted into the RA, and the balloon or balloon/stent deployed across the atrial septum. Space usually limits the feasibility of a septostomy. Static BAS is simpler with the balloon positioned half way across the atrial septum (Fig. 19.3b). A septostomy can be attempted while maintaining the position of the supporting 0.014″ wire, but it is often easier to engage the tip of the balloon within the atrial septum and then drag the balloon from the LA into the RA over the wire. Stents are deployed with approximately 4–5 mm in the RA and two thirds of the length in the LA (Fig. 19.3c, d). The stent's position is confirmed to be wholly beyond the needle tip by ultrasound and by the marker on the balloon shaft. Ideally the stent should be at least 1–2 mm proximal to the mouth of the pulmonary vein, as the LA will become smaller and the pulmonary veins less patulous after decompression. The balloon is inflated to 18–20 atmospheres (Indeflator, Abbott, Murrieta, CA, USA) to expand the stent diameter to ~3.6 mm. The balloon is then deflated and retracted within the 18G needle over the 0.014″ wire, and the whole ensemble withdrawn from the heart. Retraction of the balloon into the 18G needle after stent deployment requires considerable care, with gentle rotation, and sometimes a small amount of reinflation followed by deflation to change the balloon's profile. Excessive suction of these compliant balloons should be avoided as they may form a rigid flat "pancake" with a large diameter, making retraction more difficult. Significant pericardial effusions are drained with a 22G needle. After the procedure, the mother and fetus are observed and discharged several hours later and followed serially at our center to confirm persistent patency of the atrial septum by color mapping and PV Doppler to (or until) delivery (Figs. 19.4 and 19.5).

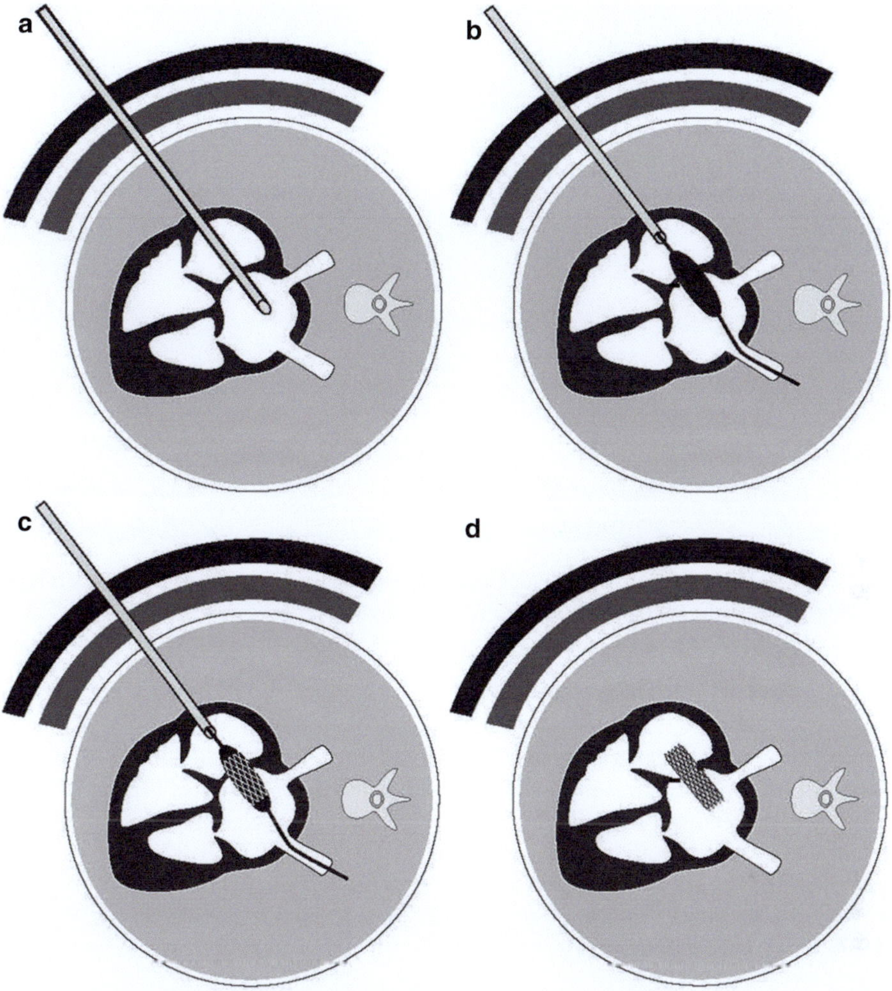

Fig. 19.3 (**a–d**) Techniques of the fetal atrial septoplasty (**b**) and atrial stenting (**c**, **d**). (**a**) The fetal position is optimal with the right atrium located superiorly. The 18G needle is advanced through the maternal abdominal wall, the uterus, the amniotic cavity, the right-sided fetal chest, the right atrium, and across the center of the atrial septum into the left atrium. (**b**) Through the lumen of the needle, the floppy 0.014″ guide wire is deployed deep in the left pulmonary vein and the premounted coronary balloon advanced. The needle is retracted into the right atrium, and the balloon deployed across the atrial septum. After positioning the balloon halfway across the atrial septum, the balloon is inflated several times to create an atrial defect. The deflated balloon is then retracted into the needle, and the needle and wire are simultaneously withdrawn. (**c**, **d**) Using the same technique as shown in (19.3**a**), the coronary stent is advanced into the left atrium. The stent should be positioned two thirds of its length in the LA and several mm proximal to the mouth of the pulmonary vein, bearing in mind that the left atrium becomes smaller, and the septum shifts in a midline position after the decompression (**c**, **d**). The balloon is inflated to 18–20 atmospheres to expand the coronary stent diameter to ~3.6 mm. The deflated balloon is retracted within the 18G needle over the 0.014″ wire, and the whole ensemble apart from the stent is withdrawn from the heart

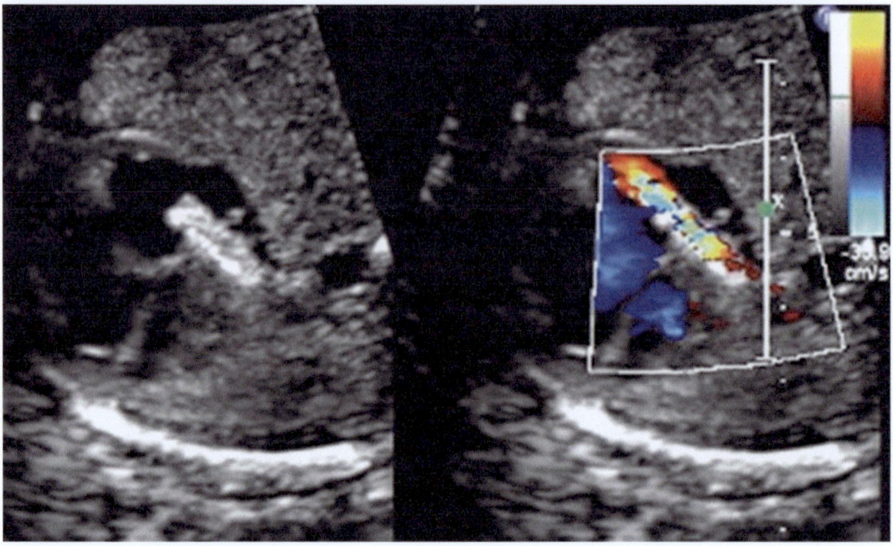

Fig. 19.4 HLHS with IAS and an optimal positioned stent allowing continuous left-right shunting

19.4 Results and Perspectives

Data is limited to the experience of a few centers with overall small number of fetuses that have undergone ultrasound-guided in utero atrial septoplasties (Table 19.2) or atrial septal stenting (Table 19.3) between 23 and 36 weeks of gestation, almost exclusively for obstructive left heart lesions [3, 13, 24, 25, 27, 33, 34, 36].

19.4.1 Atrial Septoplasty

The majority of cases reported in the literature underwent BAS as the first and only procedure. The largest experience has been reported by the Boston group in 2008 [27]. In 19 of the overall 21 attempted procedures, the intervention was considered technically successful. Fetal complications including bradycardia and pericardial or pleural effusion were frequent (38 %) and occurred irrespective of the use of the 18G or 19G cannulas (Cook Inc, Bloomington, IN, USA) or a custom-made angled cannula (ATC Technologies, Wilmington, MA, USA). In only 30 % the size of the atrial septal defect was ≥3 mm which was associated with higher postnatal oxygenation saturation and less need of neonatal septal intervention prior to surgical single ventricle palliation. However the long-term postnatal survival of these fetal atrial septoplasty cases was similar to neonates that only underwent postnatal atrial interventions in the same center [2]. The data of the overall 36 cases from four centers undergoing BAS is shown in Table 19.2. While no serious maternal complications were reported, the fetal and neonatal demise rates of 19 and 25 % were significant.

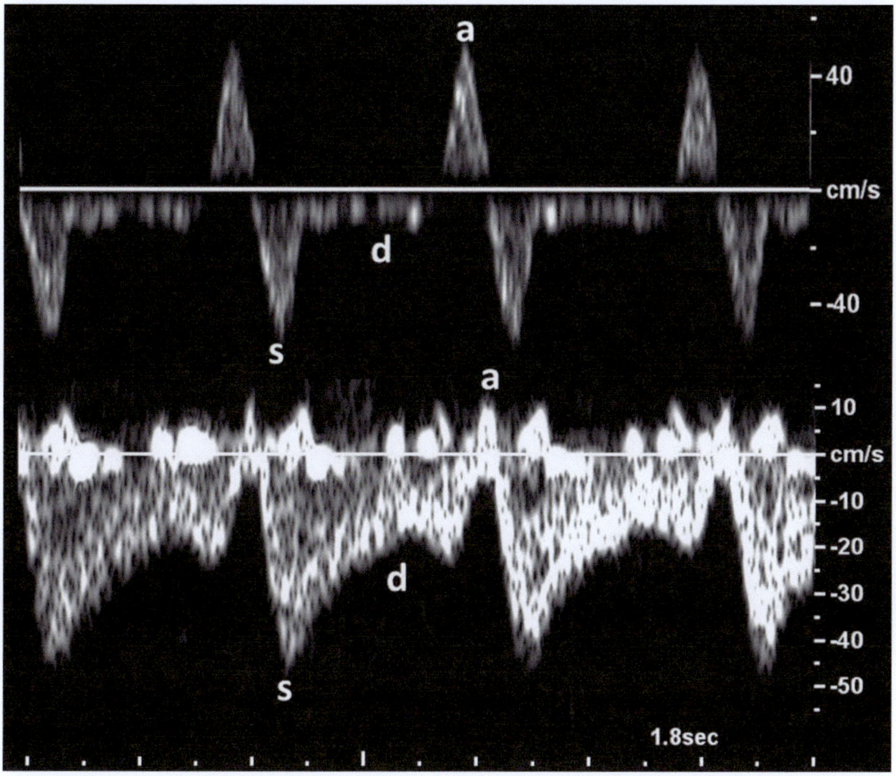

Fig. 19.5 Pulmonary vein Doppler before (*top panel*) and after (*lower panel*) atrial septal stenting of the same fetus (Fig. 19.4) confirming the left atrial decompression with normalization of the pulmonary vein Doppler following the procedure

Our own experience with BAS as the primary interventional procedure is limited to three cases, in only one fetus with evolving HLHS and a type C IAS, the post intervention atrial defect was considered sufficiently large to not require additional atrial septal stenting.

19.4.2 Atrial Septal Stenting

In fetuses with left atrial hypertension and an intact thick muscular atrial septum, we have been unable to achieve left atrial decompression by balloon septoplasty as the atrial communications have been too small and short-lived. With atrial septal stenting with currently available coronary stents, a 3.4–3.6 mm atrial communication can be reliably created with LA decompression of a greater amount and duration. In theory this may decrease fetal lung injury and possibly improve long-term outcome, but it remains uncertain if this LA decompression can be achieved early enough and for long enough in all patients with LA hypertension. Primary atrial

Table 19.2 Indications and results of fetal balloon atrial septoplasties ($n=36$)

Center	Year	Lesions	Cases	Age weeks	Technical success	ASD ≥3 mm	Additional stent	IUD	NND	Alive >1 month
Toronto [3]			3	25–28	3	1	2	0	1	2
	2015[a]	HLHS	(2)			(1)	(1)		(1)	(1)
		Tri atresia	(1)				(1)			(1)
Boston [24, 27]			26	23–36	24	6/19	1	3	8	15
	2008	HLHS	(21)		(19)	(6)	(0)	(2)	(7)	(12)
	2011	AS with MR	(5)		(5)		(1)	(1)	(1)	(3)
Bonn [36]			3	24–33	3		0	3	0	0
	2014	HLHS	(3)		(3/4)					
Sao Paolo [25]			4	26–32	4		0	1	0	3
	2014	HLHS	(4)							
Total		**ALL**	**36**		**34/37 (92 %)**	**7/22 (32 %)**	**3/36 (8 %)**	**7/36 (19 %)**	**9/36 (25 %)**	**20/36 (56 %)**

Data is shown as numbers or %. Year, year of publication, or [a]update of previous report
AS aortic stenosis, *ASD* atrial septal defect, *HLHS* hypoplastic left heart syndrome and variants, *Tri* atresia, tricuspid atresia

Table 19.3 Indications and results of fetal atrial stent procedures ($n = 19$)

Center	Year	Lesions	Cases	Age	Technical success	Stent embolization	Stent thrombosis	IUD	NND	Alive >1 month
Toronto [3]			8	28–36	7	1	1	2	1	5
	2015[a]	HLHS	(6)		(5)		(1)	(2)	(1)	(3)
		Cor triatriatum	(1)		(1)	(1)				(1)
		Tri atresia	(1)		(1)					(1)
Boston [24]			9	24–31	4	3		1	4	4
	2014	HLHS	(9)							
Bonn [36]			2	29–33	2	0	1	1	1	0
	2014	HLHS	(2)							
Total		**ALL**	**19**		**13/19 (68 %)**	**4/19 (21 %)**	**2/13 (15 %)**	**4/19 (21 %)**	**6/19 (32 %)**	**9/19 (47 %)**

Data is shown as numbers or %. Year, year of publication, or [a]update of previous report
HLHS hypoplastic left heart syndrome and variants. *Tri atresia* tricuspid atresia

stenting is a more difficult procedure than BAS with more scope for technical complications although the preliminary outcome data suggests a similar fetal complication rate compared with primary BAS. Our team first gained experience with atrial stenting in fetal lambs and use longer stents than many other centers which may explain the lower rate of technical failure and embolization in our updated patient series of 2015 (Table 19.3) [14]. Of concern has been the occurrence of partial stent obstruction several weeks after the stenting either by neointimal proliferation or protrusion of the muscle through the open cells of the stent meshwork [3]. In addition, complete stent thrombosis within 24 h of the intervention has occurred in two cases, including a patient of ours with a correctly placed stent at 36 gestational weeks. Nonetheless, most of the stented cases had persistently good flow across the stent to birth, and all neonates were stable after delivery without signs of severe hypoxia. Successful in utero LA decompression may not completely reverse lung pathology, as all of the stented HLHS cases had histological evidence of pulmonary lymphangiectasia and pulmonary vein muscularization at birth [3]. Whether the elevation in pulmonary vascular resistance persists long term is still unclear.

In *conclusion*, while fetal atrial septal interventions show promise, more experience is required to determine the clinical utility of these procedures for HLHS and other lesions that may be seriously compromised by a prematurely closed atrial septum. Fetal LA decompression is only one step in the management of this complex pathology. Outcome data beyond infancy is still largely missing although early results appear promising considering the dismal outlook of untreated fetuses with HLHS/IAS.

Acknowledgment Figure 19.3a–d was created by Jannic Jaeggi.

References

1. Kiserud T, Rasmussen S. Ultrasound assessment of the fetal foramen ovale. Ultrasound Obstet Gynecol. 2001;17:119–24.
2. Vlahos AP, Lock JE, McElhinney DB, van der Velde ME. Hypoplastic left heart syndrome with intact or highly restrictive atrial septum: outcome after neonatal transcatheter atrial septostomy. Circulation. 2004;109:2326–30.
3. Chaturvedi RR, Ryan G, Seed M, van Arsdell G, Jaeggi ET. Fetal stenting of the atrial septum: technique and initial results in cardiac lesions with left atrial hypertension. Int J Cardiol. 2013;168:2029–36.
4. Atz AM, Feinstein JA, Jonas RA, Perry SB, Wessel DL. Preoperative management of pulmonary venous hypertension in hypoplastic left heart syndrome with restrictive atrial septal defect. Am J Cardiol. 1999;83:1224–8.
5. Glatz JA, Tabbutt S, Gaynor JW, Rome JJ, Montenegro L, Spray TL, Rychik J. Hypoplastic left heart syndrome with atrial level restriction in the era of prenatal diagnosis. Ann Thorac Surg. 2007;84:1633–8.
6. Vida VL, Bacha EA, Larrazabal A, Gauvreau K, Thiagaragan R, Fynn-Thompson F, Pigula FA, Mayer Jr JE, del Nido PJ, Tworetzky W, Lock JE, Marshall AC. Hypoplastic left heart syndrome with intact or highly restrictive atrial septum: surgical experience from a single center. Ann Thorac Surg. 2007;84:581–5.

7. Vogel M, McElhinney DB, Wilkins-Haug LE, Marshall AC, Benson CB, Juraszek AL, Silva V, Lock JE, Marx GR, Tworetzky W. Aortic stenosis and severe mitral regurgitation in the fetus resulting in giant left atrium and hydrops: pathophysiology, outcomes, and preliminary experience with pre-natal cardiac intervention. J Am Coll Cardiol. 2011;57:348–55.
8. Michelfelder E, Gomez C, Border W, Gottliebson W, Franklin C. Predictive value of fetal pulmonary venous flow patterns in identifying the need for atrial septoplasty in the newborn with hypoplastic left ventricle. Circulation. 2005;112:2974–9.
9. Rychik J, Rome JJ, Collins MH, DeCampli WM, Spray TL. The hypoplastic left heart syndrome with intact atrial septum: atrial morphology, pulmonary vascular histopathology and outcome. J Am Coll Cardiol. 1999;34:554–60.
10. Taketazu M, Barrea C, Smallhorn JF, Wilson GJ, Hornberger LK. Intrauterine pulmonary venous flow and restrictive foramen ovale in fetal hypoplastic left heart syndrome. J Am Coll Cardiol. 2004;43:1902–7.
11. Photiadis J, Urban AE, Sinzobahamvya N, Fink C, Schindler E, Schneider M, Marie Brecher A, Asfour B. Restrictive left atrial outflow adversely affects outcome after the modified norwood procedure. Eur J Cardiothorac Surg. 2005;27:962–7.
12. Lowenthal A, Kipps AK, Brook MM, Meadows J, Azakie A, Moon-Grady AJ. Prenatal diagnosis of atrial restriction in hypoplastic left heart syndrome is associated with decreased 2-year survival. Prenat Diagn. 2012;32:485–90.
13. Marshall AC, van der Velde ME, Tworetzky W, Gomez CA, Wilkins-Haug L, Benson CB, Jennings RW, Lock JE. Creation of an atrial septal defect in utero for fetuses with hypoplastic left heart syndrome and intact or highly restrictive atrial septum. Circulation. 2004;110: 253–8.
14. Schmidt M, Jaeggi E, Ryan G, Hyldebrandt J, Lilly J, Peirone A, Benson L, Chaturvedi RR. Percutaneous ultrasound-guided stenting of the atrial septum in fetal sheep. Ultrasound Obstet Gynecol. 2008;32:923–8.
15. Chang AC, Wernovsky G, Kulik TJ, Jonas RA, Wessel DL. Management of the neonate with transposition of the great arteries and persistent pulmonary hypertension. Am J Cardiol. 1991;68:1253–5.
16. Kumar A, Taylor GP, Sandor GG, Patterson MW. Pulmonary vascular disease in neonates with transposition of the great arteries and intact ventricular septum. Br Heart J. 1993;69:442–5.
17. Soongswang J, Adatia I, Newman C, Smallhorn JF, Williams WG, Freedom RM. Mortality in potential arterial switch candidates with transposition of the great arteries. J Am Coll Cardiol. 1998;32:753–7.
18. Jouannic JM, Gavard L, Fermont L, Le Bidois J, Parat S, Vouhe PR, Dumez Y, Sidi D, Bonnet D. Sensitivity and specificity of prenatal features of physiological shunts to predict neonatal clinical status in transposition of the great arteries. Circulation. 2004;110:1743–6.
19. Pavlova M, Fouron JC, Drblik SP, van Doesburg NH, Bigras JL, Smallhorn J, Harder J, Robertson M. Factors affecting the prognosis of ebstein's anomaly during fetal life. Am Heart J. 1998;135:1081–5.
20. Uzun O, Babaoglu K, Ayhan YI, Moselhi M, Rushworth F, Morris S, Beattie B, Wiener J, Lewis MJ. Diagnostic ultrasound features and outcome of restrictive foramen ovale in fetuses with structurally normal hearts. Pediatr Cardiol. 2014;35:943–52.
21. Better DJ, Apfel HD, Zidere V, Allan LD. Pattern of pulmonary venous blood flow in the hypoplastic left heart syndrome in the fetus. Heart. 1999;81:646–9.
22. Seed M, Bradley T, Bourgeois J, Jaeggi E, Yoo SJ. Antenatal MR imaging of pulmonary lymphangiectasia secondary to hypoplastic left heart syndrome. Pediatr Radiol. 2009;39:747–9.
23. Divanovic A, Hor K, Cnota J, Hirsch R, Kinsel-Ziter M, Michelfelder E. Prediction and perinatal management of severely restrictive atrial septum in fetuses with critical left heart obstruction: clinical experience using pulmonary venous Doppler analysis. J Thorac Cardiovasc Surg. 2011;141:988–94.
24. Kalish BT, Tworetzky W, Benson CB, Wilkins-Haug L, Mizrahi-Arnaud A, McElhinney DB, Lock JE, Marshall AC. Technical challenges of atrial septal stent placement in fetuses with

hypoplastic left heart syndrome and intact atrial septum. Catheter Cardiovasc Interv. 2014;84:77–85.
25. Pedra SR, Peralta CF, Crema L, Jatene IB, da Costa RN, Pedra CA. Fetal interventions for congenital heart disease in Brazil. Pediatr Cardiol. 2014;35:399–405.
26. Jansz MS, Seed M, van Amerom JF, Wong D, Grosse-Wortmann L, Yoo SJ, Macgowan CK. Metric optimized gating for fetal cardiac. Magn Reson Med. 2010;64:1304–14.
27. Marshall AC, Levine J, Morash D, Silva V, Lock JE, Benson CB, Wilkins-Haug LE, McElhinney DB, Tworetzky W. Results of in utero atrial septoplasty in fetuses with hypoplastic left heart syndrome. Prenat Diagn. 2008;28:1023–8.
28. Gembruch U. Current trends of fetal echocardiography. Z Geburtshilfe Neonatol. 2012;216:111–3.
29. Arzt W, Wertaschnigg D, Veit I, Klement F, Gitter R, Tulzer G. Intrauterine aortic valvuloplasty in fetuses with critical aortic stenosis: experience and results of 24 procedures. Ultrasound Obstet Gynecol. 2011;37:689–95.
30. Rogers LS, Peterson AL, Gaynor JW, Rome JJ, Weinberg PM, Rychik J. Mitral valve dysplasia syndrome: a unique form of left-sided heart disease. J Thorac Cardiovasc Surg. 2011;142:1381–7.
31. Maeno YV, Kamenir SA, Sinclair B, van der Velde ME, Smallhorn JF, Hornberger LK. Prenatal features of ductus arteriosus constriction and restrictive foramen ovale in d-transposition of the great arteries. Circulation. 1999;99:1209–14.
32. Punn R, Silverman NH. Fetal predictors of urgent balloon atrial septostomy in neonates with complete transposition. J Am Soc Echocardiogr. 2011;24:425–30.
33. Moon-Grady AJ, Morris SA, Belfort M, Chmait R, Dangel J, Devlieger R, Emery S, Frommelt M, Galindo A, Gelehrter S, Gembruch U, Grinenco S, Habli M, Herberg U, Jaeggi E, Kilby M, Kontopoulos E, Marantz P, Miller O, Otano L, Pedra C, Pedra S, Pruetz J, Quintero R, Ryan G, Sharland G, Simpson J, Vlastos E, Tworetzky W, Wilkins-Haug L, Oepkes D. International fetal cardiac intervention registry: a worldwide collaborative description and preliminary outcomes. J Am Coll Cardiol. 2015;66:388–99.
34. Quintero RA, Huhta J, Suh E, Chmait R, Romero R, Angel J. In utero cardiac fetal surgery: laser atrial septotomy in the treatment of hypoplastic left heart syndrome with intact atrial septum. Am J Obstet Gynecol. 2005;193:1424–8.
35. Kohl T, Muller A, Tchatcheva K, Achenbach S, Gembruch U. Fetal transesophageal echocardiography: clinical introduction as a monitoring tool during cardiac intervention in a human fetus. Ultrasound Obstet Gynecol. 2005;26:780–5.
36. Herberg U, Berg C, Geipel A, Gembruch U, Breuer J. Foetal therapy: what works? Closed interatrial septum. Cardiol Young. 2014;24 Suppl 2:47–54.

Part V

Fetal Procedures: Other Treatments and Approaches

20 Perspectives on Fetal Pacing

Renato Samy Assad

20.1 Introduction

Congenital complete heart block (CHB) is now usually diagnosed in utero [1–4]. It can be isolated, i.e., with a structurally normal heart or associated with structural heart disease in the fetus (left atrial isomerism, AV septal defect, or AV discordance) [5]. Isolated congenital CHB is thought to result from the transplacental passage of maternal antibodies, anti-Rho, and anti-La [6, 7]. It is strongly associated with maternal systemic lupus erythematosus, Sjogren's syndrome, or connective tissue disorder [8–10]. The exact immunopathologic process involved remains obscure, but immunofluorescence studies have shown these antibodies sitting on the developing conduction tissue. Although fetal heart block may generate a slow heart rate of 30–50 % of normal fetal rate, this disturbance of fetal rhythm is well tolerated in the absence of complicating cardiac and systemic abnormalities or placental insufficiency [11]. The majority of the fetuses with CHB does well and progress to term and can be delivered normally. They may even continue through most of the childhood without risk and only require pacing much later in early adult life. However, a small part of the cases develops in utero heart failure, which manifests as fetal hydrops [12]. They develop pleural or pericardial effusions, ascites, and skin edema. Such fetuses are at great risk with as many as 83–100 % dying before term [13, 14]. In utero death is strongly associated with structural heart disease, endocardial fibroelastosis, and the development of fetal hydrops. It remains difficult to predict which fetuses with isolated congenital AV block will develop heart failure in utero. In a multicenter study, it has been demonstrated that fetal hydrops occurred in 22 (40 %) of the 55 fetuses diagnosed as having CHB [15]. This morbid association of diseases presented uniform fatal outcome, regardless of the presence or absence of an associated structural heart defect [16, 17].

R.S. Assad, MD, PhD
Division of Surgical Research, Heart Institute University of São Paulo, Sao Paulo, Brazil
e-mail: rsassad@cardiol.br

G. Butera et al. (eds.), *Fetal and Hybrid Procedures in Congenital Heart Diseases*, DOI 10.1007/978-3-319-40088-4_20

20.2 Fetal Therapy

Recent publication from the American College of Cardiology/American Heart Association highlights the management of fetal CHB on the basis of evidence [18]. A number of treatment modalities have been tried to prevent the development of hydrops [19]. Maternal dexamethasone has been used to try to halt the immunopathologic process [20–22]. The administration of maternal inotropes [23, 24] and sympathomimetics has been used with limited success [25, 26]. Because of the poor outcome in the fetus who is developing fetal hydrops, fetuses have been delivered electively prematurely. However, if mortality in neonatal life is examined, this is strongly associated with premature delivery (before 32 weeks), low ventricular rate, and endocardial fibroelastosis [27]. Therefore, premature delivery is not an easy option. Premature infants with complete AV block are unable to tolerate complications of being premature in the face of low heart rate and heart failure. The balance between worsening fetal hydrops and fetal demise and early planned delivery with limited survival in the perinatal period is difficult. If low-output failure and/or fetal heart rate cannot be reversed by medical treatment with positive chronotropic drugs or steroids, fetal ventricular pacing seems to be the next logical form of treatment. The arguments for trying to attempt fetal pacing are compelling. This therapeutic alternative offers some advantages. Firstly, definitive treatment can be introduced immediately after the first signs of fetal hydrops. This would allow the pregnancy to continue normally with recovery from congestive heart failure and normal fetal development until term, with stable respiratory and cardiovascular functions at delivery. Dell'Orfano et al. suggest that fetuses with CHB must be paced for at least 2–4 weeks before delivery to effectively reduce anasarca and pulmonary edema [28].

20.3 Fetal Pacing

A number of centers have attempted fetal pacing.

20.3.1 Endocardial Leads: Percutaneous Approach

Carpenter et al. attempted an in utero percutaneous approach to pacing [29]. In 1986, they attempted fetal pacing using a transabdominal, transuterine, and transthoracic route without apparent trauma to the mother or fetus. Although they were temporarily able to establish effective fetal pacing, the fetus died suddenly 4 h after placement of the ventricular pacing lead. Walkinshaw et al. also attempted a similar technique but utilizing the inferior vena cava for fetal heart access in 1994 [30]. Problems that can be foreseen with this transcutaneous transthoracic and/or transvenous approach for fetal pacing include the possibility of dislodgement of the pacing wire and potential fetal injury as the fetus moves with the wire stretching across the amniotic cavity and fetal cardiac tamponade as the wire is inserted. In addition, this approach would require maternal bed rest and would be subjected to bacterial chorioamnionitis.

20.3.2 Epicardial Leads: Maternal Laparotomy

With the ongoing experience in prenatal surgery in humans [31, 32], epicardial fetal pacing via thoracotomy has the potential for being a safer and more reliable procedure. Other groups have tried to develop the technique of open fetal surgery and an epicardial pacing approach [33–36]. However, the obvious risks here involve a maternal laparotomy, with a potential for infection, and maternal hysterotomy, with uterine irritability and premature labor, a significant morbidity to the mother. Cincinnati's group has published the longest survival of fetal pacing in a fetus of a mother with systemic lupus erythematosus, with the placement of a unipolar pacemaker via a left thoracotomy [37]. Fetal cardiac output had increased approximately 150 % compared with pre-pacemaker data. However, on postoperative day 5, sudden fetal demise was noted. The fetal pacemaker and lead were intact and in the proper location, without gross evidence of epicardial injury. The cardiac chambers were dilated, thin-walled, with diffuse evidence of endocardial fibroelastosis and dystrophic calcification. The intrauterine fetal demise seemed to be the result of chronic multi-organ failure. A concern was raised about ethical issues and indications of open fetal surgery and risks associated to the pregnancy, as well as to future fertility and pregnancies.

20.3.3 Myocardial Leads: Percutaneous Approach

A new electrode for fetal pacing has been designed with a T-shaped end that can be implanted on fetal myocardium by an 18-gauge needle (Fig. 20.1) [38]. The lead represents a modification of the temporary epicardial pacing lead commonly used after heart surgery. The main difference is that at the cardiac end, the pacing lead is cut close to the polypropylene coating, and a stainless-steel bar (5×0.5 mm) is connected to the wire, producing a T-bar, to fix to the fetal myocardium. The purpose of this shape is to keep the new lead securely anchored to the myocardium, thus

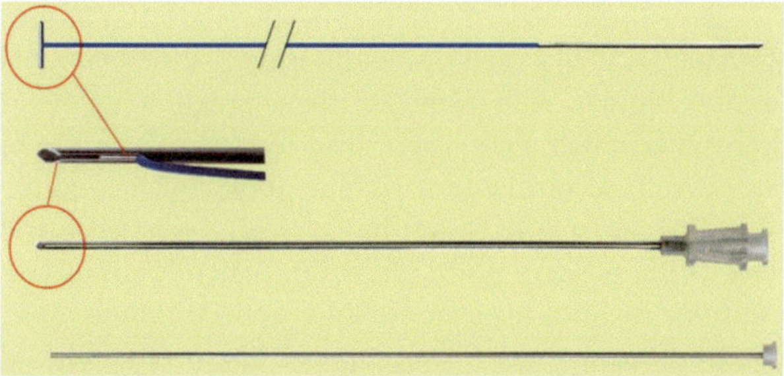

Fig. 20.1 The lead represents a modification of the temporary epicardial pacing lead commonly used after heart surgery. The cardiac end has a T-bar shape. The 18 G introducer needle has a 25° beveled tip and contains a 7 mm longitudinal side slot cut from the heel of the bevel so that this houses the T-bar until it is positioned inside the fetal heart. The use of a needle stylet is planned to eject the T-bar from the slot

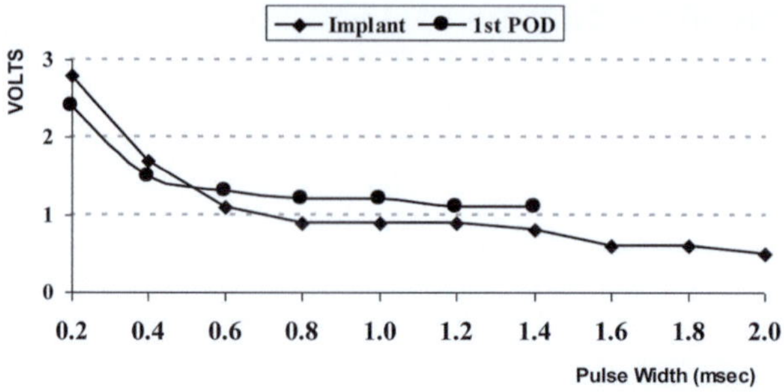

Fig. 20.2 Voltage strength-duration curves for acute myocardial stimulation threshold of a human fetus during lead implantation (implant) and on the first postoperative day (1st POD)

preventing lead dislodgment. The other end of the lead remains intact, consisting of a long straight needle. The lead length remained the original 60 cm.

This technique has been described in a 25-week old fetus with structural heart disease and congenital AV block, who was severely compromised with heart failure. The authors were able to establish pacing and implant the generator subcutaneously in the maternal abdomen. During the observed period of fetal pacing, the lead provided stable fixation with low acute thresholds, as demonstrated by the first documentation of voltage strength-duration curves of a human fetus (Fig. 20.2). However, after 36 h of ventricular pacing, the fetus developed asystole and died. Autopsy examination confirmed the presence of a major cardiac structural defect along with severe hydrops. A moderate bloody effusion was found in the pericardial sac. The authors believe that cardiac tamponade was the probable cause of death. They also speculate that a sudden fetal heart rate increase from 47 to 140 bpm may have resulted in an acid-base imbalance in the fetus as a consequence of sudden increase in myocardial oxygen consumption and cardiac output and suggested more gradual increase in rate in the postoperative course.

20.3.4 Myocardial Leads: Animal Studies

Currently, the T-shaped lead has been further improved since its initial use (Fig. 20.3) [39]. The lead is now bipolar, with a smaller diameter, allowing the use of a smaller introducer needle (20G rather than 18G). The lead consists of a bipolar parallel wire, with the negative pole insulated with blue polyethylene and the positive with red. The end of the negative pole (blue) has a small T-shaped metallic bar (4.0 × 0.4 mm). The end of the positive pole (red wire), which is slightly shorter than the negative pole, terminates in a 4.0 mm metallic tip, 5.0 mm apart from the T-bar. Lead length has also been increased from 60 to 242 cm. The other end of the lead has two long straight needles (positive and negative poles) to connect to the pulse generator.

The bipolar fetal electrode was evaluated in a fetal goat CHB model. The acute stimulation thresholds of the new fetal lead were consistently low, compatible with

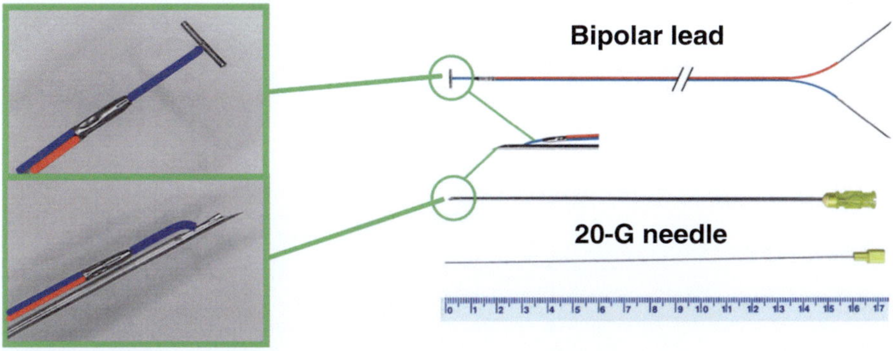

Fig. 20.3 Bipolar fetal T-bar lead consists of a parallel wire (242 cm), with the negative pole insulated with *blue* polyethylene and the positive with *red*. Superior *left panel*: The end of the negative pole (*blue*) has a small T-shaped metallic bar (4.0 × 0.4 mm). The end of the positive pole (*red wire*), which is slightly shorter than the negative pole, terminates in a 4.0 mm metallic tip, 5.0 mm apart from the T-bar. Inferior left panel: 20-G needle modified at the distal end by a 25° bevel and extension of 5.0 mm. A needle stylet was planned to eject the T-bar from the slot

safe chronic pacing during gestation. Bipolar stimulation is confined to the fetal myocardium, thus avoiding stimulation of uterine musculature and, consequently, premature uterine contractions after implantation.

An alternative way to pace hearts with CHB has been proposed by a number of laboratory groups toward replacing artificial pacemakers with a biological alternative primarily by creating ventricular sites of ectopic pacing [40–46]. Choi et al. have demonstrated the formation of an alternative AV conduction pathway in nearly one-third of the hearts implanted with engineered tissue constructs containing syngeneic fetal rat myogenic precursor cells [47, 48]. In those hearts demonstrating alternative conduction, propagation of action potentials from the atria to the ventricles was dependent on the implantation of constructs that contained viable muscle-derived cells. The authors also demonstrate that skeletal muscle-derived cells in the implants survive in the heart for the lifespan of the recipient animals, have a blood supply, and continue to express proteins important in electromechanical coupling between each other and recipient cardiomyocytes. Certainly, the ability to implant engineered tissue constructs to permanently electrically connect atrial and ventricular tissues represents an essential step for the future biological alternative to electronic pacemaker devices.

The Paris group has published a new lead for percutaneous insertion, adapted to the fetal anatomy, allowing a secured anchorage to the cardiac structures [49]. It is a unipolar and flexible lead made of a quadrifilar coil with an outer silicone insulation and a fixed screw on its distal tip (Fig. 20.4). The outer diameter of this lead is 1.0 mm (3 Fr). The length of the lead from the screw to the proximal tip is about 300 mm. The lumen is closed distally but opened proximally to accept a portion of the fully inserted stylet. The lead body is flexible when the stylet is removed. The length of penetration of the screw at the distal tip of the catheter is 1.0 mm. The study demonstrated that the unipolar lead would not be enough to generate the

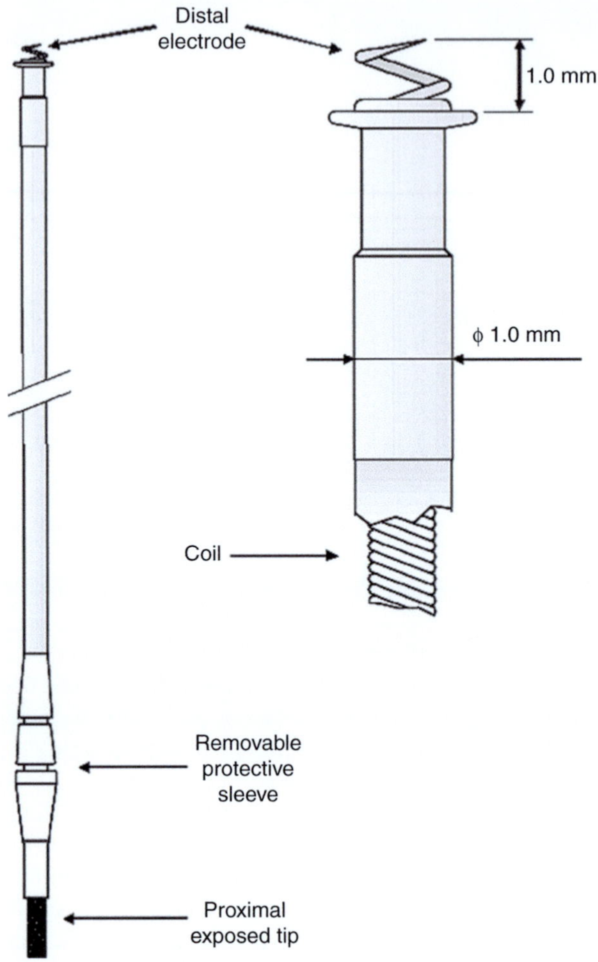

Fig. 20.4 Percutaneous fetal pacing unipolar lead, made of a quadrifilar coil with an outer silicone insulation and a fixed screw on its distal tip. The outer diameter of this lead and the length of penetration of the screw is 1.0 mm (3 Fr)

pacing and that another electrode was needed to allow pacing. To avoid the insertion of the second lead on the fetal skin that would multiply the risk of lead dislodgement with fetal movements, technical developments are hereby required to manufacture a bipolar lead.

More recently, the group of University of Southern California has developed a customized fetal single-chamber micropacemaker with a small diameter cylindrical shape (20 mm × 3 mm) that permits percutaneous implantation into a fetus through a large commonly used intrauterine cannula, capable to be deployed through a reasonably sized cannula lumen (Fig. 20.5) [50–52]. Under ultrasound guidance, the trocar and cannula are advanced from the maternal abdomen, through the uterine wall and fetal chest wall and finally, the pericardial membrane, until the tip abuts the fetal heart. The electrode is implanted on the fetal myocardium from the epicardial surface to achieve a stable anchorage in the ventricular wall. The entire pacemaker

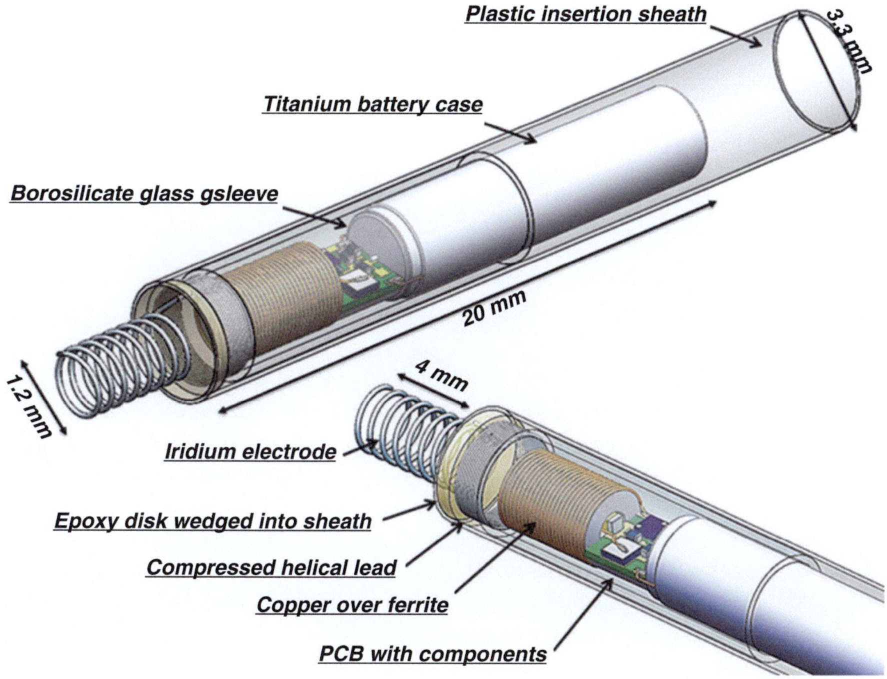

Fig. 20.5 Fetal micropacemaker system, planned to be implanted totally within the fetus, with rechargeable lithium cell. Notice the screw-in electrode tip, made from activated iridium

system was planned to be implanted within the fetus in order to avoid dislodgement and other complications from fetal motion. The functional life of the pacemaker is maintained by an implanted battery and could be extended by wireless recharging systems during patient visits in order to achieve the required duration of effective pacing. However, the stimulus parameters cannot be adjusted after implantation. The micropacemaker has been tested acutely and chronically in acute adult rabbits and chronic fetal sheep [53]. Experimental data from a strength-duration curve of the micropacemaker suggest a pacing threshold and chronaxie similar to the T-bar electrode implanted in a 25-week hydropic human fetus [38]. In a world of rapid micro- and nanotechnology development and miniaturization of devices, this prototype seems to be very promising.

20.3.5 Fetoscopic Methods: Animal Studies

Kohl et al. [54–56], VanderWall et al. [57], Estes et al. [58], and Kirchhof et al. [59], working in fetal sheep, have shown that fetal sheep can be epicardially paced using fetoscopic methods to gain direct fetal cardiac access. The authors have demonstrated that using fetoscopy, subxiphoid thoracotomy can be utilized to insert screw-in electrodes onto the fetal heart. The generator is then placed remotely subcutaneously in the maternal abdomen. Compared with open fetal surgery, fetoscopic direct fetal cardiac access may be more favorable because it avoids maternal laparotomy, hysterotomy, and fetal exteriorization, which have been accompanied by substantial decreases in fetoplacental blood flow and a poorer outcome in human fetuses with noncardiac lesions [60]. Moreover, percutaneous intra-amniotic access and uterine closure for fetoscopic surgery can be achieved reliably with little maternal and fetal morbidity in sheep [61]. However, this has not been attempted in humans.

20.4 Final Remarks

Considering the high rate of fetal demise associated with fetal hydrops with congenital AV block in utero and poor outcome of premature delivery, the way forward would appear to be fetal pacing. However, it will only be attempted in highly selective cases in which fetal mortality approaches 100 % in the absence of fetal intervention. Currently, there is no alternative effective treatment for fetuses with complete heart block who are in heart failure – apart from delivery. If, however, gestational age is <30 weeks, the additional complications of prematurity on top of hydrops mean that chances of postnatal survival are negligible. The development of a purpose-built pacing lead and the available expertise of a fetal medicine specialist, fetal cardiologist, pediatric cardiac surgeon, and electrophysiologist that can work together will optimize all and every chance of this procedure in becoming a feasible alternative to treat these high-risk fetuses.

References

1. Crowley DC, Dick M, Rayburn WF, et al. Two dimensional and M-mode echocardiographic evaluation of fetal arrhythmias. Clin Cardiol. 1985;8:1–10.
2. Achiron R, Glaser J, Gelernter I, et al. Extended fetal echocardiographic examination for detecting cardiac malformations in low risk pregnancies. Br Med J. 1992;304:671–4.
3. Benacerraf BR, Sanders SP. Fetal echocardiography. Radiol Clin North Am. 1990;28:131–47.
4. Kleinman CS, Donnerstein RL. Ultrasound assessment of cardiac function in the intact human fetus. J Am Coll Cardiol. 1985;5:84S–94.
5. Kleinman CS, Hobbins JC, Jaffe CC, et al. Echocardiographic studies of the human fetus: prenatal diagnosis of congenital heart disease and cardiac dysrhythmias. Pediatrics. 1980;65:1059–66.
6. Groves AM, Allan LD, Rosenthal E. Outcome of isolated congenital complete heart block diagnosed in utero. Heart. 1996;75(2):190–4.
7. Yamada H, Kato EH, Ebina Y, et al. Fetal treatment of congenital heart block ascribed to anti-SSA antibody: case reports with observation of cardiohemodynamics and review of the literature. Am J Reprod Immunol. 1999;42(4):226–32.
8. Richards DS, Wagman AJ, Cabaniss ML. Ascitis not due to congestive heart failure in a fetus with lupus induced heart block. Obstet Gynecol. 1990;76:957–9.
9. Buyon JP, Swersky SH, Fox HE, et al. Intrauterine therapy for presumptive fetal myocaritis with acquired heart block due to systemic lupus erythematosus. Arthritis Rheum. 1987;30:44–9.
10. Chameides L, Truex RC, Vetter V, et al. Association of maternal systemic lupus erythematosus with congenital complete heart block. N Engl J Med. 1977;297(22):1204–7.

11. Jaeggi ET, Hamilton RM, Silverman ED, et al. Outcome of children with fetal, neonatal or childhood diagnosis of isolated congenital atrioventricular block. A single institution's experience of 30 years. J Am Coll Cardiol. 2002;39(1):130–7.
12. Huhta JC, Strasburger JF, Carpenter RJ, et al. Pulsed doppler fetal echocardiography. J Clin Ultrasound. 1985;13:247–54.
13. Holsgreve W, Curry CJR, Golbus MS, et al. Investigation of nonimmune hydrops fetalis. Am J Obstet Gynecol. 1984;150:805–12.
14. Donofrio MT, Gullquist SD, Mehta ID, et al. Congenital complete heart block: fetal management protocol, review of the literature, and report of the smallest successful pacemaker implantation. J Perinatol. 2004;24(2):112–7.
15. Schimidt KG, Ulmer HE, Silverman NH, et al. Perinatal outcome of fetal complete atrioventricular block: a multicenter experience. J Am Coll Cardiol. 1991;17:1360–6.
16. Eliasson H, Sonesson S-E, Sharland G, et al. Isolated atrioventricular block in the fetus a retrospective, multinational, multicenter study of 175 patients. Circulation. 2011;124:1919–26.
17. Breur JM, Kapusta L, Stoutenbeek P, et al. Isolated congenital atrioventricular block diagnosed in utero: natural history and outcome. J Matern Fetal Neonatal Med. 2008;21:469–76.
18. Donofrio MT, Moon-Grady AJ, Hornberger LK et al.; American Heart Association Adults With Congenital Heart Disease Joint Committee of the Council on Cardiovascular Disease in the Young and Council on Clinical Cardiology, Council on Cardiovascular Surgery and Anesthesia, and Council on Cardiovascular and Stroke Nursing. Diagnosis and treatment of fetal cardiac disease: a scientific statement from the American Heart Association. Circulation. 2014;129(21):2183–242.
19. Eronen M, Heikkila P, Teramo K. Congenital complete heart block in the fetus: hemodynamic features, antenatal treatment, and outcome in six cases. Pediatr Cardiol. 2001;22(5):385–92.
20. Bierman FZ, Baxi L, Jaffe I, et al. Fetal hydrops and congenital complete heart block: response to maternal steroid therapy. J Pediatr. 1988;12:646–8.
21. Copel JA, Buyon JP, Kleinman CS. Successful in utero therapy of fetal heart block. Am J Obstet Gynecol. 1995;173:1384–90.
22. Carreira PE, Gutierrez-Larraya F, Gomez-Reino JJ. Successful intrauterine therapy with dexamethasone for fetal myocarditis an heart block in a mother with systemic lupus erythematosus. J Rheumatol. 1993;20:1204–7.
23. Anandakumar C, Biswas A, Chew SS, et al. Direct fetal therapy for hydrops secondary to congenital atrioventricular heart block. Obstet Gynecol. 1996;87:835–7.
24. Fesslova V, Vignati G, Brucato A, et al. The impact of treatment of the fetus by maternal therapy on the fetal and postnatal outcomes for fetuses diagnosed with isolated complete atrioventricular block. Cardiol Young. 2009;19:282–90.
25. Groves AMM, Allan LD, Rosenthal E. Therapeutic trial of sympathomimetics in three cases of complete heart block in the fetus. Circulation. 1995;92:3394–6.
26. Rosenthal E. Fetal heart block. In: Allan L, Hornberger L, Sharland G, editors. Textbook of fetal cardiology. 1st ed. London: Greenwich Medical Media; 2000. p. 438–51.
27. Abrams ME, Meredith KS, Kinnard P. Hydrops fetalis: a retrospective review of cases reported to a large national database and identification of risk factors associated with death. Pediatrics. 2007;120:84–9.
28. Dell' Orfano J, Chou HA, Park DA, et al. The monolithic fetal pacemaker: prototype lead design for closed thorax deployment. Pacing Clin Electrophysiol. 2003;26(4 pt 1):805–11.
29. Carpenter Jr RJ, Strasbuerger JF, Garson A, et al. Fetal ventricular pacing for hydrops secondary to complete atrioventricular block. J Am Coll Cardiol. 1986;8:1434–6.
30. Walkinshaw SA, Welch CR, McCormack J. In utero pacing for fetal congenital heart block. Fetal Diagn Ther. 1994;9:183–5.
31. Longaker MT, Golbus MS, Filly RA, et al. Maternal outcome after open fetal surgery. A review of the first 17 human cases. JAMA. 1991;265:737–41.
32. Hisaba WJ, Cavalheiro S, Almodim CG, et al. Intrauterine myelomeningocele repair postnatal results and follow-up at 3.5 years of age--initial experience from a single reference service in Brazil. Childs Nerv Syst. 2012;28(3):461–7.

33. Assad RS, Jatene MB, Moreira LF, et al. Fetal heart block: a new experimental model to assess fetal pacing. Pacing Clin Electrophysiol. 1994;17:1256–63.
34. Silverman NH, Kohl T, Harrison MR, et al. Experimental fetal surgery in the animal model and in the human fetus. In: Momma K, Imai Y, editors. Proceedings of the Second World Congress of Pediatric Cardiology and Cardiac Surgery. Armonk: Futura Publishing Co; 1998. p. 622–3.
35. Crombleholme TM, Harrison MR, Longaker MT. Complete heart block in fetal lambs, I technique and acute physiological response. J Pediatr Surg. 1990;25:587–93.
36. Scagliotti D, Shimokochi DD, Pringle KC. Permanent cardiac pacemaker implant in the fetal lamb. Pacing Clin Eletrophysiol. 1987;10:1253–61.
37. Eghtesady P, Michelfelder EC, Knilans TK, et al. Fetal surgical management of congenital heart block in a hydropic fetus: lessons learned from a clinical experience. J Thorac Cardiovasc Surg. 2011;141(3):835–7.
38. Assad RS, Zielinsky P, Kalil R, et al. New lead for in utero pacing for fetal congenital heart block. J Thorac Cardiovasc Surg. 2003;126(1):300–2.
39. Assad RS, Thomaz PG, Valente AS, et al. Experimental assessment of a new electrode for fetal pacing. Braz J Cardiovasc Surg. 2006;21(3):272–82.
40. Ruhparwar A, Tebbenjohanns J, Niehaus M, et al. Transplanted fetal cardiomyocytes as cardiac pacemaker. Eur J Cardiothorac Surg. 2002;21:853–7.
41. Miake J, Marban E, Nuss HB. Biological pacemaker created by gene transfer. Nature. 2002; 419:132–3.
42. Potapova I, Plotnikov A, Lu Z, et al. Human mesenchymal stem cells as a gene delivery system to create cardiac pacemakers. Circ Res. 2004;94:952–9.
43. Plotnikov AN, Sosunov EA, Qu J, et al. Biological pacemaker implanted in canine left bundle branch provides ventricular escape rhythms that have physiologically acceptable rates. Circulation. 2004;109:506–12.
44. Qu J, Plotnikov AN, Danilo Jr P, et al. Expression and function of a biological pacemaker in canine heart. Circulation. 2003;107:1106–9.
45. Xue T, Cho HC, Akar FG, et al. Functional integration of electrically active cardiac derivatives from genetically engineered human embryonic stem cells with quiescent recipient ventricular cardiomyocytes: insights into the development of cell-based pacemakers. Circulation. 2005;111:11–20.
46. Kehat I, Khimovich L, Caspi O, et al. Electromechanical integration of cardiomyocytes derived from human embryonic stem cells. Nat Biotechnol. 2004;22:1282–9.
47. Sill B, Alpatov IV, Pacak CA, et al. Implantation of engineered tissue in the rat heart (Video Article). J Vis Exp. 2010. (www.jove.com/video/1139) 28(e1139):1–2.
48. Choi YH, Stamm C, Hammer PE, et al. Cardiac conduction through engineered tissue. Am J Pathol. 2006;169(1):72–85.
49. Boudjemline Y, Rosenblatt J, de La Villeon G, et al. Development of a new lead for in utero fetal pacing. Prenat Diagn. 2010;30(2):122–6.
50. Zhou L, Chmait R, Bar-Cohen Y, et al. Percutaneously injectable fetal pacemaker: electrodes, mechanical design and implantation. Conf Proc IEEE Eng Med Biol Soc. 2012;2012:6600–3.
51. Nicholson A, Chmait R, Bar-Cohen Y, et al. Percutaneously injectable fetal pacemaker: electronics, pacing thresholds, and power budget. Conf Proc IEEE Eng Med Biol Soc. 2012;2012: 5730–3.
52. Loeb GE, Zhou L, Zheng K. Design and testing of a percutaneously implantable fetal pacemaker. Ann Biomed Eng. 2013;41(1):17–27.
53. Bar-Cohen Y, Loeb GE, Pruetz JD, et al. Preclinical testing and optimization of a novel fetal micropacemaker. Heart Rhythm. 2015;12(7):1683–90.
54. Kohl T, Strumper D, Witteler R, et al. Fetoscopic direct fetal cardiac access in sheep: an important experimental milestone along the route to human fetal cardiac intervention. Circulation. 2000;102:1602–4.
55. Kohl T, Szabo Z, Suda K, et al. Fetoscopic and open transumbilical fetal cardiac catheterization in sheep. Potential approaches for human fetal cardiac intervention. Circulation. 1997;95(4):1048–53.

56. Kohl T, Witteler R, Strumper D, et al. Operative techniques and strategies for minimally invasive fetoscopic fetal cardiac interventions in sheep. Surg Endosc. 2000;14(5):424–30.
57. VanderWall KJ, Meuli M, Szabo Z, et al. Percutaneous access to the uterus for fetal surgery. J Laparoendosc Surg. 1996;6:S65–7.
58. Estes JM, MacGillivary TE, Hedrick MH, et al. Fetoscopic surgery for the treatment of congenital anomalies. J Pediatr Surg. 1992;27(8):950–4.
59. Kirchhof P, Kohl T, Eckardt L, et al. Simultaneous in utero assessment of AV nodal and ventricular electrophysiologic parameters in the fetal sheep heart. Basic Res Cardiol. 2001; 96(3):251–7.
60. Kohl T, McElhinney DB, Farrel J, et al. Impact of fetoscopic versus open fetal surgery on fetoplacental blood flow and outcome in human fetuses. Eur Heart J. 1999;20:644A.
61. Kohl T, Szabo Z, Suda K, et al. Percutaneous fetal access and uterine closure for fetoscopic surgery. Lessons learned from 16 consecutive procedures in pregnant sheep. Surg Endosc. 1997;11(8):819–24.

Alternative Vascular Access in Fetus

21

Guiti Milani and Younes Boudjemline

21.1 Introduction

Fetal echocardiography leads to the development of antenatal diagnosis [1]. In antenatal cardiology, proofs of evolution of congenital defect have been made: serial scans performed on fetuses with aortic valve disease demonstrated poor evolution of the left ventricle in some cases, leading to the concept of evolving hypoplastic left heart syndrome [2–4].

The first report of in utero treatment of these fetuses in order to avoid progression of the disease is more than 30 years old [5].

Until now in utero procedures remain challenging for several reasons: the definite proof of efficiency of in utero treatment remains to be given, avoiding maternal mortality and morbidity is mandatory, avoiding fetal mortality is important, and access to the fetus is difficult.

Thanks to the development of minimally invasive techniques and continued animal experiments, fetal interventional therapy is evolving with current low rate of morbidity and mortality [6]. Careful selection of fetuses' candidates for treatment improves results [7]. This review will focus on possible access for fetal interventions.

G. Milani, MD
Cardiologie Pédiatrique, Centre de Référence Malformations Cardiaques Congénitales Complexes – M3C, Necker Hospital for Sick Children, Assistance Publique des Hôpitaux de Paris, Paris, France

Y. Boudjemline, MD, PhD (✉)
Cardiologie Pédiatrique, Centre de Référence Malformations Cardiaques Congénitales Complexes – M3C, Necker Hospital for Sick Children, Assistance Publique des Hôpitaux de Paris, Paris, France

Université Paris V Descartes, Paris, France
e-mail: yboudjemline@yahoo.fr

G. Butera et al. (eds.), *Fetal and Hybrid Procedures in Congenital Heart Diseases*, DOI 10.1007/978-3-319-40088-4_21

21.2 Cordocentesis

Ultrasound-guided cordocentesis was first described in 1983 by Daffos et al. [8]. The procedure involves percutaneous access to the fetal vascular compartment to draw fetal blood for cytological, biochemical, and cytogenetic studies; it is also used for fetal transfusion in cases of fetal anemia due to maternofetal alloimmunization. Furthermore, it allows perfusion of therapeutic agents to the fetus for sedation analgesia during any invasive therapy such as in utero intracardiac interventions. The risk of fetal loss related to the cordocentesis is estimated around 1 %. Some authors have investigated the possibility to use this access for intracardiac procedure. Kohl et al. described transumbilical fetal cardiac catheterization in sheep [9]. All fetuses died secondary to dissection, total thrombosis of umbilical vein, or blood loss after sheath dislodgment or removal. The length of the umbilical cord and its highly tortuous course make progression with a guide very difficult and dangerous. The translation of cordonal cardiac catheterization to a human fetus seems inconceivable at present; its interest lies in the simplicity of ultrasound guidance, but its morbidity and mortality rates in animals are close to 100 %.

21.3 Cardiocentesis

Percutaneous, per utero, fetal, transthoracic, direct ventricular access was proposed as an alternative to cordonal access for fetal transfusion in cases of maternofetal rhesus alloimmunization when cordonal access was technically impossible or after failure of cordocentesis [10]. Cardiocentesis is performed with local anesthesia of maternal skin and direct needle puncture of the fetal chest wall to enter the fetal heart. Besides technical problems such as difficult access with varying fetal lie and catheter/balloon fragmentation, the rate of fetal loss is estimated at around 6 %. Current indications are fetal reduction in dichorionic twin pregnancies if one of the fetuses satisfies indication for termination of pregnancy and treatment of fetus with severe congenital heart disease. Cardiac interventions are currently performed through this access [11].

It requires experience in percutaneous puncture, under ultrasound guidance. Good positioning of the fetus is mandatory before puncture. Procedure should not be done if position is not ideal.

Because vascular access of the fetus remains a challenge, some authors have investigated alternative approaches to the fetal heart. Fetoscopic approach and transhepatic access have been reported.

21.4 Fetoscopic Access

Kohl et al. described fetoscopic access in a fetal sheep: with three to four trocars percutaneously placed in the uterus and video fetoscopic equipment, they achieved a limited thoracotomy to obtain minimally invasive, direct, fetal cardiac access [12].

This approach was tested on fetal sheep for fetal cardiac pacing or antegrade fetal cardiac catheterization. The technique was feasible. But, many complications were reported: fetal death, maternal death by sepsis, and technical complications, such as bleeding of the puncture site, and technical difficulty in identifying the subxiphoid region were also noted. Fetoscopic access has some advantages compared with maternal hysterectomy. Because it is highly invasive compared to direct transventricular access, this approach is presently not used in humans for cardiac procedures.

21.5 Transhepatic Access

The technical deadlock in performing transumbilical fetal cardiac catheterization led to the suggestion of transhepatic access [13]. Transhepatic catheterization can be safely performed in children in cases of blocked venous access [14].

Feasibility of fetal cardiac catheterization using a transhepatic ultrasound-guided puncture of the intra-abdominal veins in the fetal lamb was demonstrated allowing anterograde catheterization of the fetal heart [13, 15]. The aim was to reproduce the conditions of catheterization using Seldinger's technique as it is done in the postnatal period and to improve fetal tolerance. In addition, it was hypothesized that the bleeding related to vessel puncture would be well tolerated because bleeding would appear in the peritoneal space. The peritoneum allows reabsorption of red blood cells in fetus. The feasibility of anterograde, echocardiography-guided cardiac catheterization through a transhepatic approach of the intra-abdominal fetal vessels was tested in fetal lambs. Access to the subdiaphragmatic portion of the inferior vena cava was performed by ultrasound guidance via a transhepatic approach. A guide was placed into the subhepatic vein, and cardiac catheterization was performed according to Seldinger's technique, allowing the heart chambers to be reached in all cases, with atrial or ventricular pacing and/or ballooning of the pulmonary valve. Three out of ten fetuses died after the procedure, and five fetuses were born at term, with an autopsy showing no significant cardiac or peritoneal injury. The simplicity of the procedure, with its shallow learning curve, has successfully lowered complication rates in subsequent studies. In the future, this method could become an alternative to percutaneous transventricular catheterization. However, variations in fetal positions and hepatic vein diameter add to the challenges; the latter limits this method to the second part of pregnancy when a needle can be safely inserted (Fig. 21.1).

Conclusion

Cardiac intervention is presently performed through transventricular access. This approach leads to serious morbidity and mortality in particular because of obligatory pericardial bleeding. Alternative access such as cordonal or transhepatic access has been recently reported in animals with interesting results. Human experience is still pending.

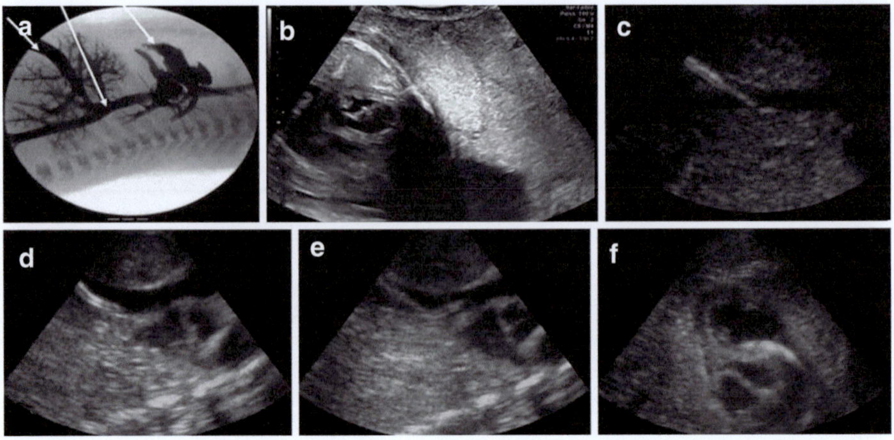

Fig. 21.1 (**a**) Possible vascular access to the heart is shown: umbilical cord, transhepatic access, and direct transventricular puncture. (**b**) Human case of direct ventricular access. (**c–f**) Pictures showing transhepatic access (**c**) and the advance of a coronary catheter from inferior vena cava (**d**) to the main pulmonary artery (**e, f**)

References

1. Kovalchin JP, Silverman NH. The impact of fetal echocardiography. Pediatr Cardiol. 2004;25:299–306.
2. Trines J, Hornberger LK. Evolution of congenital heart disease in utero. Pediatr Cardiol. 2004;25:287–98.
3. Hornberger LK, Need L, Benacerraf BR. Development of significant left and right ventricular hypoplasia in the second and third trimester fetus. J Ultrasound Med. 1996;15:655–9.
4. Hornberger LK, Sanders SP, Rein AJ, Spevak PJ, Parness IA, Colan SD. Left heart obstructive lesions and left ventricular growth in the mid trimester fetus: a longitudinal study. Circulation. 1995;92:1531–8.
5. Maxwell D, Allan L, Tynan MJ. Balloon dilatation of the aortic valve in the fetus: a report of two cases. Br Heart J. 1991;65:256–8.
6. Tworetzky W, Wilkins-Haug L, Jennings R, van der Velde M, Marshall A, Marx G, Colan S, Benson C, Lock J, Perry S. Balloon dilation of severe aortic stenosis in the fetus potential for prevention of hypoplastic left heart syndrome candidate selection, technique, and results of successful intervention. Circulation. 2004;110:2125–31.
7. Mäkikallio K, McElhinney DB, Levine JC, et al. Fetal aortic valve stenosis and the evolution of hypoplastic left heart syndrome: patient selection for fetal intervention. Circulation. 2006;113:1401–5.
8. Daffos F, Capella-Pavlovsky M, Forestier F. Direct collection of fetal blood from the umbilical vein under echography. First results, prospects. Presse Med. 1983;12:1017.
9. Kohl T, Szabo Z, Suda K, Petrossian E, Ko E, Kececioglu D, Moore P, Silverman NH, Harrison MR, Chou TM, Hanley FL. Fetoscopic and open transumbilical fetal cardiac catheterization in sheep: potential approaches for human fetal cardiac intervention. Circulation. 1997;95:1048–53.
10. Moise Jr KJ. Management of rhesus alloimmunization in pregnancy. Obstet Gynecol. 2008;112:164–76.

11. McElhinney D, Tworetzky W, Lock J. Current status of fetal cardiac intervention. Circulation. 2010;121:1256–63.
12. Kohl T, Strumper D, Witteler R, Merschhoff G, Alexiene R, Callenbeck C, Asfour B, Reckers J, Aryee S, Vahlhaus C, Vogt J, Van Aken H, Scheld HH. Fetoscopic direct fetal cardiac access in sheep: an important experimental milestone along the route to human fetal cardiac intervention. Circulation. 2000;102:1602–4.
13. Jouannic JM, Boudjemline Y, Benifla JL, Bonnet D. Transhepatic ultrasound-guided cardiac catheterization in the fetal lamb. A new approach for cardiac interventions in fetuses. Circulation. 2005;111:736–41.
14. Shim D, Lloyd TR, Cho KJ, et al. Transhepatic cardiac catheterization in children: evaluation of efficacy and safety. Circulation. 1995;92:1526–30.
15. Edwards A, Veldman A, Nitsos I, Chan Y, Brew N, Teoh M, Menahem S, Schranz D, Wong F. A percutaneous fetal cardiac catheterization technique for pulmonary valvuloplasty and valvulotomy in a mid-gestation lamb model. Prenat Diagn. 2015;35:74–80.

Part VI

Introductory Aspects in Hybrid Procedures

Physician's Perspective

22

John P. Cheatham

What do we mean by "hybrid"? According to Webster's Revised Unabridged Dictionary (1996), hybrid\hy "brid"\, N. {L. hybrida, hibrida, (BIOL.)} is "the offspring of the union of two distinct species; an animal or plant produced from the mixture of two species." Some would argue that the interventional cardiologist and the cardiothoracic surgeon are definitely two different species. They think "differently." They act "differently." They dress "differently." They are certainly paid "differently." As an interventional cardiologist, we are always interested in new treatments, always ready to test and try a new device or technique, and are always self-confident. Our cardiothoracic surgical colleagues usually believe that "if things aren't broke, don't try and fix them"; once a surgical technique is mastered, they are reluctant to change it and are even more self-confident.

However, occasionally a cardiothoracic surgeon comes along and challenges the interventional cardiologist to think "outside the box," which is what happened in our Heart Center. The collaborative team's goals are to reduce morbidity and mortality, to reduce the cumulative impact of multiple interventions over the lifetime of a patient, to improve quality of life, to deliver more efficient and cost-effective care, and to encourage teamwork. In the congenital heart disease world, it is much easier to develop hybrid strategies than in the adult cardiovascular world. We are routinely using a multidisciplinary team approach, while this was not true in the adult world. The main interventional procedures in adult CV medicine used to be percutaneous coronary interventions (PCI) procedures, where cardiac surgery, anesthesia, or imaging was seldom involved. Not until transcatheter aortic valve replacement (TAVR) became available and forced the adult team to work together did the word "hybrid" enter into their vocabulary. Now, the "buzz word" in adult CV medicine is structural heart disease (SHD), and everyone wants to be a member of the team.

J.P. Cheatham, MD, FAAP, FACC, MSCAI
The Heart Center, Nationwide Children's Hospital, Pediatrics & Internal Medicine,
The Ohio State University, Columbus, OH, USA
e-mail: John.Cheatham@nationwidechildrens.org

G. Butera et al. (eds.), *Fetal and Hybrid Procedures in Congenital Heart Diseases*, DOI 10.1007/978-3-319-40088-4_22

So let us look at some of the procedures that a hybrid approach would benefit the interventional cardiologist and the patient. The surgeon can provide vascular access to complete a complex interventional procedure. As an example, the critically ill neonate with low cardiac output, aortic obstruction with multi-organ failure is a poor surgical candidate upon presentation. However, a simple carotid cutdown by the surgeon allows the interventional cardiologist to use whatever materials are necessary, regardless of the French size needed to deliver them, i.e., cutting balloon angioplasty with or without stent therapy for middle thoracic aortic coarctation or balloon aortic valvuloplasty in extreme premature neonate. Another example is for the surgeon to provide per-ventricular access through a small substernal incision to perform a quick balloon pulmonary valvuloplasty in an extreme premature neonate weighing only 700 g with no venous access and renal failure (Fig. 22.1a, b).

Another example is how the surgeon can help the interventional cardiologist treat an infant with a large muscular VSD (MVSD) and heart failure. Many times the only surgical option available in these sick infants is to perform a pulmonary artery band as the initial palliative procedure. Otherwise, attempting to surgically close a single or multiple large MVSDs in neonates is high risk with a great likelihood of leaving residual flow. From the pivotal study using the Amplatzer MVSD occluder (SJM, Minneapolis, MN) in the USA, if the infant was less than or equal to 5.2 kg or some say less than 8–10 kg, percutaneous device closure had high morbidity and possible mortality. However, with the CT surgeon providing perventricular access and with transesophageal echo guidance, most, if not all, muscular VSDs can be closed using the device without cardiopulmonary bypass (CPB) (Fig. 22.2a, b). This procedure requires special skills of the "interventional" echocardiographer. They provide the "loops" for the surgeons and fluoroscopy for the interventional cardiologists. It is a very rewarding procedure and usually results in eliminating heart failure [1].

The next major hybrid procedure that has benefited both the interventional cardiologist and CT surgeon is intraoperative stent therapy. The interventional cardiologist faces challenges of delivering stents percutaneously to pulmonary arteries in small patients. The CT surgeon faces challenges of exposure to the pulmonary arteries and cannot easily see distally in order to perform patch repair. The hybrid approach to PA stenting benefits both disciplines as well as the patient [2]. In some instances, the procedure may be performed off CPB (Fig. 22.3a–c), while others may require CPB for the surgical correction of additional defects. The use of endoscopic evaluation before and after PA stent therapy offers advantages in the hybrid OR (Fig. 22.4a–c). Regardless, with the advent of hybrid operative suites, like ours at Nationwide Children's Hospital, these combined procedures can be performed more easily. In addition, exit angiography using a permanent single-plane FPD can easily be performed to not only assess surgical results immediately post-repair but can also confirm intraoperative stent therapy (Fig. 22.5a, b) [3]. This applies to the more common procedure of intraoperative pulmonary artery stenting but also in the more rare case of intraoperative aortic stenting. Furthermore, 3D rotational angiography (3DRA) can now be performed in hybrid operative suites and provides additional information compared to a single-plane angiogram. The 3DRA gives a more

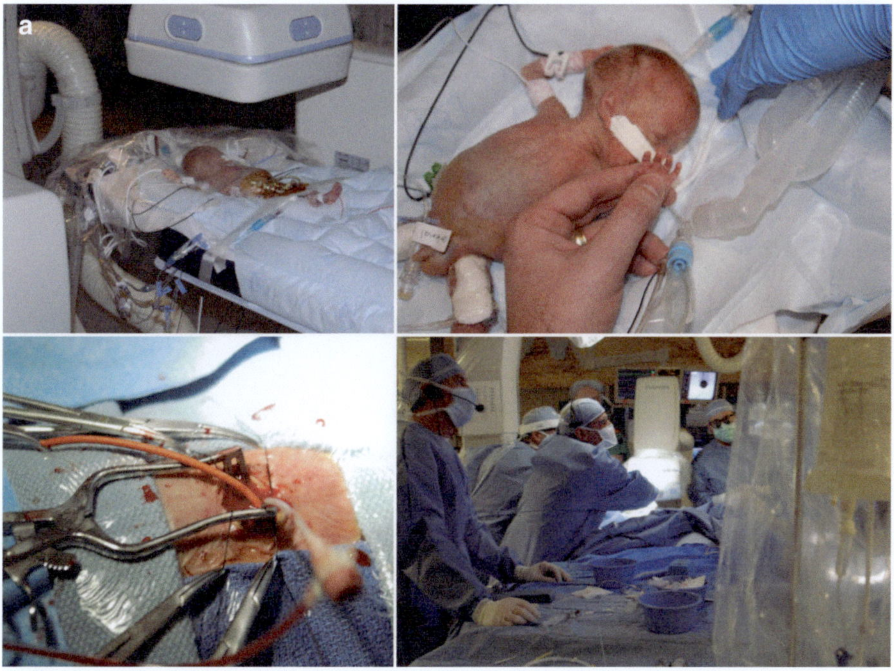

Fig. 22.1 In (**a**), a 700 g premature neonate with severe PVS, renal failure, ascites, and no vascular access presented a challenge for therapy. A per-ventricular hybrid approach to insert the sheath to allow balloon pulmonary valvuloplasty was the answer. In (**b**), the balloon procedure was successful, and this extreme premature neonate survived and was eventually discharged home

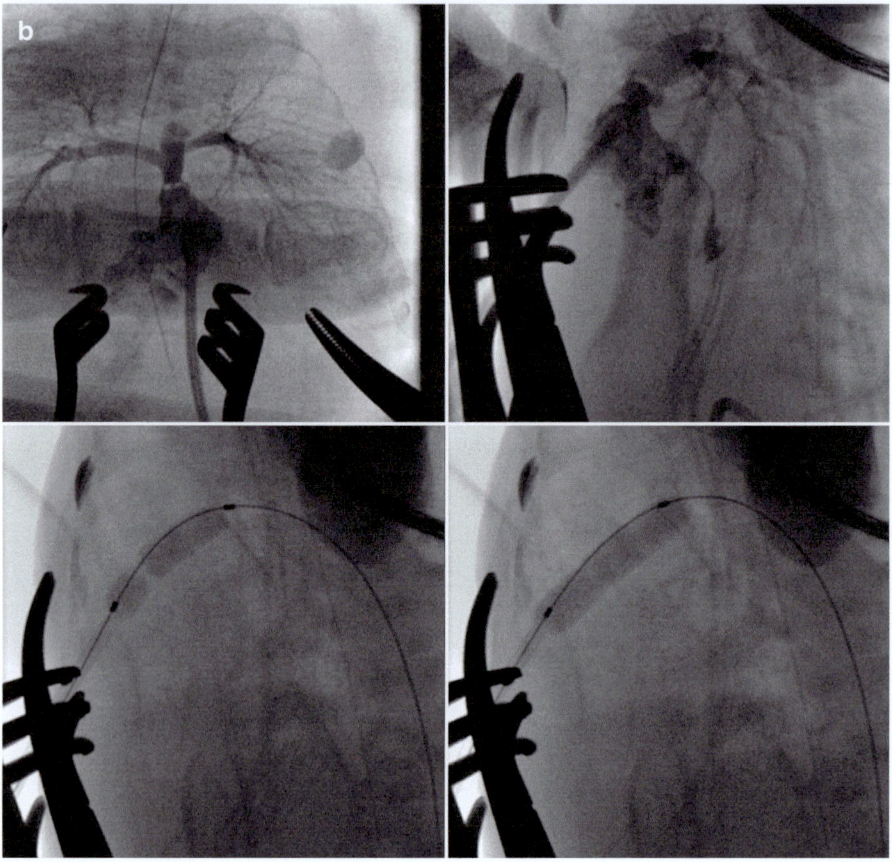

Fig. 22.1 (continued)

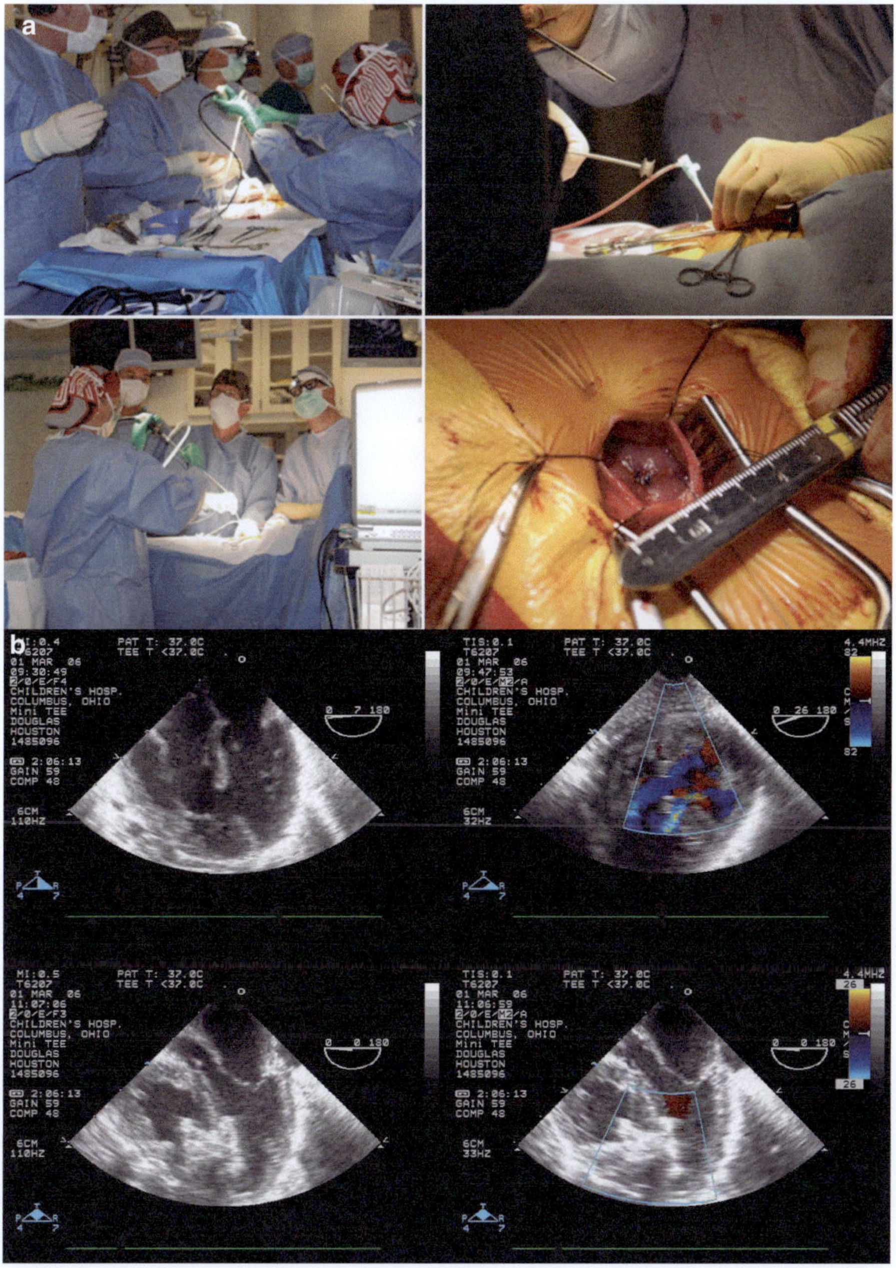

Fig. 22.2 In (**a**), the hybrid team of the CT surgeon and interventionalist is seen preparing a perventricular approach to close a large MVSD in a 2 kg premature infant. In (**b**), the sheath is introduced across the defect and an 8 mm Amplatzer MVSD occluder delivered without difficulty

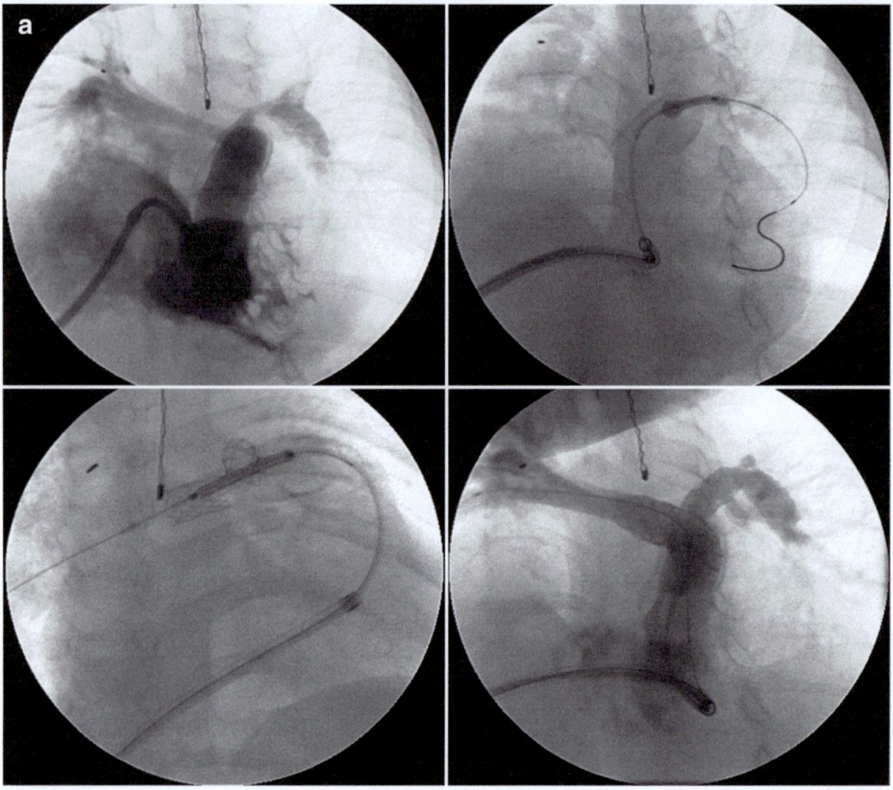

Fig. 22.3 In (**a**), an angiogram is shown that demonstrates complex PA stenoses bilaterally after truncus arteriosus repair. The patient also had no central venous access! In (**b**), after transhepatic cardiac catheterization was performed and demonstrated the RV-PA conduit, the CT surgeon performed direct transthoracic needle puncture into the conduit to provide a second access point for "PA rehabilitation." In (**c**), kissing stents were delivered to the RPA branches and CBA performed on the LPA. CPB was avoided in this patient

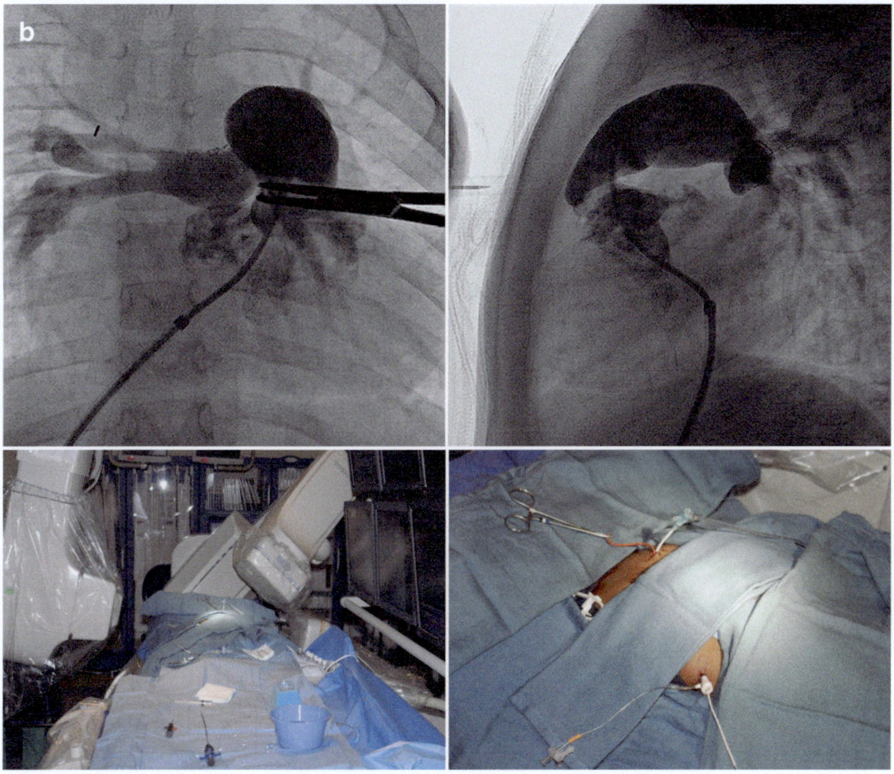

Fig. 22.3 (continued)

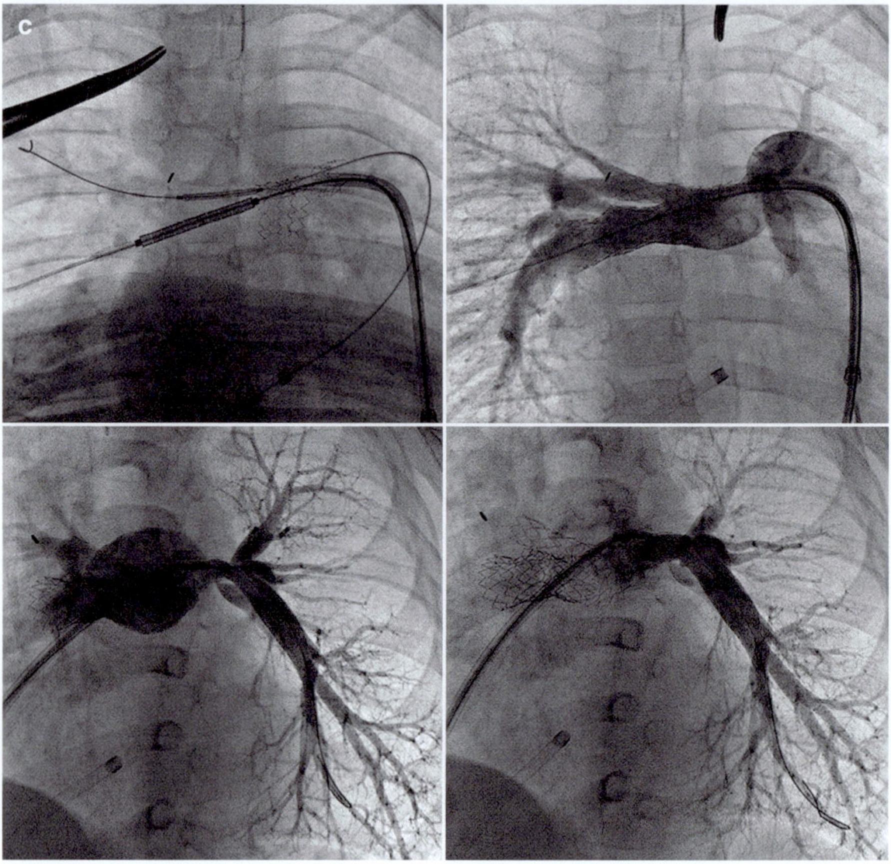

Fig. 22.3 (continued)

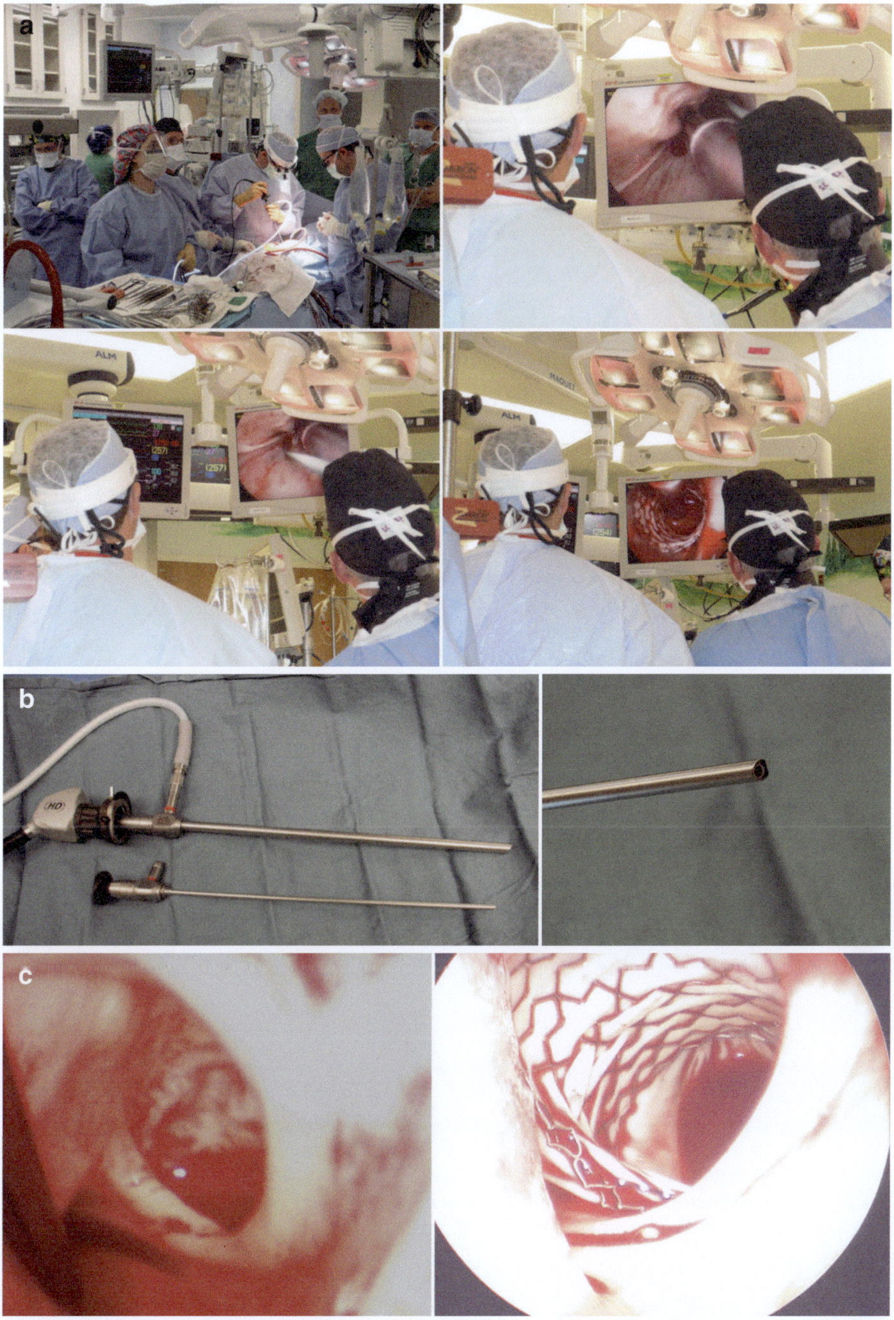

Fig. 22.4 Sometimes CPB is necessary. In (**a**), the hybrid OR is seen with the CT surgical and interventional teams imaging the PAs through an endoscope. In (**b**), the small endoscopic camera is shown. The pre- and post-stent endoscopic images of the proximal LPA stenosis are nicely shown in (**c**)

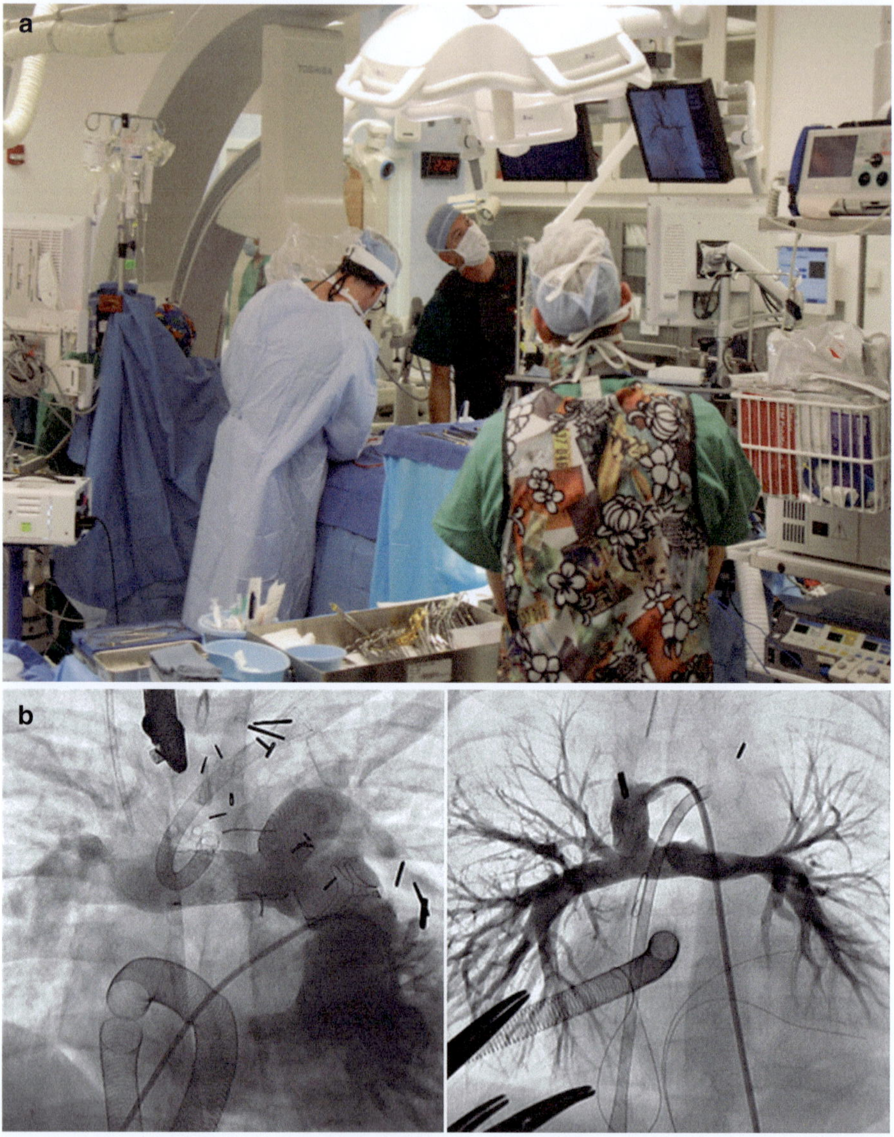

Fig. 22.5 Exit angiography is easily performed in a hybrid cardiac OR suite as demonstrated in (**a**). In (**b**), an exit angiogram after PVR and PA stents is seen in the *left panel*, while the *right panel* shows a nice result after comprehensive stage II repair for HLHS

robust assessment of anatomy, as well as define the best view for an intervention. If intraoperative PA stenting is being performed on CPB, one can also use endoscopic camera evaluation of the anatomy, both pre- and post-stent therapy.

The most talked about hybrid procedure that has benefited both the interventional cardiologist and CT surgeon is the hybrid approach to hypoplastic left heart syndrome, which is discussed in more detail elsewhere in this book. Instead of the complex Norwood/Sano procedure performed in the newborn on cardiopulmonary bypass with or without circulatory arrest, the surgeon can place right pulmonary artery and left pulmonary Gore-Tex bands within 30–40 min off cardiopulmonary bypass and with immediate improvement of hemodynamics, resulting in a 10 mmHg rise in systolic BP and a 10% fall in O2 saturations. The interventional cardiology team can then come into the hybrid suite to place the patent ductus arteriosus (PDA) stent through a direct approach via a purse-string that the surgeon provides in the proximal main pulmonary artery above the pulmonary valve leaflets. Using fluoroscopy in the hybrid suite, the placement of the PDA stent takes 15–20 min and causes no hemodynamic consequences compared to percutaneous delivery of the same PDA stent. This method of delivery can cause hemodynamic instability by crossing the tricuspid valve and pulmonary valve with a stiff guidewire and sheath, causing TR and PR. In a hybrid approach, the stent is easily placed using fluoroscopy and commonly using a lateral projection.

The next arena for a hybrid approach is the delivery of transcatheter heart valves. This likely started with the transapical delivery of the Edwards SAPIEN transcatheter heart valve for TAVR. Soon we learned that a per-ventricular approach to deliver a transcatheter pulmonary valve off cardiopulmonary bypass was very easy and quickly performed [4]. There will be more discussion of this technique elsewhere in this book. This has now evolved into the hybrid delivery of transcatheter mitral valves, as well as to close paravalve leaks around bioprosthetic/mechanical mitral valve replacement. This hybrid approach lessens the risk for the patient and allows an easier access and procedure for both the CT surgeon and the interventional cardiologist.

So, from the interventional cardiologist's viewpoint, a hybrid approach has simplified the procedure, allowed innovative approaches, and minimized the morbidity of the procedure. This is the future of the treatment of complex congenital heart disease, so everyone needs to be on board. You do not need a specialized hybrid suite to perform these procedures. You need a collaborative team who see no limitations in possibilities.

References

1. Pedra CA, et al. Per-ventricular device closure of congenital muscular ventricular septal defects. Expert Rev Cardiovasc Ther. 2010;8(5):663–74.
2. Holzer RJ, et al. "Hybrid" stent delivery in the pulmonary circulation. J Invasive Cardiol. 2008;20(11):592–8.
3. Holzer RJ, et al. Completion angiography after cardiac surgery for congenital heart disease: complementing the intraoperative imaging modalities. Pediatr Cardiol. 2009;30(8):1075–82.
4. Phillips AB, et al. Development of a novel hybrid strategy for transcatheter pulmonary valve placement in patients following transannular patch repair of tetralogy of fallot. Catheter Cardiovasc Interv. Off J Soc Card Angiogr Interv. 2015;87:403–10.

23 Parents' Perspective on the Hybrid Approach

Sharon L. Cheatham

For the purpose of this chapter, the focus will be on the hybrid approach for hypoplastic left heart syndrome (HLHS). The diagnosis of HLHS can be devastating for parents, whether diagnosed prenatally or after birth. A fetal diagnosis of HLHS may present families with a difficult decision regarding possible termination, albeit the fetal diagnosis is confirmed at an early enough gestation. Parents may consider termination, comfort care only following birth due to a lethal diagnosis, primary transplant, or three-staged surgical palliation. If the diagnosis is made following birth, parents may be in a state of shock, physically and mentally exhausted from the birth. At the same time, they are trying to comprehend the medical explanation of a complex form of congenital heart disease, as well as the surgical options presented to them. Alternatively, comfort care only may be offered. Family counseling provided by the cardiologist and cardiothoracic surgeon may have a tremendous influence on not only the decision but also the pathway to surgical management.

Few studies in the literature have evaluated the psychosocial and financial effect, or impact on families, when a newborn is diagnosed with HLHS. The published qualitative studies focus on HLHS babies who have undergone the traditional staged Norwood or Norwood-Sano procedure. The parents' perspective on the hybrid approach to managing infants with HLHS, and the psychosocial impact, have not been well reported. No matter which pathway is undertaken for palliation or comfort care, a family's life is changed forever.

A web-based survey on the Pediatric Heart Network showed different management options that are recommended based on institution and patient characteristics. Two hundred United States (US) cardiologists participated in the survey. US East Coast and Midwest respondents were more likely to recommend the traditional Norwood procedure (54 % and 60 %, respectively), and the US South and West respondents favored the Norwood with Sano modification (73 % and 82 %,

S.L. Cheatham, PhD, ACNP-BC, FSCAI
The Heart Center, Nationwide Children's Hospital, Columbus, OH, USA
e-mail: Sharon.Cheatham@nationwidechildrens.org

G. Butera et al. (eds.), *Fetal and Hybrid Procedures in Congenital Heart Diseases*, DOI 10.1007/978-3-319-40088-4_23

respectively). Both were recommended over comfort care only, hybrid palliation, or cardiac transplant for patients with an intact atrial septum ($p<0.05$), moderate to severe tricuspid regurgitation ($p<0.05$), or birth weight less than 2 kg ($p<0.05$). Comfort care only was preferred in low-birth-weight infants over hybrid palliation or cardiac transplantation ($p<0.05$), as well as over any other palliation for infants born premature less than 30 weeks' gestation, chromosomal abnormalities, or end-organ dysfunction ($p<0.05$) [1].

How the diagnosis and information are presented to parents is extremely important. Parents need and expect honesty, empathy, and compassion during delivery of this diagnosis and therapeutic options. The parent-physician relationship may be stressed during this time with the delivery of such a devastating diagnosis. The information needs to be presented in layman's terms, avoiding too much clinical jargon and utilizing pictures to help provide a clear understanding of the severity of the disease and possible surgical options. On the other hand, parents may be looking for advocacy for termination of the pregnancy. Family values and morals, as well as religion, may play an integral role in the decision-making process. Parents appreciate open communication, understanding and respect, and a willingness to help them make the right decision for their baby. Parents often grieve the loss of not having a normal healthy baby, afraid to bond, with fear of their baby dying. Their world has been torn apart. Qualitative studies show parents are devastated with the diagnosis and reportedly were the "worst time of their lives" [2].

Once the parents and the cardiothoracic surgeon come to a decision on palliation, and the hybrid pathway is chosen, Hybrid Stage I is performed. Having seen a HLHS baby who is postoperative the Norwood procedure laying in a bed next to the baby who had Hybrid Stage I, the family after hybrid palliation felt fortunate being able to hold and interact with their baby. On the other hand, they remain fearful for the "big" second stage surgery and survival. Once again, mixed emotions prevail.

During the interstage period, the time between stage I and stage II palliation, parents are faced with other stressors. The goal is to reach four to six months of age and approximately six kilograms (kg) before undergoing the big open heart Comprehensive Stage II procedure. Therefore, parents' focus is now on feeding issues and weight gain, as well as oxygen saturations and work of breathing. Following Hybrid Stage I and prior to discharge, single-ventricle patients who underwent the hybrid procedure are usually enrolled in a home monitoring program where the caregiver or parent perform daily weights and documentation of daily caloric formula intake, as well as daily pulse oximetry oxygen saturations to assess potential complications [3–8]. Home monitoring may reduce mortality [9], however may increase parental stress. Data is reviewed weekly. Any breach in established criteria is to be reported by parents in a timely fashion, and the cardiologist determines if further assessment or admission to the hospital is necessary. Close monitoring is recommended in the outpatient cardiology clinic every one to two weeks. These clinic visits should review the feeding history and home monitoring data, as well as perform a physical examination, an electrocardiogram, and an echocardiogram. A nutritionist, as well as a physical or occupational therapist are often included in the single-ventricle team. These frequent clinic visits are usually long and burdensome for families. Prolonged hospitalization, as well as frequent and long clinic visits, impact family dynamics. This is time taken away from other children or work responsibilities. Usually one parent needs to relinquish their work to become the primary caretaker. This, coupled with accumulating hospital bills, places a tremendous financial stress on families. In a study measuring anxiety/stress levels of parents/caregivers of children with single-ventricle physiology who underwent a hybrid procedure, significant correlations were noted between anxiety/stress scores and caregiver's gender, caregiver's age, caregiver's level of education, percent of time a caregiver spent feeding the child, if caregivers were taking medications for anxiety, and if the child was seen in the emergency room during the interstage period. There was no correlation of anxiety/stress scores with caregiver's race, child's underlying cardiac diagnosis, age of child, route of feeding during the interstage period, birth order, or number of children in the family, relationship status, or distance from the hospital [10].

Following the staged surgical palliative procedures, particularly Hybrid Stage I and Comprehensive Stage II, a common concern of parents is "Will my child be normal?" or "Will my child be delayed (developmentally)?" The first published study on neurodevelopmental outcomes in infants with HLHS and other univentricular hearts, who underwent hybrid palliation versus the Norwood procedure, showed no significant difference in mortality at one year of age. Psychomotor development index and mental development index scores were similar in the hybrid and the Norwood group. Both were significantly lower than the norm at one year of age, particularly with motor impairment [11].

In a more recent study, investigators studied early motor, language, and intellectual development of infants with HLHS after Hybrid Stage I palliation. At 6 months of age, there was a statistically significant difference between the HLHS group and the normal age-matched control group in fine and gross motor skills ($p=0.049$). However, there was no significant difference for cognitive and receptive and expressive language at 6 months. This is important information for parents where occupational and physical therapy can provide early intervention to help educate and aid parents to assist in the development of gross and fine motor skills of their infant [12].

Parents concerns are realistic and justified. From the impact of the initial diagnosis to the stressful interstage period and Comprehensive Stage II, to finally Fontan completion, parents are fearful of their child not surviving, and if they do, what will the neurodevelopmental outcomes be for their future. Healthcare providers need to better support patients and families from the initial diagnosis, whether a fetal or postnatal diagnosis. All options need to be explained to parents free of bias, despite the struggle some cardiologists and cardiothoracic surgeons may have presenting certain options. Every single-ventricle patient should be enrolled in a home monitoring program with 24/7 availability and access to support from the single-ventricle cardiac team. Every family should receive psychosocial support and counseling. The financial burden alone warrants assistance with frequent evaluations, echocardiograms, hospital admissions, cardiac surgeries, and interventional cardiac catheterization procedures. Family financial resources are often exhausted throughout early childhood for financial burdens do not end with the third-staged surgery. Care providers need to continue to evaluate neurodevelopment throughout childhood, providing interventions and support for the best possible outcomes.

In our institution, the hybrid approach for HLHS is offered at equipoise with the Norwood or Norwood-Sano procedure. Reports from Nationwide Children's Hospital in Columbus, Ohio [13], and the team from Giessen, Germany [14], prefer the hybrid approach, not only the cardiothoracic surgery and interventional teams but the parents' preference as well.

References

1. Yates AR, et al. Initial counseling prior to palliation for hypoplastic left heart syndrome. Congenit Heart Dis. 2011;6(4):347–58.
2. Cantwell-Bartl AM, Tibballs J. Psychosocial responses of parents to their infant's diagnosis of hypoplastic left heart syndrome. Cardiol Young. 2015;25(6):1065–73.
3. Ghanayem NS, Cava JR, Jaquiss RD, Tweddell JS. Home monitoring of infants after stage one palliation for hypoplastic left heart syndrome. Semin Thorac Cardiovasc Surg Pediatr Card Surg Annu. 2004;7:32–8.
4. Ghanayem NS, Hoffman GM, Mussatto KA, Cava JR, Frommelt PC, Rudd NA, et al. Home surveillance program prevents interstage mortality after the Norwood procedure. J Thorac Cardiovasc Surg. 2003;126(5):1367–77.
5. Ghanayem NS, Tweddell JS, Hoffman GM, Mussatto K, Jaquiss RD. Optimal timing of the second stage of palliation for hypoplastic left heart syndrome facilitated through home monitoring, and the results of early cavopulmonary anastomosis. Cardiol Young. 2006;16 Suppl 1:61–6.
6. Hehir DA, Cooper DS, Walters EM, Ghanayem NS. Feeding, growth, nutrition, and optimal interstage surveillance for infants with hypoplastic left heart syndrome. Cardiol Young. 2011;21 Suppl 2:59–64.
7. Miller-Tate H, Stewart J, Allen R, Husain N, Rosen K, Cheatham JP, et al. Interstage weight gain for patients with hypoplastic left heart syndrome undergoing the hybrid procedure. Congenit Heart Dis. 2013;8(3):228–33.
8. Rudd NA, Frommelt MA, Tweddell JS, Hehir DA, Mussatto KA, Frontier KD, Slicker JA, Bartz PJ, Ghanayem NS. Improving interstage survival after Norwood operation: outcomes from 10 years of home monitoring. J Thorac Cardiovasc Surg. 2014;148(4):1540–7.
9. Hansen JH, Furck AK, Petko C, Buchholz-Berdau R, Voges I, Scheewe J, Rickers C, Kramer HH. Use of surveillance criteria reduces interstage mortality after the Norwood operation for hypoplastic left heart syndrome. Eur J Cardiothorac Surg. 2012;41(5):1013–8.
10. Stewart J, Dempster R, Allen R, Miller-Tate H, Dickson G, Fichtner S, Principe AJ, Fonseca R, Nicholson L, Cua CL. Caregiver anxiety due to interstage feeding concerns. Congenit Heart Dis. 2015;10(2):E98–106. doi:10.1111/chd.12257.
11. Knirsch W, Liamlahi R, Hug MI, et al. Mortality and neurodevelopmental outcome at 1 year of age comparing hybrid and Norwood procedures. Eur J Cardiothorac Surg. 2012;42(1):33–9.
12. Cheatham SL, Carey H, Chisolm JL, Heathcock JC, Steward D. Early results of neurodevelopment following hybrid stage I for hypoplastic left heart syndrome. Pediatr Cardiol. 2015;36(3):685–91.

13. Galantowicz M, Cheatham JP, Phillips A, Cua CL, Hoffman TM, Hill SL, et al. Hybrid approach for hypoplastic left heart syndrome: intermediate results after the learning curve. Ann Thorac Surg. 2008;85(6):2063, 70; discussion 2070–1.
14. Schranz D, Bauer A, Reich B, Steinbrenner B, Recla S, Schmidt D, et al. Fifteen-year single center experience with the "Giessen Hybrid" approach for hypoplastic left heart and variants: current strategies and outcomes. Pediatr Cardiol. 2015;36(2):365–73.

The Hybrid Catheterization Laboratory 24

Ralf J. Holzer

24.1 Introduction

Hybrid procedures encompass the procedural cooperation between cardiothoracic surgeon and interventional cardiologist. These procedures include therapies such as hybrid palliation of hypoplastic left heart syndrome, perventricular VSD closure, and intraoperative stent placement [1–6]. An increasing number of centers have been embracing hybrid therapies [7], with the most important ingredient for the success of a hybrid program being the attitude of the interventional and surgical team, embracing a collaborative approach and being able to "think outside the box" when combining surgical and interventional techniques. While hybrid procedures can be performed with the right attitude and a portable c-arm, having a dedicated hybrid cardiac catheterization suite definitely reduces the difficulties in performing these procedures. It is therefore important to consider carefully whether to upgrade a cath lab to a dedicated hybrid catheterization suite.

24.2 The Hybrid Cardiac Catheterization Laboratory

Many of the design elements that are considered for a hybrid cardiac catheterization laboratory would also be considered for a new stand-alone cath lab. These includes an improved space utilization, pan/tilt/zoom cameras, and a dedicated routing solution, as well as strategically placed monitors at various locations within the catheterization laboratory, so that all relevant aspects of the procedure can be viewed from any position necessary. These are important design decisions not necessarily limited

R.J. Holzer, MD, MSc, FSCAI
Cardiac Catheterization & Interventional Therapy, Division Chief Cardiology (Acting), Sidra Cardiovascular Center of Excellence, Sidra Medical and Research Center, PO Box 26999, Doha, Qatar
e-mail: rholzer@sidra.org

G. Butera et al. (eds.), *Fetal and Hybrid Procedures in Congenital Heart Diseases*, DOI 10.1007/978-3-319-40088-4_24

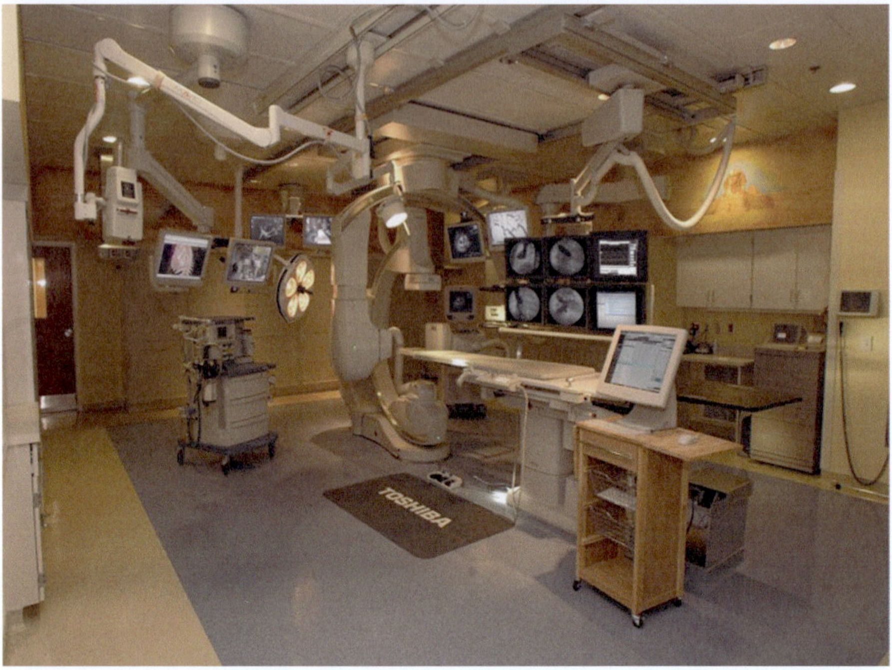

Fig. 24.1 Hybrid catheterization suite (hybrid catheterization laboratory at Nationwide Children's Hospital)

to a hybrid suite but also required for a modern stand-alone catheterization laboratory. The setup of the control room does not differ significantly between a hybrid suite and a modern non-hybrid cath suite. It will accommodate the usual monitoring and (post-processing) workstations and provide a free and unobstructed view to the procedural area, which is supplemented by images that are routed to the appropriate monitors from integrated pan/tilt/zoom cameras. The control room also usually houses the hardware of the routing solution.

So how does a hybrid cath lab (Fig. 24.1) differ from a modern newly designed stand-alone cath lab? First and foremost, a hybrid cath lab should usually be a lot bigger than a standard surgical operating room, with many modern hybrid labs having a floor space of at least 900–1,200 square feet. Size certainly does matter when it comes to a hybrid cath lab, as a variety of equipment will need to be accommodated. Besides the standard biplane imaging equipment, cardiac anesthesia, and all the other diagnostic and imaging tools frequently utilized during cardiac catheterization procedures (IVUS, ICE, TEE, RF, hemodynamic system, pressure wire, Angiojet, etc.), a hybrid catheterization laboratory will need to be able to accommodate the complete surgical setup including trays, additional members of staff (surgical team, scrub nurses, perfusionists), cardiopulmonary bypass and/or ECMO, electrocautery, fiber-optic light sources, and others.

In addition, there is a need for at least one additional set of gases (ideally three sets), to accommodate the cardiopulmonary bypass and/or ECMO circuits. Furthermore, the electrical power outlets need to be appropriate to accommodate all the surgical and catheter equipments that are being used in the catheterization laboratory. Storage solutions need to be easily movable so that the entire room can be cleaned appropriately and without difficulties.

Ceiling-mounted booms are ideal for housing many of the needed equipment. However, it is important to clearly understand the location where any type of equipment may be needed, so that the booms can reach to the appropriate positions while not obstructing a necessary passage that may be required, for example, for TEE or IVUS. Also, it is crucial to make sure that staff is still able to move and access the patient if and when all the relevant equipment is in place. Some devices lend themselves to be mounted on equipment booms (such as defibrillator, surgical gases, some cameras, electrocautery), while others may be either freestanding or ceiling or wall mounted (such as contrast injector and some cameras). Monitors will be required in front of the interventionists, at the head end, behind the interventionists to facilitate viewing for the cardiothoracic surgeon, as well as strategically in other positions of the lab so that the important parts of the procedure can be visualized from any location with the hybrid suite.

In addition to the aforementioned, a hybrid lab has to conform to operating room standards, including a monolithic ceiling design, appropriate temperature, and humidity control, as well as more than 13 air exchanges per hour. Infection control is important, and therefore an induction room will have important benefits (in particular in a pediatric center where parents may accompany a patient). Equally, a scrub sink should be placed so it can be used prior to entering the hybrid cath lab. While surgical attire is not required in the control room during standard catheterization procedures, this will be mandatory if and when a hybrid procedure is being performed. For this purpose it is important to have a room in front of the control room, where surgical masks, head and shoe covers, and bunny suits are available for those visitors that may want to enter the control room during hybrid procedures without entering the procedure room itself. If more than one catheterization laboratory is present in the same institution, it is of benefit to have a lockable door between the two cath labs, thereby avoiding the need to treat the adjacent control room as a sterile area when a hybrid procedure is being performed in the other lab.

An important consideration for the hybrid suite is the cath table itself. Ideally it should be able to tilt right- and leftward, as well as being able to move into a head or foot-down position. Furthermore, the table needs to be securely lockable so that it is not easily unlocked during the surgical component of a hybrid procedure.

For surgical hybrid suites (Fig. 24.2), many design considerations are somewhat different to those taken for a hybrid catheterization suite [8]. Some important considerations are centered on creating a shielded area within the operating room, as well as making sure that the degree of lead lining of the walls is sufficient to meet the requirements for fixed, ceiling-mounted c-arm installations by the relevant state. In addition, many surgical hybrid suites may just utilize a single-plane system, which requires notably less floor space than a biplane system. Furthermore, the ceiling may need to

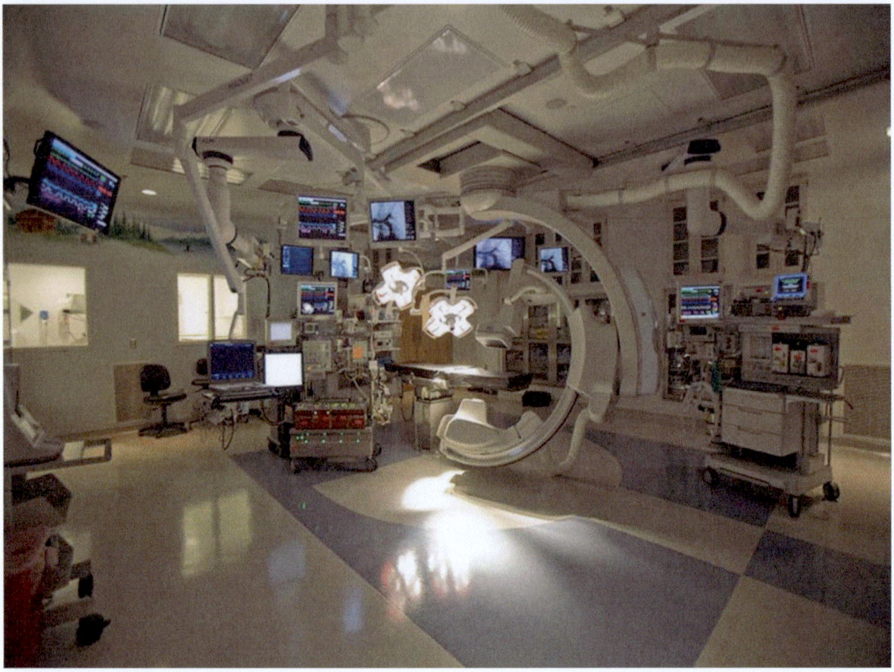

Fig. 24.2 Hybrid operating suite (hybrid operating suite at Nationwide Children's Hospital)

be reinforced to be able to accommodate a fixed installed c-arm. The surgical table should be carbon fiber and lightweight to facilitate appropriate imaging.

24.3 Summary

Given the many considerations that need to be taken into account, it is essential to have all stakeholders involved in the design process at an early stage (cath and surgical team, facilities, biomedical engineering, administration, etc.). While there are many common issues that need to be solved for installation of a hybrid suite, the process is often somewhat institution specific, and the individual requirements and details may vary. Also, converting existing cath labs to a hybrid suite may pose different challenges than starting with a completely fresh installation [9]. In general, many of the decisions that need to be made (such as routing) are not unique to a hybrid suite, but would also need to be considered for a stand-alone catheterization laboratory.

References

1. Michel-Behnke I, Akintuerk H, Marquardt I, et al. Stenting of the ductus arteriosus and banding of the pulmonary arteries: basis for various surgical strategies in newborns with multiple left heart obstructive lesions. Heart. 2003;89(6):645–50.

2. Galantowicz M, Cheatham JP. Lessons learned from the development of a new hybrid strategy for the management of hypoplastic left heart syndrome. Pediatr Cardiol. 2005;26(2):190–9.
3. Galantowicz M, Cheatham JP. Fontan completion without surgery. Semin Thorac Cardiovasc Surg Pediatr Card Surg Annu. 2004;7:48–55.
4. Bacha EA, Cao QL, Starr JP, Waight D, Ebeid MR, Hijazi ZM. Perventricular device closure of muscular ventricular septal defects on the beating heart: technique and results. J Thorac Cardiovasc Surg. 2003;126(6):1718–23.
5. Bacha EA, Cao QL, Galantowicz ME, et al. Multicenter experience with perventricular device closure of muscular ventricular septal defects. Pediatr Cardiol. 2005;26(2):169–75.
6. Hjortdal VE, Redington AN, de Leval MR, Tsang VT. Hybrid approaches to complex congenital cardiac surgery. Eur J Cardiothorac Surg. 2002;22(6):885–90.
7. Holzer R, Marshall A, Kreutzer J, et al. Hybrid procedures: adverse events and procedural characteristics—results of a multi-institutional registry. Congenit Heart Dis. 2010;5(3):233–42.
8. Bonatti J, Vassiliades T, Nifong W, et al. How to build a cath-lab operating room. Heart Surg Forum. 2007;10(4):E344–8.
9. Hirsch R. The hybrid cardiac catheterization laboratory for congenital heart disease: from conception to completion. Catheter Cardiovasc Interv: Off J Soc Cardiac Angiogr Interv. 2008;71(3):418–28.

Part VII

Hypoplastic Left Heart Syndrome (HLHS)

Hypoplastic Left Heart Syndrome: Natural and Surgical History

25

Ina Michel-Behnke

25.1 Natural History

The spectrum of left heart hypoplasia has its extremes from a diminutive left ventricle and mitral/aortic atresia at one end to those classified as hypoplastic left heart complex [1–3] where pre- and postnatal interventions might achieve a biventricular circulation. This chapter is focused on the understanding of hypoplastic left heart syndrome (HLHS) as a lesion with the morphology and physiology of a severely underdeveloped left ventricle and outflow as the dominant findings.

Occurrence of HLHS within congenital heart disease is 2–3 % with a tendency of lower prevalence over the last decade [4]. Due to its severity, the newborns die in 95 % in the first days or weeks. Prenatal diagnosis is commonly made at 18–24 weeks of gestation within screening programs for the fetal heart. Underdevelopment of the left ventricle and aorta can be detected earlier, but due to physiological and anatomical changes later in pregnancy as left ventricular growth occurs, endocardial fibroelastosis and premature closure of the foramen ovale among others allow planning of postnatal therapeutic strategies only at later stages and longitudinal follow-up [5, 6].

25.1.1 Transition from Fetal to Postnatal Circulation

Onset of symptoms occurs when the arterial duct and the foramen ovale are closing, in the first days of life. As a duct-dependent lesion with a left ventricle unable to support the systemic circulation, discontinuation of a right-to-left shunt through the arterial duct initiates heart failure and metabolic acidosis. In the presence of aortic atresia with retrograde perfusion of the coronaries, myocardial performance

I. Michel-Behnke
Pediatric Heart Center Vienna, Vienna, Austria
e-mail: ina.michel-behnke@meduniwien.ac.at

G. Butera et al. (eds.), *Fetal and Hybrid Procedures in Congenital Heart Diseases*, DOI 10.1007/978-3-319-40088-4_25

deteriorates at this stage. The pale-cyanotic newborn with weak or absent femoral pulses, edema, and tachypnea represents the hemodynamic changes of increased systemic afterload of the closing arterial duct.

Besides the open arterial duct, mixing at the atrial level through an atrial septal defect (ASD) is mandatory for survival. Restriction of the interatrial communication or even premature closure during pregnancy has been accounted for development of HLHS [7] and moreover for secondary arterialization of the pulmonary veins, constituting the most fatal group concerning postnatal treatment options [8–10]. Limitation of a left-to-right atrial blood flow consequently increases left atrial pressure and decreases egress of pulmonary venous drainage that further worsens cyanosis and respiratory distress preceding circulatory collapse.

Having said that, unrestricted ASDs in HLHS expose the heart to a high-volume load, pulmonary overcirculation, and congestive heart failure. Diagnosis in this group of neonates can be missed early after birth, as oxygen saturation may be in the 90s until they deteriorate showing up with tachypnea and hepatomegaly and edema. The two phenotypes and their pathophysiology are depicted in Fig. 25.1. If the clinical signs are misinterpreted as neonatal sepsis or cardiogenic shock, death occurs usually in the first days of life.

25.2 Surgical History

Evidence from in vivo experiments that prostaglandin E infusion is able to maintain ductal patency [11] and successful application in neonates with duct-dependent pulmonary or systemic circulation [12–16] cleared the way for surgical treatment of cyanotic congenital heart disease [CHD] and thus also for HLHS.

25.2.1 Univentricular Palliation

The first successful attempts to build a systemic circulation supported by the right ventricle by reconstruction of the aortic arch, connecting the occasionally diminutive ascending aorta with the pulmonary trunk together with atrial septectomy and provision of pulmonary perfusion by a modified Blalock-Taussig (BT) shunt, were undertaken by Norwood and colleagues in the 1980s. After the initial learning curve, early mortality in a larger series at CHOP of 104 patients within 2 years was 39 % (30 early, 11 late). Fate of the palliative surgery was contributed to limited perioperative interventions, hypoxemia, and aortic arch obstructions [17–21]. Since then many institutions worldwide with variable success pursued the concept. It turned out that besides improvement of surgical techniques, the balance of pulmonary and systemic circulation (Qp/Qs) and avoiding coronary steal play a key role to reduce early and interstage mortality.

The complications inherent with BT shunts either by obstruction or by induction of pulmonary overflow and thereby causing steal from the myocardial perfusion result from the physiology of the shunt flow throughout the whole cardiac cycle, i.e.,

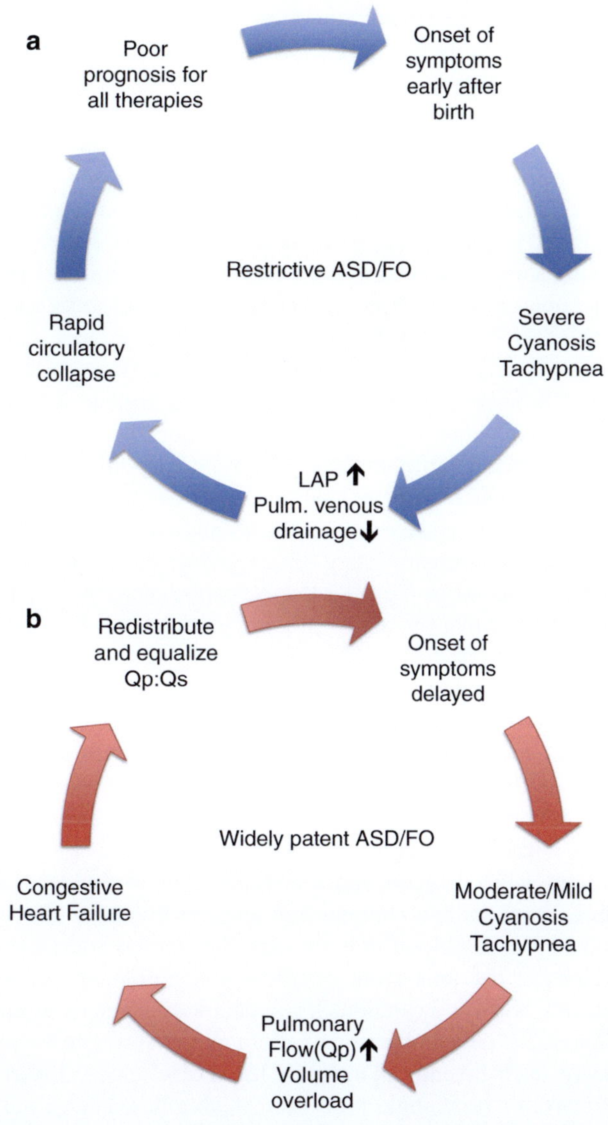

Fig. 25.1 Clinical phenotypes of hypoplastic left heart syndrome. The neonate with restrictive atrial septal defect(ASD)/foramen ovale(FO) presents early and cyanotic after birth with rapid hemodynamic decline (**a**), while a widely open interatrial communication can mask the diagnosis with mildly decreased saturations and delayed onset of heart failure (**b**). Irrespective of the ASD/FO, worsening occurs as the arterial duct closes

systole and diastole. As about 70 % of coronary perfusion occurs in diastole, pressures must not fall below the critical threshold.

Thus surgeons rediscovered the initial idea of William Norwood of a RV-PA shunt, and it was Shunji Sano in 2003 who promoted a non-valved 4–5 mm PTFE tube connecting the RV to the main pulmonary artery [22, 23]. Early hospital mortality decreased considerably and was attributed to higher diastolic pressures and less pulmonary runoff. Perioperative management became easier not only in high volume centers. Survival rates in controlled case series revealed 89–93 % in the RV-PA shunt versus 53–72 % after BT shunt [22, 24, 25]. Conflicting data with no difference in early hospital mortality were reported [26–28].

While the advantages of the RV-PA shunts within the first stage of the palliative track are obvious, the impact on long-term outcome had to be determined. The largest series investigating survival after the second and third operation, i.e., partial and total cavopulmonary connection, has been undertaken in a multicenter randomized prospective trial with 555 cases [29]. Death at 1 year of age or heart transplantation as primary end points were in favor for the RV-PA shunt (26 % vs. 36 %) but equalized during the total follow-up of 32 ± 11 months. While satisfactory pulmonary artery growth was achieved in either the RV-PA or the BT shunt, potential disadvantages as myocardial scar followed by arrhythmia and ventricular dysfunction have been investigated and argued to reduce the beneficial aspects of the postoperative management on the long run [30–33]. Interstage complications and mortality have been related to myocardial dysfunction, coronary artery disease, tricuspid regurgitation, aortic arch obstruction, and shunt stenosis, the latter one occurring more frequently after RV-PA shunt than after BT shunt placement [34–36]. Suggestions on when and how to repair the tricuspid valve and modified techniques of aortic arch reconstruction aimed at improving and preserving performance of the systemic right ventricle until volume unloading at the time of Glenn operation is achieved [37–40].

In the 1990s, the idea of joining the experience of surgeons and pediatric cardiologists brought up the hybrid approach for HLHS. Based on the experience of Gibbs [41] to maintain ductal patency by stent implantation together with bilateral pulmonary artery banding, this concept was elaborated mainly by two groups in the USA (Mark Galantowicz, surgeon, and John Cheatham, cardiologist) and Germany (Hakan Akinturk, surgeon, and Dietmar Schranz, cardiologist) [42–46]. The strategy to secure the systemic blood flow through the stented arterial duct and at the same time protecting the lung from overflow and pulmonary hypertension was applied to high-risk Norwood candidates and enabled the teams to move an extensive surgery beyond the neonatal period or alternatively to bridge the patient to heart transplantation or even biventricular repair for HLHC cases. Either sequentially (Giessen, Germany) or in a single procedure (Columbus, USA), the surgical and transcatheter interventions were installed.

While after the classical Norwood or Sano modification of aortic reconstruction, the bidirectional superior cavopulmonary connection does not differ from other single-ventricle repairs; the hybrid approach is followed by the comprehensive stage II surgery that combines the cavopulmonary connection of the SVC to the RPA together with the components of stage I, i.e., aortic arch reconstruction and dissection of the pulmonary artery, to rebuild the systemic RV outlet. Several modifications and adjustments from other institutions have been suggested, including a reversed BT shunt for protection of coronary perfusion [47, 48]. Comparative studies between the Norwood/Sano procedures versus hybrid procedure emerged from all over the world and elaborated the individual patient-specific decision for either approach [49–53].

Whatever type of palliation is applied, a home surveillance program for reduced morbidity and mortality turned out to be essential after hospital discharge [54–59].

25.2.2 Biventricular Repair and Heart Transplantation

Besides the collaborative surgical-interventional approach, efforts have been put in the recruitment of the hypoplastic left ventricle by relief of inflow and outflow tract obstruction added by resection of endocardial fibroelastosis [60], keeping in mind the limited ability for hyperplasia rather than hypertrophy within the cellular signaling within LV development [2].

Leonard Bailey from Loma Linda (USA) initiated the surgical history of heart transplantation [HTX] in HLHS in 1985 shortly after the reports of Norwood [61]. The special requirements of enlargement of the hypoplastic aortic arch during transplantations are challenging. Due to high wait-list mortality, primary transplantation is performed mostly in those neonates not eligible for Norwood or hybrid-type palliations like significant tricuspid regurgitation, severe dysfunction of the right ventricle, or coronary fistula and stenoses. Outcome of heart transplantation early or late after failure of surgical palliation is comparable to non-CHD-HTX [62] but requires adjustment of surgical techniques [63].

In summary, progress of prenatal screening, intensive care management, and refinements of surgical techniques have improved survival and quality of life for children with HLHS. The therapeutic portfolio for those brought to birth includes the option for:

- Comfort care management
- Staged functional univentricular palliation (Norwood/Sano/Hybrid)
- Primary cardiac transplantation

The offers to patients with HLHS are very much influenced by the attitude of caregivers as early as during detection in fetuses. Counseling is influenced by personal experience, actual published results of palliative surgery and heart transplantation, associated genetic disorders as well as neurodevelopmental outcome, and finally ethical aspects [64, 65].

References

1. Tchervenkov CI, Jacobs JP, Weinberg PM, Aiello VD, Béland MJ, Colan SD, Elliott MJ, Franklin RCG, Gaynor JW, Krogmann ON, Kurosawa H, Maruszewski B, Stellin G. The nomenclature, definition and classification of hypoplastic left heart syndrome. Cardiol Young. 2006;16:339–68.
2. Hickey EJ, Caldarone CA, McCrindle BW. Left ventricular hypoplasia. J Am Coll Cardiol. 2012;59:S43–54.

3. Kearney DL. The pathological spectrum of left-ventricular hypoplasia. Semin Cardiothorac Vasc Anesth. 2013;17:105–16.
4. Egbe A, Uppu S, Lee S, Stroustrup A, Ho D, Srivastava S. Temporal variation of birth prevalence of congenital heart disease in the United States. Congenit Heart Dis. 2015;10:43–50.
5. Yagel S, Weissman A, Rotstein Z, Manor M, Hegesh J, Anteby E, Lipitz S, Achiron R. Congenital heart defects: natural course and in utero development. Circulation. 1997; 96:550–5.
6. Cole CR, Eghtesady P. The myocardial and coronary histopathology and pathogenesis of hypoplastic left heart syndrome. Cardiol Young. 2016;26(1):19–29.
7. Gardiner HM. Response of the fetal heart to changes in load: from hyperplasia to heart failure. Heart. 2005;91:871–3.
8. Taketazu M, Barrea C, Smallhorn JF, Wilson GJ, Hornberger LK. Intrauterine pulmonary venous flow and restrictive foramen ovale in fetal hypoplastic left heart syndrome. J Antimicrob Chemother. 2004;43:1902–7.
9. Vlahos AP, Lock JE, McElhinney DB, van der Velde ME. Hypoplastic left heart syndrome with intact or highly restrictive atrial septum: outcome after neonatal transcatheter atrial septostomy. Circulation. 2004;109:2326–30.
10. Hoque T, Richmond M, Vincent JA, Bacha E, Torres A. Current outcomes of hypoplastic left heart syndrome with restrictive atrial septum: a single-center experience. Pediatr Cardiol. 2013;34:1181–9.
11. Sharpe GL, Larsson KS. Studies on closure of the ductus arteriosus. X. In vivo effect of prostaglandin. Prostaglandins. 1975;9:703–19.
12. Graham TP, Atwood GF, Boucek RJ. Pharmacologic dilatation of the ductus arteriosus with prostaglandin E1 in infants with congenital heart disease. South Med J. 1978;71:1238–46.
13. Olley PM, Coceani F, Bodach E. E-type prostaglandins: a new emergency therapy for certain cyanotic congenital heart malformations. Circulation. 1976;53:728–31.
14. Heymann MA, Berman W, Rudolph AM, Whitman V. Dilatation of the ductus arteriosus by prostaglandin E1 in aortic arch abnormalities. Circulation. 1979;59:169–73.
15. Lang P, Freed MD, Rosenthal A, Castaneda AR, Nadas AS. The use of prostaglandin E1 in an infant with interruption of the aortic arch. J Pediatr. 1977;91:805–7.
16. Yabek SM, Mann JS. Prostaglandin E1 infusion in the hypoplastic left heart syndrome. Chest. 1979;76:330–1.
17. Norwood WI, Kirklin JK, Sanders SP. Hypoplastic left heart syndrome: experience with palliative surgery. Am J Cardiol. 1980;45:87–91.
18. Norwood WI, Lang P, Casteneda AR, Campbell DN. Experience with operations for hypoplastic left heart syndrome. J Thorac Cardiovasc Surg. 1981;82:511–9.
19. Norwood WI, Lang P, Hansen DD. Physiologic repair of aortic atresia-hypoplastic left heart syndrome. N Engl J Med. 1983;308:23–6.
20. Pigott JD, Murphy JD, Barber G, Norwood WI. Palliative reconstructive surgery for hypoplastic left heart syndrome. Ann Thorac Surg. 1988;45:122–8.
21. Norwood WI. Hypoplastic left heart syndrome. Ann Thorac Surg. 1991;52:688–95.
22. Sano S, Ishino K, Kawada M, Arai S, Kasahara S, Asai T, Masuda Z-I, Takeuchi M, Ohtsuki S-I. Right ventricle-pulmonary artery shunt in first-stage palliation of hypoplastic left heart syndrome. J Thorac Cardiovasc Surg. 2003;126:504–9; discussion 509–10.
23. Sano S, Ishino K, Kawada M, Honjo O. Right ventricle-pulmonary artery shunt in first-stage palliation of hypoplastic left heart syndrome. Semin Thorac Cardiovasc Surg Pediatr Card Surg Annu. 2004;7:22–31.
24. Pizarro C, Malec E, Maher KO, Januszewska K, Gidding SS, Murdison KA, Baffa JM, Norwood WI. Right ventricle to pulmonary artery conduit improves outcome after stage I Norwood for hypoplastic left heart syndrome. Circulation. 2003;108 Suppl 1:II155–60. Lippincott Williams & Wilkins.
25. Mair R, Tulzer G, Sames E, Gitter R, Lechner E, Steiner J, Hofer A, Geiselseder G, Gross C. Right ventricular to pulmonary artery conduit instead of modified Blalock-Taussig shunt

improves postoperative hemodynamics in newborns after the norwood operation. J Thorac Cardiovasc Surg. 2003;126:1378–84.
26. Mahle WT, Cuadrado AR, Tam VKH. Early experience with a modified Norwood procedure using right ventricle to pulmonary artery conduit. Ann Thorac Surg. 2003;76:1084–8; discussion 1089.
27. Tabbutt S, Dominguez TE, Ravishankar C, Marino BS, Gruber PJ, Wernovsky G, Gaynor JW, Nicolson SC, Spray TL. Outcomes after the stage I reconstruction comparing the right ventricular to pulmonary artery conduit with the modified Blalock Taussig shunt. Ann Thorac Surg. 2005;80:1582–90; discussion 1590–1.
28. Azakie A, Martinez D, Sapru A, Fineman J, Teitel D, Karl TR. Impact of right ventricle to pulmonary artery conduit on outcome of the modified Norwood procedure. Ann Thorac Surg. 2004;77:1727–33.
29. Ohye RG, Sleeper LA, Mahony L, Newburger JW, Pearson GD, Lu M, Goldberg CS, Tabbutt S, Frommelt PC, Ghanayem NS, Laussen PC, Rhodes JF, Lewis AB, Mital S, Ravishankar C, Williams IA, Dunbar-Masterson C, Atz AM, Colan S, Minich LL, Pizarro C, Kanter KR, Jaggers J, Jacobs JP, Krawczeski CD, Pike N, McCrindle BW, Virzi L, Gaynor JW. Pediatric Heart Network Investigators. Comparison of shunt types in the Norwood procedure for single-ventricle lesions. N Engl J Med. 2010;362:1980–92.
30. Kolcz J, Skladzien T, Kordon Z, Rudzinski A, Skalski J. Impact of right ventricle-pulmonary artery conduit placement on pulmonary artery development after the Norwood procedure in hypoplastic left heart syndrome. Eur J Cardiothorac Surg. 2012;42:218–23; discussion 223–4. Oxford University Press.
31. Frommelt PC, Sheridan DC, Mussatto KA, Hoffman GM, Ghanayem NS, Frommelt MA, Tweddell JS. Effect of shunt type on echocardiographic indices after initial palliations for hypoplastic left heart syndrome: Blalock-Taussig shunt versus right ventricle-pulmonary artery conduit. J Am Soc Echocardiogr. 2007;20:1364–73.
32. Ghanayem NS, Jaquiss RDB, Cava JR, Frommelt PC, Mussatto KA, Hoffman GM, Tweddell JS. Right ventricle–to–pulmonary artery conduit versus blalock-taussig shunt: a hemodynamic comparison. Ann Thorac Surg. 2006;82:1603–10.
33. Ohye RG, Ludomirsky A, Devaney EJ, Bove EL. Comparison of right ventricle to pulmonary artery conduit and modified Blalock-Taussig shunt hemodynamics after the Norwood operation. Ann Thorac Surg. 2004;78:1090–3.
34. Bartram U, Grünenfelder J, Van Praagh R. Causes of death after the modified Norwood procedure: a study of 122 postmortem cases. Ann Thorac Surg. 1997;64:1795–802.
35. Nathan M, Williamson AK, Mayer JE, Bacha EA, Juraszek AL. Mortality in hypoplastic left heart syndrome: Review of 216 autopsy cases of aortic atresia with attention to coronary artery disease. J Thorac Cardiovasc Surg. 2012;144:1301–6.
36. Sharma V, Deo SV, Huebner M, Dearani JA, Burkhart HM. In search of the ideal pulmonary blood source for the Norwood procedure: a meta-analysis and systematic review. Ann Thorac Surg. 2014;98:142–50.
37. Bautista-Hernandez V, Brown DW, Loyola H, Myers PO, Borisuk M, del Nido PJ, Baird CW. Mechanisms of tricuspid regurgitation in patients with hypoplastic left heart syndrome undergoing tricuspid valvuloplasty. – PubMed – NCBI. J Thorac Cardiovasc Surg. 2014;148:832–40.
38. Ruzmetov M, Welke KF, Geiss DM, Fortuna RS. Outcomes of tricuspid valve repair in children with hypoplastic left heart syndrome. J Card Surg. 2014;29:698–704.
39. Fraser CD, Mee RB. Modified Norwood procedure for hypoplastic left heart syndrome. Ann Thorac Surg. 1995;60:S546–9.
40. Mery CM, Guzmán-Pruneda FA, Carberry KE, Watrin CH, McChesney GR, Chan JG, Adachi I, Heinle JS, McKenzie ED, Fraser CD. Aortic arch advancement for aortic coarctation and hypoplastic aortic arch in neonates and infants. Ann Thorac Surg. 2014;98:625–33.
41. Gibbs JL, Wren C, Watterson KG, Hunter S, Hamilton JR. Stenting of the arterial duct combined with banding of the pulmonary arteries and atrial septectomy or septostomy: a new approach to palliation for the hypoplastic left heart syndrome. Br Heart J. 1993;69:551–5.

42. Akintuerk H, Michel-Behnke I, Valeske K, Mueller M, Thul J, Bauer J, Hagel K-J, Kreuder J, Vogt P, Schranz D. Stenting of the arterial duct and banding of the pulmonary arteries: basis for combined Norwood stage I and II repair in hypoplastic left heart. Circulation. 2002;105:1099–103.
43. Akintürk H, Michel-Behnke I, Valeske K, Mueller M, Thul J, Bauer J, Hagel K-J, Schranz D. Hybrid transcatheter-surgical palliation: basis for univentricular or biventricular repair: the Giessen experience. Pediatr Cardiol. 2007;28:79–87.
44. Michel-Behnke I, Akintuerk H, Marquardt I, Mueller M, Thul J, Bauer J, Hagel KJ, Kreuder J, Vogt P, Schranz D. Stenting of the ductus arteriosus and banding of the pulmonary arteries: basis for various surgical strategies in newborns with multiple left heart obstructive lesions. Heart. 2003;89:645–50.
45. Galantowicz M, Cheatham JP, Phillips A, Cua CL, Hoffman TM, Hill SL, Rodeman R. Hybrid approach for hypoplastic left heart syndrome: intermediate results after the learning curve. Ann Thorac Surg. 2008;85:2063–70; discussion 2070–1.
46. Galantowicz M, Cheatham JP. Lessons learned from the development of a New hybrid strategy for the management of hypoplastic left heart syndrome. Pediatr Cardiol. 2005;26:190–9.
47. Caldarone CA, Benson LN, Holtby H, Van Arsdell GS. Main pulmonary artery to innominate artery shunt during hybrid palliation of hypoplastic left heart syndrome. J Thorac Cardiovasc Surg. 2005;130:e1–2.
48. Caldarone CA, Benson L, Holtby H, Li J, Redington AN, Van Arsdell GS. Initial experience with hybrid palliation for neonates with single-ventricle physiology. Ann Thorac Surg. 2007;84:1294–300.
49. Brescia AA, Jureidini S, Danon S, Armbrecht E, Fiore AC, Huddleston CB. Hybrid versus Norwood procedure for hypoplastic left heart syndrome: contemporary series from a single center. J Thorac Cardiovasc Surg. 2014;147:1777–82.
50. Bacha EA. Individualized approach in the management of patients with hypoplastic left heart syndrome (HLHS). Semin Thorac Cardiovasc Surg Pediatr Card Surg Annu. 2013;16:3–6.
51. Pizarro C, Davies RR, Woodford E, Radtke WA. Improving early outcomes following hybrid procedure for patients with single ventricle and systemic outflow obstruction: defining risk factors. Eur J Cardiothorac Surg. 2015;47:995–1001.
52. Malik S, Bird TM, Jaquiss RDB, Morrow WR, Robbins JM. Comparison of in-hospital and longer-term outcomes of hybrid and Norwood stage 1 palliation of hypoplastic left heart syndrome. J Thorac Cardiovasc Surg. 2015;150:474–80.e2.
53. Schranz D, Bauer A, Reich B, Steinbrenner B, Recla S, Schmidt D, Apitz C, Thul J, Valeske K, Bauer J, Müller M, Jux C, Michel-Behnke I, Akintürk H. Fifteen-year single center experience with the 'Giessen Hybrid' approach for hypoplastic left heart and variants: current strategies and outcomes. Pediatr Cardiol. 2015;36:365–73. Springer US.
54. Ghanayem NS, Hoffman GM, Mussatto KA, Cava JR, Frommelt PC, Rudd NA, Steltzer MM, Bevandic SM, Frisbee SS, Jaquiss RDB, Litwin SB, Tweddell JS. Home surveillance program prevents interstage mortality after the Norwood procedure. J Thorac Cardiovasc Surg. 2003;126:1367–77.
55. Ghanayem NS, Cava JR, Jaquiss RDB, Tweddell JS. Home monitoring of infants after stage one palliation for hypoplastic left heart syndrome. Semin Thorac Cardiovasc Surg Pediatr Card Surg Annu. 2004;7:32–8.
56. Knirsch W, Bertholdt S, Stoffel G, Stiasny B, Weber R, Dave H, Prêtre R, von Rhein M, Kretschmar O. Clinical course and interstage monitoring after the Norwood and hybrid procedures for hypoplastic left heart syndrome. Pediatr Cardiol. 2014;35:851–6. Springer US.
57. Hansen JH, Furck AK, Petko C, Buchholz-Berdau R, Voges I, Scheewe J, Rickers C, Kramer H-H. Use of surveillance criteria reduces interstage mortality after the Norwood operation for hypoplastic left heart syndrome. Eur J Cardiothorac Surg. 2012;41:1013–8. Oxford University Press.

58. Dobrolet NC, Nieves JA, Welch EM, Khan D, Rossi AF, Burke RP, Zahn EM. New approach to interstage care for palliated high-risk patients with congenital heart disease. J Thorac Cardiovasc Surg. 2011;142:855–60.
59. Miller-Tate H, Stewart J, Allen R, Husain N, Rosen K, Cheatham JP, Galantowicz M, Cua CL. Interstage weight gain for patients with hypoplastic left heart syndrome undergoing the hybrid procedure. Congenit Heart Dis. 2013;8:228–33.
60. Emani SM, McElhinney DB, Tworetzky W, Myers PO, Schroeder B, Zurakowski D, Pigula FA, Marx GR, Lock JE, del Nido PJ. Staged left ventricular recruitment after single-ventricle palliation in patients with borderline left heart hypoplasia. J Am Coll Cardiol. 2012;60:1966–74.
61. Bailey LL. Role of cardiac replacement in the neonate. J Heart Transplant. 1985;4:506–9.
62. Murtuza B, Dedieu N, Vazquez A, Fenton M, Burch M, Hsia T-Y, Tsang VT, Kostolny M. Results of orthotopic heart transplantation for failed palliation of hypoplastic left heart. Eur J Cardiothorac Surg. 2013;43:597–603. Oxford University Press.
63. Hosseinpour A-R, González-Calle A, Adsuar-Gómez A, Cuerpo G, Greco R, Borrego-Domínguez JM, Ordoñez A, Wallwork J. Surgical technique for heart transplantation: a strategy for congenital heart disease. Eur J Cardiothorac Surg. 2013;44:598–604. Oxford University Press.
64. Murtuza B, Elliott MJ. Changing attitudes to the management of hypoplastic left heart syndrome: a European perspective. Cardiol Young. 2011;21 Suppl 2:148–58.
65. Mavroudis C, Mavroudis CD, Farrell RM, Jacobs ML, Jacobs JP, Kodish ED. Informed consent, bioethical equipoise, and hypoplastic left heart syndrome. Cardiol Young. 2011;21 Suppl 2:133–40.

The Engineering Perspective

26

Giovanni Biglino, Silvia Schievano, Tain-Yen Hsia, and Andrew M. Taylor

Experimental and computational models can provide insight into complex congenital heart defects [1–5], including single ventricle physiology [6–10], with the advantage of performing parametric studies [11–14]. Numerical simulations of the hybrid procedure for palliation of hypoplastic left heart syndrome (HLHS) are feasible, as demonstrated by four studies cited here, and can provide valuable understanding, such as variations in systemic and cerebral oxygen delivery or changes in ventricular energetics comparing the hybrid approach vs. the traditional Norwood procedure.

One study [15] employed a finite-element analysis approach to compare the hybrid palliation with the traditional stage 1 Norwood operation, using either a modified Blalock–Taussig (mBT) or a right ventricle-to-pulmonary artery shunt, i.e. the Sano modification. The hybrid model included a 7-mm ductal stent and bilateral pulmonary artery (PA) bands (2 mm in diameter). The advantage of the computational approach in this case is that different Norwood models were coupled, with a multiscale approach, to an identical lumped parameter network that summarised the remainder of the circulation – in a sense performing the three different procedures virtually on the same representative patient. These simulations predicted that for the hybrid palliation there was an increased pulmonary-to-systemic flow ratio and lower cardiac output, as well as reduced total systemic and cerebral oxygen delivery. The same group expanded this engineering insight into the hybrid Norwood procedure by simulating pulmonary artery banding variations between 1.5 and 3.5 mm, investigating the effects of retrograde aortic arch hypoplasia and obstruction, and testing for a range of aortic arch diameters (2–5 mm) and coarctation severities (2.5–5 mm). This work [16, 17] concluded that retrograde aortic arch hypoplasia or obstruction could lead to suboptimal cerebral and coronary perfusion, based on simulation results. An

G. Biglino (✉) • S. Schievano • T.-Y. Hsia • A.M. Taylor
Institute of Cardiovascular Science, University College London & Cardiorespiratory Unit, Great Ormond Street Hospital for Children, NHS Foundation Trust, London, UK
e-mail: g.biglino@ucl.ac.uk

G. Butera et al. (eds.), *Fetal and Hybrid Procedures in Congenital Heart Diseases*, DOI 10.1007/978-3-319-40088-4_26

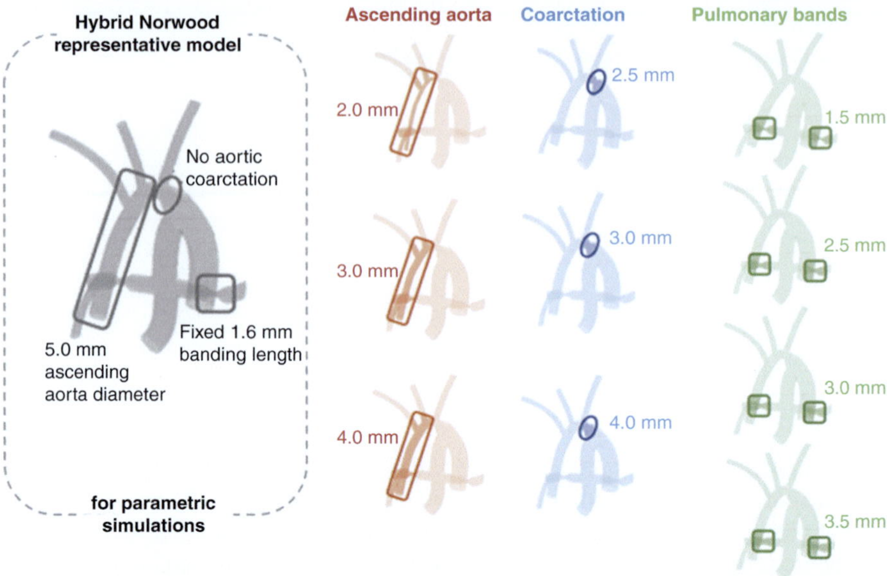

Fig. 26.1 A representation of the use of a parametric approach to study the hybrid Norwood in a representative 3D model. The 3D model (which is coupled to a lumped parameter network summarising the remainder of the circulation) is set with representative values (e.g. no aortic coarctation, 5-mm ascending aorta diameter, pulmonary artery banding of 1.6 mm length), and the incremental changes in ascending aorta diameter, coarctation diameter and pulmonary banding diameter are implemented, generating a range of scenarios (Image modified from Baker et al. [17])

indication was also made that accurate adjustments to pulmonary artery banding might improve interstage physiology in HLHS patients treated with the hybrid approach (Fig. 26.1).

Another study [18] also employed multiscale modelling, coupling 3D hybrid Norwood geometries with a lumped parameter model and testing the concomitant presence of aortic arch stenosis (90 % severity) and a preventive reverse Blalock–Taussig shunt on coronary and carotid flows, by comparing four idealised realistic models, i.e. with/without narrowing on the aortic arch and with/without the additional shunt. Computational fluid dynamics (CFD) highlighted that the shunt counterweighted the effect of the stenosis, but also indicated areas of flow recirculation and stagnation that might be associated with thrombogenic risk.

A fourth study [19] focused on ventricular energetics in the hybrid Norwood scenario, again with a numerical modelling approach (i.e. time-varying elastance model + modified three-element Windkessel model), comparing the hybrid procedure with the Sano modification (right ventricle-to-pulmonary artery shunt). Computational results suggest, in this case, that the hybrid Norwood increases systolic pressure-volume area, leading to impaired mechanical efficiency.

The title of this last interesting study – "Hybrid stage I palliation for hypoplastic left heart syndrome has no advantage on ventricular energetics: a theoretical analysis" – pertinently summarises both a major limitation and an important advantage of numerical models. On the one hand, it can be misleading to draw strong conclusions (in this case, one approach having no advantage over another) based on simulations that, albeit sophisticated and sometimes validated, do not account for a multitude of real-life phenomena (e.g. concomitant medications, baroreceptor adaptations, other comorbidities), which can also be counterproductive in terms of clinical translation of these tools. Clinicians will correctly reject strong affirmations based on grossly simplified models, despite their technical complexity and refinement from an engineering point of view. Whilst on the other hand, these same models offer the possibility of exploring hypothetical scenarios – "a theoretical analysis" – by essentially allowing us to explore what might have happened to a "patient" (in the above cases, geometries with realistic dimensions and realistic boundary conditions for palliated HLHS) if minimal and incremental (parametric) changes were performed, e.g. varying the size of a shunt and/or increasing the degree of a stenosis, whilst keeping the haemodynamic parameters constant. In turn, this can provide insight into mechanisms that are not intuitive, precisely because of all the other elements happening simultaneously. Such additional insight could lead to innovative solutions, which are generated in this idealised/theoretical framework, also offering the possibility of optimising solutions in a mathematical sense [20]. This is in part what one of the above-mentioned studies [18] attempted, by testing the additional presence of the prophylactic reverse BT shunt, providing preliminary evidence towards its beneficial presence and potential risks. Indeed, in other instances ideas that can impact surgical strategies have been generated based on modelling solutions, even in the specific context of HLHS, i.e. the Y-graft baffle for Fontan completion [21–23]. It should not be excluded therefore that modelling could not only provide insight into such complex and small patients, otherwise difficult to acquire in vivo (e.g. streamlines from CFD, wall shear stress values, parametric changes), but could possibly be employed to inform and even refine the procedure itself.

From an engineering perspective, modelling the hybrid Norwood requires us to take the following variables into account: aortic arch stiffness and dimensions, dimensions of the patent ductus arteriosus (PDA), structural properties and dimensions of the stent in the PDA, and size of pulmonary artery bands. The single ventricle can be approximated by a lumped parameter model, and differences between 0D and 3D models have been explored even specifically for the hybrid Norwood [24], or could also be simulated including its morphology, wall thickness and intraventricular flows [10].

At present, computational simulations can offer clinically relevant information, such as:

- *Structural simulations* relevant for stenting the ductus, including information on stresses acting on the vessel wall
- *Flow visualisation* where other techniques such as 4D cardiovascular magnetic resonance (CMR) imaging are still technically challenging, particularly

considering the small dimension and fast heart rate of these patients, who are unlikely to remain still for several minutes

- *Optimisation data*, such that the theoretically best solution could be identified in terms of dimensions (e.g. of PA bands); this has been well exemplified precisely in the context of patients with Norwood physiology by a study that used an optimisation approach to investigate mBT shunt placement and diameter [20]

Computational models, however, are still lacking important information, such as:

- When simulating the Norwood procedure, aortic distensibility should be taken into account, whether the aortic arch is surgically reconstructed (i.e. traditional Norwood) or not (i.e. hybrid Norwood), possibly even including local changes in distensibility, and this is feasible by means of a fluid–structure interaction (FSI) approach, which is more challenging computationally.
- True multiscale phenomena (e.g. thrombus formation) could be included in the simulations, by accounting phenomena at a cellular level and coupling these with the global hemodynamic variables, rendering the models themselves more realistic.
- Accounting for growth in these very young patients, who then progress in their palliation pathway, which might be achieved by means of statistical shape analysis, as used, for example, to look at growth and remodelling in other congenital scenarios [25].

Moreover, experimental (bench top) experiments have been developed for HLHS, including patient-specific anatomical models post-Norwood procedure with mBT shunt [26, 27] and Sano modification [28]. An experimental model of the hybrid Norwood would require the additional presence of the patent ductus arteriosus (PDA) stent and PA bands; therefore, a distensible phantom would be indicated [29]. To our knowledge, an experimental model of the hybrid Norwood has not been presented yet.

In conclusion, engineering modelling can indeed be a powerful tool for investigating complex physiologies, but should always be strictly validated and guided by a multidisciplinary conversation between clinicians (cardiologists, surgeons, imagers) and modellers in a virtuous circle of reciprocal education.

References

1. Xenos M, Karakitsos D, Labropoulos N, Tassiopoulos A, Bilfinger TV, Bluestein D. Comparative study of flow in right-sided and left-sided aortas: numerical simulations in patient-based models. Comput Methods Biomech Biomed Engin. 2015;18(4):414–25.
2. DeCampli WM, Argueta-Morales IR, Divo E, Kassab AJ. Computational fluid dynamics in congenital heart disease. Cardiol Young. 2012;22(6):800–8.
3. Ladisa Jr JF, Taylor CA, Feinstein JA. Aortic coarctation: recent developments in experimental and computational methods to assess treatments for this simple condition. Prog Pediatr Cardiol. 2010;30(1):45–9.

4. Celestin C, Guillot M, Ross-Ascuitto N, Ascuitto R. Computational fluid dynamics characterization of blood flow in central aorta to pulmonary artery connections: importance of shunt angulation as a determinant of shear stress-induced thrombosis. Pediatr Cardiol. 2015;36(3):600–15.
5. Goubergrits L, Riesenkampff E, Yevtushenko P, Schaller J, Kertzscher U, Hennemuth A, Berger F, Schubert S, Kuehne T. MRI-based computational fluid dynamics for diagnosis and treatment prediction: clinical validation study in patients with coarctation of aorta. J Magn Reson Imaging. 2015;41(4):909–16.
6. Slesnick TC, Yoganathan AP. Computational modeling of Fontan physiology: at the crossroads of pediatric cardiology and biomedical engineering. Int J Cardiovasc Imaging. 2014;30(6):1073–84.
7. Bossers SS, Cibis M, Gijsen FJ, Schokking M, Strengers JL, Verhaart RF, Moelker A, Wentzel JJ, Helbing WA. Computational fluid dynamics in Fontan patients to evaluate power loss during simulated exercise. Heart. 2014;100(9):696–701.
8. Haggerty CM, Restrepo M, Tang E, de Zélicourt DA, Sundareswaran KS, Mirabella L, Bethel J, Whitehead KK, Fogel MA, Yoganathan AP. Fontan hemodynamics from 100 patient-specific cardiac magnetic resonance studies: a computational fluid dynamics analysis. J Thorac Cardiovasc Surg. 2014;148(4):1481–9.
9. Corsini C, Baker C, Kung E, Schievano S, Arbia G, Baretta A, Biglino G, Migliavacca F, Dubini G, Pennati G, Marsden A, Vignon-Clementel I, Taylor A, Hsia TY, Dorfman A; Modeling of Congenital Hearts Alliance (MOCHA) Investigators. An integrated approach to patient-specific predictive modeling for single ventricle heart palliation. Comput Methods Biomech Biomed Engin. 2014;17(14):1572–89
10. de Vecchi A, Nordsletten DA, Remme EW, Bellsham-Revell H, Greil G, Simpson JM, Razavi R, Smith NP. Inflow typology and ventricular geometry determine efficiency of filling in the hypoplastic left heart. Ann Thorac Surg. 2012;94(5):1562–9.
11. Pekkan K, Dasi LP, Nourparvar P, Yerneni S, Tobita K, Fogel MA, Keller B, Yoganathan A. In vitro hemodynamic investigation of the embryonic aortic arch at late gestation. J Biomech. 2008;41(8):1697–706.
12. Dubini G, de Leval MR, Pietrabissa R, Montevecchi FM, Fumero R. A numerical fluid mechanical study of repaired congenital heart defects. Application to the total cavopulmonary connection. J Biomech. 1996;29(1):111–21.
13. Bove EL, de Leval MR, Migliavacca F, Guadagni G, Dubini G. Computational fluid dynamics in the evaluation of hemodynamic performance of cavopulmonary connections after the Norwood procedure for hypoplastic left heart syndrome. J Thorac Cardiovasc Surg. 2003;126(4):1040–7.
14. Migliavacca F, Pennati G, Dubini G, Fumero R, Pietrabissa R, Urcelay G, Bove EL, Hsia TY, de Leval MR. Modeling of the Norwood circulation: effects of shunt size, vascular resistances, and heart rate. Am J Physiol Heart Circ Physiol. 2001;280(5):H2076–86.
15. Hsia TY, Cosentino D, Corsini C, Pennati G, Dubini G, Migliavacca F; Modeling of Congenital Hearts Alliance (MOCHA) Investigators. Use of mathematical modeling to compare and predict hemodynamic effects between hybrid and surgical Norwood palliations for hypoplastic left heart syndrome. Circulation. 2011;Sep 13;124 Suppl 11:S204–10.
16. Corsini C, Cosentino D, Pennati G, Dubini G, Hsia TY, Migliavacca F. Multiscale models of the hybrid palliation for hypoplastic left heart syndrome. J Biomech. 2011;44(4):767–70.
17. Baker CE, Corsini C, Cosentino D, Dubini G, Pennati G, Migliavacca F, Hsia TY; Modeling of Congenital Hearts Alliance (MOCHA) Investigators. Effects of pulmonary artery banding and retrograde aortic arch obstruction on the hybrid palliation of hypoplastic left heart syndrome. J Thorac Cardiovasc Surg. 2013;146(6):1341–8.
18. Ceballos A, Argueta-Morales IR, Divo E, Osorio R, Caldarone CA, Kassab AJ, Decampli WM. Computational analysis of hybrid Norwood circulation with distal aortic arch obstruction and reverse Blalock-Taussig shunt. Ann Thorac Surg. 2012;94(5):1540–50.
19. Shimizu S, Kawada T, Une D, Shishido T, Kamiya A, Sano S, Sugimachi M. Hybrid stage I palliation for hypoplastic left heart syndrome has no advantage on ventricular energetics: a theoretical analysis. Heart Vessels. 2014 Nov 29. [Epub ahead of print].

20. Moghadam ME, Migliavacca F, Vignon-Clementel IE, Hsia TY, Marsden AL; Modeling of Congenital Hearts Alliance (MOCHA) Investigators. Optimization of shunt placement for the Norwood surgery using multi-domain modeling. J Biomech Eng. 2012;134(5):051002.
21. Marsden AL, Bernstein AJ, Reddy VM, Shadden SC, Spilker RL, Chan FP, Taylor CA, Feinstein JA. Evaluation of a novel Y-shaped extracardiac Fontan baffle using computational fluid dynamics. J Thorac Cardiovasc Surg. 2009;137(2):394–403.e2
22. Yang W, Vignon-Clementel IE, Troianowski G, Reddy VM, Feinstein JA, Marsden AL. Hepatic blood flow distribution and performance in conventional and novel Y-graft Fontan geometries: a case series computational fluid dynamics study. J Thorac Cardiovasc Surg. 2012;143(5):1086–97.
23. Yang W, Chan FP, Reddy VM, Marsden AL, Feinstein JA. Flow simulations and validation for the first cohort of patients undergoing the Y-graft Fontan procedure. J Thorac Cardiovasc Surg. 2015;149(1):247–55.
24. Young A, Gourlay T, McKee S, Danton MH. Computational modelling of the hybrid procedure in hypoplastic left heart syndrome: a comparison of zero-dimensional and three-dimensional approach. Med Eng Phys. 2014;36(11):1549–53.
25. Mansi T, Voigt I, Leonardi B, Pennec X, Durrleman S, Sermesant M, Delingette H, Taylor AM, Boudjemline Y, Pongiglione G, Ayache N. A statistical model for quantification and prediction of cardiac remodelling: application to tetralogy of Fallot. IEEE Trans Med Imaging. 2011;30(9):1605–16.
26. Biglino G, Corsini C, Schievano S, Dubini G, Giardini A, Hsia TY, Pennati G, Taylor AM; Mocha Collaborative Group. Computational models of aortic coarctation in hypoplastic left heart syndrome: considerations on validation of a detailed 3D model. Int J Artif Organs. 2014;37(5):371–81.
27. Biglino G, Giardini A, Baker C, Figliola RS, Hsia TY, Taylor AM, Schievano S; MOCHA Collaborative Group. In vitro study of the Norwood palliation: a patient-specific mock circulatory system. ASAIO J. 2012;58(1):25–31.
28. Biglino G, Giardini A, Baker C, Figliola RS, Hsia TY, Taylor AM, Schievano S; MOCHA Collaborative Group. Implementing the Sano modification in an experimental model of first-stage palliation of hypoplastic left heart syndrome. ASAIO J. 2013;59(1):86–9.
29. Biglino G, Verschueren P, Zegels R, Taylor AM, Schievano S. Rapid prototyping compliant arterial phantoms for in-vitro studies and device testing. J Cardiovasc Magn Reson. 2013;15:2.

General Principles of the Hybrid Approach in Hypoplastic Left Heart Syndrome

27

Darren P. Berman and John P. Cheatham

27.1 Introduction

Congenital heart disease remains the most common form of birth defect and occurs in ~1 % of all live births. Hypoplastic left heart syndrome (HLHS) occurs in 2–3/10,000 live births in the USA [1]. It was uniformly fatal through the 1970s until the Norwood surgical palliation was proposed in 1980 [2]. When done properly, this operation, and its Sano modification, achieves a tenuous but stable circulation as a first step in palliation for HLHS. Less traumatic neonatal palliation has since been pursued as an alternative to the Norwood operation. Gibbs et al. first described neonatal stenting of the arterial duct combined with pulmonary artery banding and atrial septectomy or septostomy as an alternative palliation for HLHS in 1993 [3]. Since that time hundreds of articles have been published describing variations on technique and outcomes from this so-called hybrid approach to HLHS.

Irrespective of preference or approach, successful neonatal palliation for HLHS necessitates three objectives: (1) controlling or limiting pulmonary blood flow, (2) providing reliable and adequate systemic perfusion, and (3) assuring unrestricted flow of pulmonary venous blood return from the left atrium into the right atrium. The driving principal of the hybrid Stage 1 approach to HLHS is to achieve these objectives in a less invasive way with hopefully less morbidity and mortality (Fig. 27.1).

D.P. Berman (✉)
The Heart Center, Nationwide Children's Hospital, Columbus, OH, USA
e-mail: Darren.Berman@nationwidechildrens.org

J.P. Cheatham
Pediatrics & Internal Medicine, The Ohio State University, Columbus, OH, USA

G. Butera et al. (eds.), *Fetal and Hybrid Procedures in Congenital Heart Diseases*, DOI 10.1007/978-3-319-40088-4_27

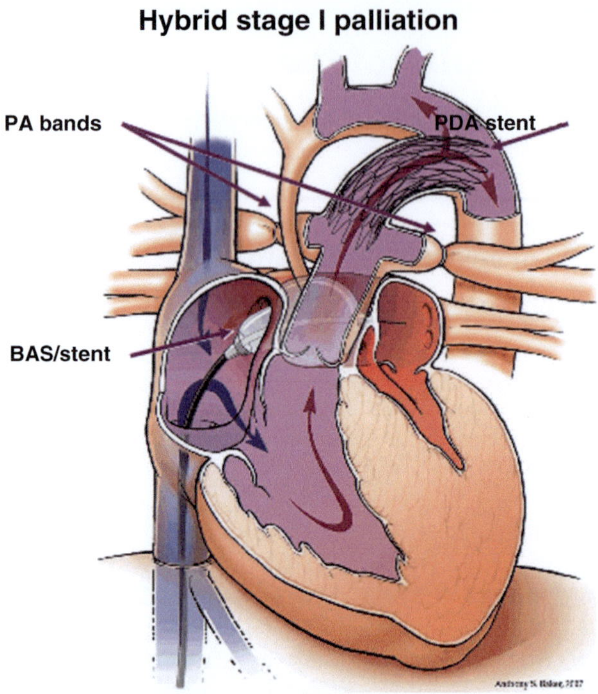

Fig. 27.1 Schematic of stage 1 hybrid palliation for HLHS. Note the pulmonary artery bands on both the left and right pulmonary arteries placed proximal to take off the upper lobe branches, the stent within the arterial duct, and the septostomy catheter representing decompression of the left atrium

27.2 Controlling or Limiting Pulmonary Blood Flow

As the newborn with HLHS transitions away from fetal circulation, pulmonary vascular resistance drops dramatically and pulmonary blood flow increases. The hybrid approach to HLHS relies on branch pulmonary artery banding to decrease and control the amount of pulmonary blood flow. While there were initial transcatheter attempts to accomplish this with internal flow restrictors, externally placed bands is the general approach in the current era. This requires a median sternotomy and dissecting free each of the branch pulmonary arteries. Surgically fashioned circumferential bands, typically made from Gore-Tex, are sewn around each of the pulmonary arteries. The band size typically varies between 3.0 and 3.5 mm depending on the patient size and goal length of palliation (Fig. 27.2). The larger the band, the less the restriction to pulmonary blood flow, at times leading to relative pulmonary overcirculation and associated clinical symptoms of tachypnea, poor feeding, and poor weight gain. The tighter the band, the lower

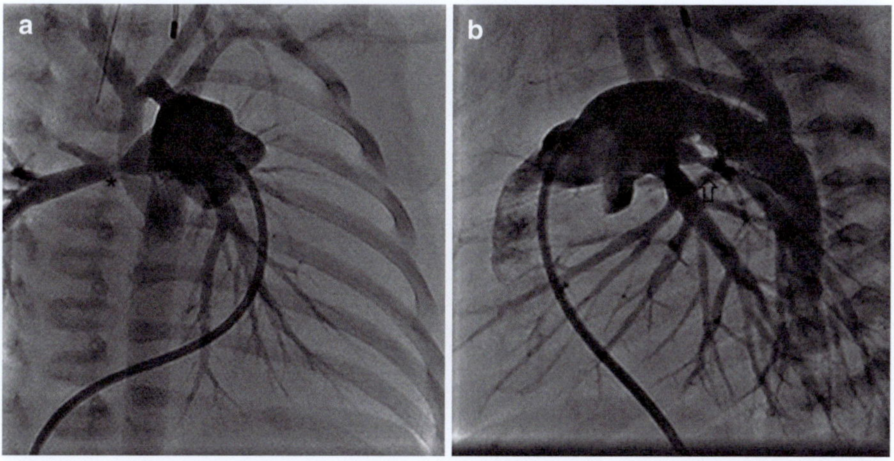

Fig. 27.2 A neonate born with HLHS undergoing catheterization 8 days after PA banding and ductal stenting for planned balloon atrial septostomy. An antegrade angiogram performed in the main pulmonary artery profiles, the RPA band (*) with RAO angulation of the frontal flat panel (**a**), and the LPA band (*arrow*) with LAO angulation on the lateral front panel (**b**)

the systemic saturation as pulmonary blood flow is limited. Finding this balance is part of the art of the hybrid procedure for neonates with HLHS.

27.3 Adequate Systemic Perfusion

Neonates born with HLHS are dependent on right to left shunting via the arterial duct for maintaining adequate systemic perfusion. When the diagnosis goes unrecognized, ductal closure ensues and profound cardiogenic shock develops as all end organs are hypoperfused. Without the initiation of prostaglandin E1 (PGE1) to maintain ductal patency, death is almost universal. Prenatal or early postnatal diagnosis of HLHS is now relatively common. As such, PGE1 is started immediately after birth or shortly thereafter as a temporizing way to maintain adequate systemic perfusion. Because long-term PGE1 infusion is associated with significant side effects, a more permanent and reliable solution is needed to maintain ductal patency. As Gibbs first described in 1993 [3], ductal stenting replaces the need for PGE1. The shunt through the arterial duct is obligatorily from right to left in systole with, at times, significant left to right "steal" into the pulmonary vasculature as the pulmonary vascular resistance continues to decrease. In the most severe forms of HLHS involving aortic atresia, both coronary artery and cerebral perfusion is completely dependent on the retrograde filling of the aortic arch (Fig. 27.3).

The timing of ductal stenting varies by institution. While some may approach this percutaneously as a separate procedure from the banding of the pulmonary

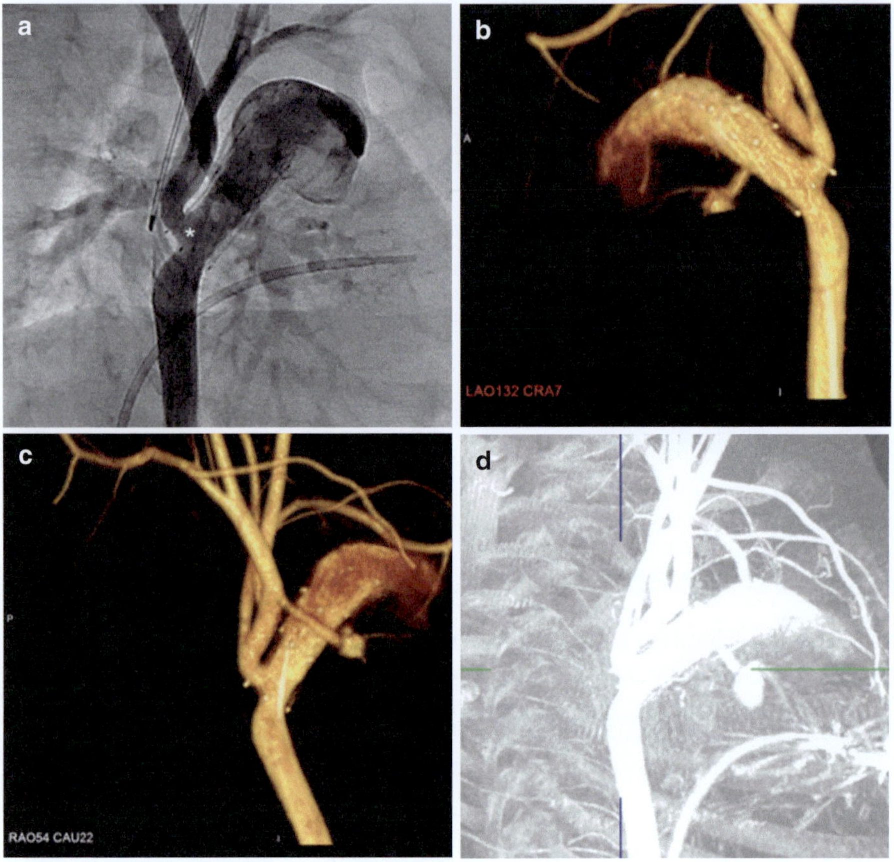

Fig. 27.3 While the stented arterial duct can typically be seen adequately with an antegrade angiogram in the main pulmonary artery, if concerns arise for retrograde filling of the hypoplastic aortic arch, a retrograde angiogram (**a**) or 3D rotational angiogram (**b**, **c**) with CT-like tomographic images (**d**), can be utilized to help profile this area. Note the angle and take off the retrograde arch (*)

arteries, it can easily be done in the same setting of the pulmonary artery bands via the median sternotomy and in concert with one's surgical colleagues. In either scenario, it is essential that the entire length of the arterial duct be covered appropriately by the stent(s). Uncovered ductal tissue on either end of the duct will constrict once off PGE1, increasing afterload on an already stressed right ventricle as well as compromising systemic perfusion both to the retrograde arch (brain and coronary arteries) and to the descending aorta. The deleterious effects of this may not be recoverable depending on the timing of recognition and severity of the insult.

Needless to say, a successful first stage hybrid palliation for HLHS depends on appropriate stenting of the arterial duct and close surveillance of retrograde arch perfusion during the interstage period. This is never truer when dealing with the severest forms of HLHS, namely, the aortic atresia type.

27.4 Assuring Unrestricted Flow of Pulmonary Venous Return into the Right Atrium

Neonates born with HLHS typically have a relatively unrestricted atrial communication, allowing oxygenated pulmonary venous return to reach the right atrium and sufficiently mix with systemic venous return. Rarely, the atrial septum is highly restrictive at birth and even more rarely completely intact. These scenarios require urgent and at times emergent intervention and thankfully deviate from the norm.

When dealing with a stable newborn on PGE1, the systemic saturation and mean Doppler gradient across the atrial septum will inform the degree of true restriction at the atrial level. While the echo mean Doppler gradient may increase over the first several days of life, this is often in association with and due to the decreasing pulmonary vascular resistance and increasing amount of pulmonary blood flow and subsequent return to the left atrium. An increasing echo Doppler gradient in conjunction with decreasing systemic saturations should alert the clinician to increasing the restriction to flow at the atrial septal level.

Part of a successful hybrid stage 1 palliation is creation of a reliable unrestrictive communication that will remain so until stage 2 reconstruction. While this may have required surgical atrial septectomy, in some of the original descriptions of this approach, with current technologies, a durable and reliable atrial septal communication can be created with a balloon atrial septostomy. For a number of reasons, including size of the left atrium, location of the defect within the atrial septum, and initial size of the atrial septal defect, this step of hybrid stage 1 palliation can be technically challenging. Specific techniques and timing of this portion of stage 1 palliation are discussed separately and reflect the experience and knowledge gained over the many years of taking on this approach to HLHS palliation.

Conclusion

All three objectives for successful palliation of the vulnerable newborn with HLHS can be accomplished less invasively via the hybrid stage 1 procedure. No single approach, either hybrid or Norwood, eliminates the fragile interstage period where the slightest change to a tenuously balanced circulation can lead to potentially irreversible myocardial and other end organ damage. Interstage monitoring is essential for this patient population to help minimize these risks. Hybrid stage 1 palliation offers an acceptable method for managing the fragile newborn with HLHS. With appropriate outpatient monitoring, it delays the inevitable complex semilunar amalgamation and aortic reconstruction to the outside of the neonatal period where it is combined with pulmonary artery band removal, ductal stent removal, atrial septectomy, and cavopulmonary anastomosis into the so-called comprehensive stage 2.

References

1. Reller MD, Strickland MJ, Riehle-Colarusso T, Mahle WT, Correa A. Prevalence of congenital heart defects in metropolitan Atlanta, 1998–2005. J Pediatr. 2008;153(6):807–13.
2. Norwood WI, Kirklin JK, Sanders SP. Hypoplastic left heart syndrome: experience with palliative surgery. Am J Cardiol. 1980;45(1):87–91.
3. Gibbs JL, Wren C, Watterson KG, Hunter S, Hamilton JR. Stenting of the arterial duct combined with banding of the pulmonary arteries and atrial septectomy or septostomy: a new approach to palliation for the hypoplastic left heart syndrome. Br Heart J. 1993;69(6):551–5.

Hypoplastic Left Heart Syndrome: The Giessen Approach – History, Technique, and Results

28

Dietmar Schranz and Hakan Akintuerk

28.1 Introduction

Patients with small left heart belong to a spectrum of a wide variety of possible combinations of hypoplastic heart structures. The treatment of newborns with hypoplastic left heart syndrome (HLHS) follows a well-established classical three-step algorithm for most institutions worldwide [1–4]. In Giessen, the hybrid approach was developed as a primary palliation for newborns with HLHS and later on for patients with hypoplastic left heart complex (HLHC). The hybrid procedure has moved from a rescue approach to an alternative modality of a Norwood palliation [4–7]. The "Giessen hybrid" stage I consists of surgical bilateral pulmonary artery banding (bPAB) combined with percutaneous stenting of the arterial duct and atrial septum manipulation, if necessary. The lessons learned by the hybrid strategy for the treatment of HLHS, HLHC, and variants have added a novel impulse for treating selected patients with cardiovascular failure beyond the neonatal period [8–10]. In our center meanwhile all types of HLHS and variants are treated with the modified Giessen hybrid strategy [4, 11]. Since June 1998 almost 200 patients received the Giessen hybrid stage I procedure as an initial approach. The physiological objectives of the hybrid approach are similar as for the classical Norwood procedure by alternative techniques in controlling pulmonary blood flow, whereas unobstructed systemic perfusion is maintained via an open arterial duct. This strategy involves off-pump bilateral pulmonary artery banding (bPAB) and interventional stenting or continuous prostaglandin therapy of the ductus arteriosus mostly, but not exclusively performed in the neonatal period (hybrid stage I). Aortic arch reconstruction using cardiopulmonary bypass combined with a superior cavo-pulmonary connection summarized as comprehensive stage II or as indicated a biventricular correction

D. Schranz, MD (✉) • H. Akintuerk, MD
Pediatric Heart Center, Justus-Liebig University Clinic,
Feulgenstr. 12, Giessen 30385, Germany
e-mail: dietmar.schranz@paediat.med.uni-giessen.de

G. Butera et al. (eds.), *Fetal and Hybrid Procedures in Congenital Heart Diseases*, DOI 10.1007/978-3-319-40088-4_28

is deferred until the age of 4–8 months [6, 10]. In our institution hybrid therapy has initially been proposed to overcome obvious drawbacks of the classical Norwood operation and aims to improve survival and outcome for these patients in a less invasive way [4, 7]. The hybrid approach could be established as a highly effective treatment in particular for newborns with cardiovascular collapse and even for premature babies or neonates to small for gestational age [4].

In recent years hybrid treatment has moved to an alternative modality in a growing number of institutions globally but usually applied to high-risk patients in comparison with the classical Norwood palliation so far [12–15]. Therefore, it has to be emphasized that there are substantial differences in the patient selection, the operative and medical treatment strategies, and the detailed further management of the patients who undergo hybrid palliation with an impact on early and late outcomes. The presented data of hybrid stage I therapy performed for all types of HLHS, HLHC, and variants was applied in a standard manner with very few variations based on our learning curve and due to novel developments of material for duct stenting and IAS manipulation [4, 7, 10, 11]. Within the last decade, the surgical technique of bilateral pulmonary banding was changed, as described at first by Galantowicz et al. [3]. In addition, manipulations of the atrial septum were perfromed if necessary.

28.2 Giessen Hybrid Features

Since in Giessen in June 1998, the first HLHS neonate was treated by bPAB as a rescue approach; further 192 patients received a hybrid stage I approach as an initial palliation until October 2015. The first patient, Brandon, meanwhile 17 years old, was borne with HLHS and unrestricted atrial septum defect. After a couple of postnatal days, he was admitted to our institution in a cardiogenic shock with lactate acidosis due to pulmonary runoff and systemic low cardiac output. By utilizing the hybrid approach with first bPAB, he entirely recovered and received consecutively in the same year the first comprehensive stage II operation worldwide followed by Fontan completion two years later [10].

Considering the retrospective analysis of our experience with hybrid stage I over the last 15 [4, 7] nowadays 17 years [11], three groups of patients could be differentiated, those with the postnatal option of a univentricular palliation (HLHS-group I) or biventricular repair (HLHC-group II) and a small group of patients, who received hybrid stage I procedure for primarily listing to cardiac transplantation or for compassionate therapy in agreement with the parents decision (group III). Additionally, retrospective data collection included postnatal variables and admission, operative and postoperative variables, as well as follow-up information obtained during the 17-year observational period.

Based on the institutional experience, an admission of each patient is classified concerning anatomic features and risk factors. HLHS is morphologically subdivided in mitral and/or aortic atresia or stenosis, respectively. Neonates with HLHS, but even HLHC, remain stable as long as a parallel circulation is balanced or still in part assured. It has to be considered that about 6 % of HLHS patients have a complete intact atrial septum at birth and up to 22 % a severely restrictive atrial septum, which is associated with an increased rate of mortality [16, 17]. Additionally, the HLHS patients have to be classified in order to adjust the complexity according to specific patient and procedural characteristics prior to initial hybrid stage I palliation. Risk factors are examined for their potential influence on procedure-related mortality which includes age, prematurity, birth weight, weight at surgery, multiple pregnancies, prenatal diagnosis, lowest pre-operative pH, organ dysfunction, and, in addition to the exact cardiac diagnosis of HLHS or variant with or without the presence of aortic atresia, genetic or chromosomal abnormality; we recommend to calculate the comprehensive Aristotle score in term if the neonate would receive a Norwood palliation [18]. In HLHC patients the exact cardiac diagnosis has to be determined in assessment of an early corrective or Norwood-like palliation before hybrid procedure is considered. In case of a decision for hybrid approach, the time and mode of the follow-up corrective surgery is hypothesized not at least for fair parental counseling, which has to include the current operative mortality for the staged procedure of hybrid strategy [4, 7, 11].

28.3 Diagnostic Tools

28.3.1 Fetal Echocardiography

The outlook for newborns with hypoplastic left heart (HLH) has substantially improved over the last decade. However, differences in outcome among various anatomical subgroups are still described. In Giessen a strong fetal diagnostic and prenatal therapeutic program improved the outcome of all congenital heart defects most prominent in the group of HLHS and HLHC. Even highly dedicated diagnosis is carried out. In this context, prenatal assessment of ventriculocoronary connections and ventricular endocardial fibroelastosis (EFE) in hypoplastic left heart did not limit the results of surgical-interventional palliation and short-term outcome. We could find that EFE predominantly occurred in the subgroup of MS/AA and MA/AA and in those cases with aortic valve stenosis and evolving HLH. The overall hospital survival on an intention-to-treat basis was 91.2 % (52/57 newborns). Hospital survival was 91 % for the subgroup of cases with MS/AA and for all other anatomical subgroups [19].

In summary, prenatal diagnostics allows to offer hybrid approach with low procedural mortality and with high success rate. For neonates born with HLHS and HLHC at the University of Giessen, cardiogenic shock becomes a rarity over the last decade; only two patients with complete obstructive interatrial septum and lymphangiectasia could postnatally not be treated with long-term success despite cardiac transplantation in one of them. Considering our animal studies the use of self-expnadable stents (Sinus-SuperFlex-DS, Optimed, Germany) are currently our stents of choice to unload left atrial pressure, even by transhepatic access [20].

28.3.2 Neonatal Echocardiography: Magnetic Resonance Imaging

The anatomic diagnosis of HLHS and HLHC and the cardiovascular function are based on the immediately performed two-dimensional echocardiography. Magnetic resonance imaging (MRI) and heart catheterization are added for analysis of special anatomical and functional details. The presence of aortic valve atresia or annulus hypoplasia or absence of the left ventricle and a duct-dependent systemic circulation with or without retrograde flow in the aortic arch should be evaluated as well as the atrioventricular valve(s) and right (left) ventricular function. Obstruction of one or all pulmonary venous connections and even a stenosis within an anomaly of return have to be treated, if a significant mean gradient greater than 5–8 mmHg is present on Doppler interrogation at the level of the interatrial septal communication or anomalous pulmonary venous connection.

Cardiac magnetic resonance imaging (*CMRI*) becomes an important tool in neonatal period to analyze exactly the aortic arch and the junction of duct to descending aorta as well as to exclude myocardial perfusion deficits. The CMRI is in particular of high interest prior to comprehensive stage II and for diagnostic reasons before Fontan completion. In concert of a lot of answered questions, the persistence of aortopulmonary collateral flow, its relation to pulmonary artery size, as well as influence on ventricular dimensions can optimally visualized by CMRI [21].

28.3.3 Surgical-Interventional Aspects of the Hybrid Stage I

In terms of the physiopathology, hybrid approach consisting of bilateral pulmonary banding (bPAB), percutaneous duct stenting, or in some long-term prostaglandin infusion and atrio-septostomy including stent placement is performed for lung protection, preserving adequate systemic perfusion and unloading of the left atrium, respectively.

Bilateral pulmonary arterial banding is performed by median sternotomy followed by subtotal thymectomy and limited cranial pericardiotomy of 3–4 cm in length. Two pieces of 3.5 mm PTFE tube are cut in about 1.5–2 mm width for bPAB in patients with body weight above 2.5 kg and 3 mm PTFE bands in lower weight. The bands are fixed by using a 6/0 Prolene suture. Pericardial space is washed out with normothermic saline before closure of the pericardial space in that the pericardial ends are reapproximated completely with a running 6/0 PDS suture to limit adhesions at comprehensive stage II operation. Following these algorithms intrapericardial adhesions do not complicate or prolong comprehensive stage II operation.

Stenting of the ductus arteriosus is carried out in all patients by percutaneous transcatheter approach utilizing 4 F sheath for femoral vein or artery access, since novel designed self-expandable Sinus-SuperFlex-DS stents with the CE mark for duct stenting in newborns' (OptiMed, Karlsruhe, Germany) duct are stented mostly from the arterial access [4, 11]. After the initial learning curve, heart catheterization for duct stenting and atrial septum manipulation is routinely performed in sedated patients, when surgical bilateral pulmonary artery banding (bPAB) is already finished and the patient extubated. In high-urgency patients, parts of stage I should be performed considering the reason for the patient's deterioration: surgical bPAB in case of a pulmonary runoff, duct stenting if the duct remained obstructed despite prostaglandin infusion, or interventions to solve life-threatening atrial septal or pulmonary vein obstructions [22, 23]. Stent size and positioning within the duct is based on a right lateral oblique 30° and 90° lateral angiogram, which can be done by hand injection of contrast medium through a 4 F Judkins or 4 F multipurpose catheters positioned in the pulmonary trunk and/or descending aorta, respectively. Initially, the different types of balloon-expandable stents were used for stenting the duct. Since 2006 nearly exclusively self-expandable sinus-Repo delivered through 5 F femoral sheath was used. Currently Sinus-SuperFlex-DS stents (OptiMed, Karlsruhe, Germany) are certificated with CE mark; they are deliverable through 4 F sheath and available in widths of 7, 8, 9, and 10 mm and lengths of 12, 15, 18, 20, and 24 mm, respectively. The choice of stents is largely influenced by the ductal anatomy and the morphology of the ductal-aortic junction. Additional narrowed aortic isthmus or aortic coarctation is treated, if necessary by 9×5 or 6 mm Sinus-Repo self-expandable stents. Therefore, flow acceleration or narrowing of the color Doppler jet is not per se considered a contraindication for stenting among patients with aortic atresia (for further details [24, 25, 26]).

The adequacy of the atrial septal communication is determined on echocardiographic and by invasive hemodynamic data. If the atrial septal communication is found to be restrictive or even absent, a balloon atrial septostomy or deployment of an atrial septal stent currently even exclusively with a Sinus-SuperFlex-DS (15×8 mm) is performed; in some, stenting is performed after reopening the atrial septum by Brockenbrough or alternatively by high-frequency technique. Even, an obstructed total anomalous venous return can be connected by catheter technique [23]. Considering the persistence of a parallel circulation after hybrid stage I, routinely the patients are discharged home on chronic treatment with 1×0.1–(0.2) mg/kg bisoprolol and lisinopril, respectively; medication of digoxin and furosemide is routinely avoided. The main two indications to combine both drugs are to reduce oxygen consumption by avoiding unnecessary high heart rate and consecutively breath rate and to reduce systemic vascular resistance without endangering perfusion pressures; blocking of the neurohumoral activation reduces diastolic left-right shunt across the stented duct (Fig. 28.1).

Outpatient follow-up prior to stage II is routinely performed at 1–2-week intervals or earlier depending on the clinical condition; it includes historical information of the parents in particular how the baby is breathing during sleep, weight gain development, systolic and diastolic mean blood pressure measurements at the right arm and of the leg, which is not used by catheterization before, and pulse oximetry at arm and one leg (HLHC); after these mandatory

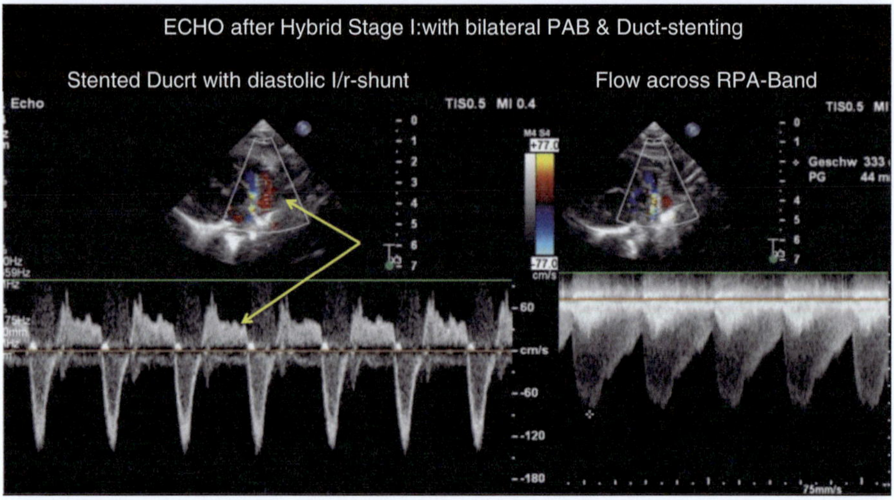

Fig. 28.1 Depicts the 2D color echocardiography of the diastolic reflow through a just implanted duct stent; additional Doppler flows show the systolic and diastolic flow pattern through the stented duct as well as across the banded right pulmonary artery

information, echocardiographic data are obtained. Patients with a hybrid approach are not referred for elective complete invasive hemodynamic and angiographic evaluation, but if a hemodynamic issue is suspected. CMRI is used, additionally to echocardiography assessment, if any unanswered diagnostic question remains open; it has to be noticed that for CMRI and elective heart catheterizations, only sedated and spontaneous breathing patients are examined, while general anesthesia is routinely avoided (Fig. 28.2).

Since 2002, as hybrid stage II was first time described by Akintuerk et al. [10], several modifications were preformed and adapted mostly based on the patient's anatomical condition. In case of an innominate subclavian artery, the artery wall is used for aortic arch reconstruction in some patients [4, 6, 11]. Additionally, some patients underwent comprehensive stage II not only without circulatory but even without cardiac arrest [4]. The stage II surgical reconstruction consisted of amalgamation of the proximal ascending aorta with the main pulmonary artery, removal or resection of the ductus/stent complex, aortic arch reconstruction, atrial septectomy, removal of the branch pulmonary artery bands with routine angioplasty or left pulmonary artery stenting in one, and superior cavo-pulmonary connection; left bidirectional Glenn is performed if a left SVC without a bridging vein is present. Considering completion of stage III in terms of Fontan circulation, a total cavo-pulmonary connection is performed without circulatory or cardiac arrest by utilizing an extracardiac conduit in most but not all with surgical fenestration. Transcatheter fenestration is performed, if necessary [26, 27]. The variants of biventricular repair are described in part previously, as well as the surgical technique of heart transplantation (HTX) with the special aspects of the morphology in patients with HLHS [6, 7, 28].

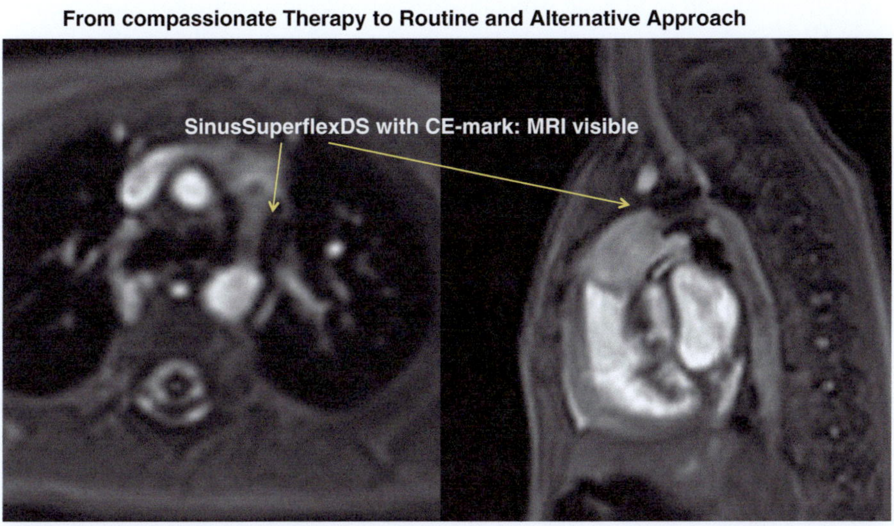

Fig. 28.2 Shows magnetic resonance imaging of the visible self-expandable Sinus-SuperFlex-DS positioned in the arterial duct in sagittal and coronary plane. Not at least based on the technical improvements, the hybrid developed from a rescue to a first-line approach in neonates with HLHS

28.3.4 Critical Patients

At least four different kinds of features are described in HLHS, HLHC, and variants:

I. HLHS with extreme hypoplastic ascending aorta without V connection to the aortic arch
II. HLHS with restrictive and/or complete obstructed atrial septum or obstructed total anomalous pulmonary venous return (TAPVR)
III. HLHS with myocardial dysfunction with or without presence of coronary sinusoids, fistulae, or dysplastic tricuspid valve
IV. HLHC with similar critical anatomical or functional issues (I–III), but in particular with residual diastolic dysfunction of the sub-aortic left or even right (ccTGA) ventricle

28.3.5 Results

Our 15-year follow-up data and further updated results are published and in press, respectively [4, 7, 11]. Between June 1998 and October 2015 meanwhile, 193 patients with the diagnosis of HLHS, HLHC, and variants received a surgical-interventional hybrid stage I in the Pediatric Heart Center Giessen. Among the group of 193 patients, a cohort of 41 patients who have been defined to have borderline/hypoplastic left ventricular structures and seven patients with the initial diagnosis of HLHS were later amenable to receive a biventricular circulation after hybrid stage I procedure [4]. Comfort care was provided in eight patients on the basis of a family decision to abandon any therapeutic measure. 137 patients were palliated with the Giessen hybrid stage I procedure for a univentricular palliation or a primary heart transplantation ($n=8$). No patient is excluded due to complicated preoperative status such as cardiopulmonary shock or syndromatic features without an explicit family decision. Median age of patients at hybrid stage I was 6 days (0–237). Median weight at hybrid stage I procedure was 3.2 kg (1.2–7).

Operative mortality has been defined 30-day mortality postoperatively. Interstage mortality is defined for patients who died between 30 days postoperatively and the following stage of palliation. Re-interventions are defined as any surgical or interventional procedure that was required due to a cardiac or hemodynamic problem.

Figure 28.3 shows a flow chart of the number of patients at different stages, operative and interstage deaths during hybrid palliation.

Median follow-up time after hybrid stage I palliation ($n=129$) is 4.8 years (0–17.5). A comprehensive stage II operation has still to be performed in four patients, and Fontan completion is planned in 26 patients. The number of patients who underwent HTX was two and three patients after hybrid stage I and after comprehensive stage II, respectively. These patients are alive. Another two patients were listed for HTX late following Fontan operation and died on the waiting list. Two patients received HTX after Fontan completion, but both died in the follow-up.

So far, the overall mortality of all patients receiving Giessen hybrid stage I, including the eight patients with comfort therapy, is 19.6 %. The overall unadjusted cumulative operative and interstage mortality of all patients with univentricular strategy is 19.3 % (25 of 129 patients) during a 17-year follow-up. Operative mortalities were 2.2 %, 4.8 %, and 0 % at hybrid stage I, for comprehensive stage II and Fontan completion, respectively. Estimated survival of all patients who underwent hybrid stage I procedure is 79.1 % at 10-year follow-up. Similarly, patients who were directed to univentricular palliation or HTX after Giessen hybrid stage I ($n=129$) had a survival estimate of 78 % at 10-year follow-up. Birth weight (<2.5 kg) had no significant impact on survival [4, 11]. Additionally, five patients with HLHS and concomitant total anomalous pulmonary venous connection are most recently alive. Three patients received Fontan operation, one patient received biventricular correction and one patient is still awaiting Fontan operation. The Achilles heel of the hybrid approach is the fate of the left pulmonary artery; we analyzed the effect with and without stenting of the growth and size of the pulmonary arteries [11]. The freedom from pulmonary artery intervention at 1-year follow-up is 55 % and decreases at 10- and 15-year follow-up to 35 %. When the rate of interventions is separately analyzed between the years of initial experience 1998–2007 in comparison with recent practice between 2008 and 2015, no significant difference in the total number and the probability of freedom from intervention was detected. Before the year 2004 we had used a high number of aortic and pulmonary homografts for aortic reconstruction and were faced with the problem of extensive

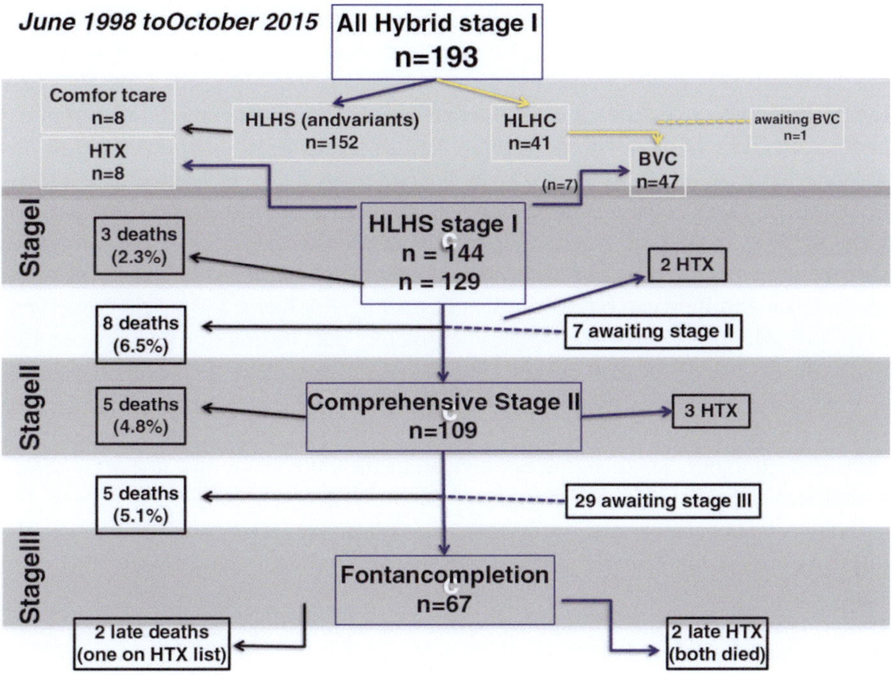

Fig. 28.3 Flow chart of patients at different stages, operative and interstage deaths during hybrid palliation

calcifications during the Fontan completion. The use of the curved porcine xenograft for the aortic arch reconstruction resulted in a non-calcified aortic arch, which eased the surgical preparation at the Fontan completion. A re-intervention on the aortic arch after the comprehensive stage II operation was needed in 17 %. These technical details are important issues with the need for continuous improvement by worldwide knowledge exchange. However at the end, the individualized quality of life, in particular the neurological outcome, and the long-term follow-up will tell us the full truth in the future.

28.4 Summary

Prenatal diagnosis of prenatally HLHS and HLHC improves the postnatal management. Neonates are not further admitted in cardiogenic shock because of severe obstruction of the arterial duct, pulmonary runoff in unrestricted interatrial communication, or by severe atrial septum restriction. Surgical options are based on a three-staged procedure or heart transplantation (HTX). Independent of the improvements of surgical, interventional, and intensive care for newborns with HLHS, the parents have to decide for classical Norwood stage I, surgical-interventional treatment (hybrid stage I) and HTX, or compassionate therapy after an intense repetitive communication. Hybrid stage I is a lifesaving procedure in particular to high-risk HLHS patients. Presupposed, the pediatric heart team is familiar with a hybrid strategy and with any surgical and interventional step of the approach. Only then, the hybrid approach gives the chance to avoid neonatal high-risk operations, utilizing cardiopulmonary bypass with or without cardiac arrest. Hybrid approach per se has not to be associated with mortality. From the current available techniques and materials at least in Europe, there is almost no reason for death from the procedural point of view, as it was in the past, when the hybrid procedure started [5, 29]. Considering the parts of the whole hybrid approach, we are convinced that most causes of postnatal cardiovascular failure can be easliy solved by a single or orchestral surgical-interventional procedure. In case of prostaglandin refractory duct obstruction with consecutive metabolic acidosis, percutaneous duct stenting is the treatment of choice; in systemic low cardiac output due to pulmonary runoff, surgical bPAB is the most effective measure; for a restrictive or intact atrial septum, pulmonary venous decompression by catheter techniques has to be recommended at the immediate and first step before completing hybrid stage I. We emphasize that the outcome of newborns with HLHS is strictly dependent on straightforward decision-making and based on the goal to offer an effective but "gentile medicine" in terms of minimal invasiveness [30].

Perspective Hybrid stage I will be performed in a spontaneous breathing, well-sleeping newborn by percutaneous transcatheter technique. The surgeon will focus on a comprehensive stage II while preparing for stage III, so that even the transcatheter Fontan completion can be performed again in an only sedated patient. Bacha and Hijazi [31] mentioned years ago that becoming a "learning leader" is a condition sine qua non to achieve satisfactory results. In Columbus and Giessen, the surgeons and pediatric cardiologists made the decisions to change their classical programs for favoring hybrid stage I approach in most with HLHS or univentricular variants. In Giessen the hybrid stage I approach is additionally used for newborns with HLHC to postpone a high-risk operation from the neonatal period to late infancy with augmenting the options and to avoid an initial decision for a univentricular strategy.

References

1. Ohye RG, Sleeper LA, Mahony L, Newburger JW, Pearson GD, Lu M, et al. Comparison of shunt types in the Norwood procedure for single-ventricle lesions. N Engl J Med. 2010;362:1980–92.
2. Iannettoni MD, Bove EL, Mosca RS, Lupinetti FM, Dorostkar PC, Ludomirsky A, et al. Improving results with first-stage palliation for hypoplastic left heart syndrome. J Thorac Cardiovasc Surg. 1994;107:934–40.
3. Galantowicz M, Cheatham JP, Phillips A, Cua CL, Hoffman TM, Hill SL, et al. Hybrid approach for hypoplastic left heart syndrome: intermediate results after the learning curve. Ann Thorac Surg. 2008;85:2063–70.

4. Schranz D, Bauer A, Reich B, Steinbrenner B, Recla S, Schmidt D, et al. Fifteen-year single center experience with the "Giessen Hybrid" approach for hypoplastic left heart and variants: current strategies and outcomes. Pediatr Cardiol. 2015;36:365–73.
5. Michel-Behnke I, Akintuerk H, Marquardt I, Mueller M, Thul J, Bauer J, Hagel KJ, Kreuder J, Vogt P, Schranz D. Stenting of the ductus arteriosus and banding of the pulmonary arteries: basis for various surgical strategies in newborns with multiple left heart obstructive lesions. Heart. 2003;89(6):645–50.
6. Akinturk H, Michel-Behnke I, Valeske K, Mueller M, Thul J, Bauer J, et al. Hybrid transcatheter-surgical palliation: basis for univentricular or biventricular repair: the Giessen experience. Pediatr Cardiol. 2007;28(2):79–87.
7. Yerebakan C, Murray J, Valeske K, Thul J, Elmontaser H, Mueller M, et al. Long-term results of biventricular repair after initial Giessen hybrid approach for hypoplastic left heart variants. J Thorac Cardiovasc Surg. 2015;149(4):1112–20.
8. Latus H, Apitz C, Schmidt D, Müller M, Bauer J, Akintuerk H, Schneider M, Schranz D. Potts shunt and atrial septostomy in pulmonary hypertension caused by left ventricular disease. Ann Surg. 2013;96(1):317–9.
9. Latus H, Yerebakan C, Schranz D, Akintuerk H. Right ventricular failure from severe pulmonary hypertension after surgery for shone complex: back to fetal physiology with reducting, atrioseptectomy, and bilateral pulmonary arterial banding. J Thorac Cardiovasc Surg. 2014;148:e226–8.
10. Akintuerk H, Michel-Behnke I, Valeske K, Mueller M, Thul J, Bauer J, Hagel KJ, Kreuder J, Vogt P, Schranz D. Stenting of the arterial duct and banding of the pulmonary arteries: basis for combined Norwood stage I and II repair in hypoplastic left heart. Circulation. 2002;105(9):1099–103.
11. Yerebakan C, Valeske K, Elmontaser H, Yörüker U, Mueller M, Thul J, Mann V, Latus H, Villanueva A, Hofmann K, Schranz D, Akintuerk H. Hybrid therapy for hypoplastic left heart syndrome – myth, alternative or standard? J Thorac Cardiovasc Surg. 2016;151(4): 1112–23.
12. Baba K, Kotani Y, Chetan D, Chaturvedi RR, Lee KJ, Benson LN, et al. Hybrid versus Norwood strategies for single-ventricle palliation. Circulation. 2012;126:S123–31.
13. Davies RR, Radtke WA, Klenk D, Pizarro C. Bilateral pulmonary arterial banding results in an increased need for subsequent pulmonary artery interventions. J Thorac Cardiovasc Surg. 2014;147:706–12.
14. Saiki H, Kurishima C, Masutani S, Tamura M, Senzaki H. Impaired cerebral perfusion after bilateral pulmonary arterial banding in patients with hypoplastic left heart syndrome. Ann Thorac Surg. 2013;96:1382–8.
15. Pizarro C, Davies RR, Woodford E, Radtke WA. Improving early outcomes following hybrid procedure for patients with single ventricle and systemic outflow obstruction: defining risk factors. Eur J Cardiothorac Surg. 2015;47(6):995–1000.
16. Rychik J, Rome JJ, Collins MH, DeCampli WM, Spray TL. The hypoplastic left heart syndrome with intact atrial septum: atrial morphology, pulmonary vascular histopathology and outcome. J Am Coll Cardiol. 1999;34:554–60.
17. McElhinney DB, Tworetzky W, Lock JE. Current status of fetal cardiac intervention. Circulation. 2010;121:1256–63.
18. Lacour-Gayet F, Clarke DR. Aristotle committee. The Aristotle method: a new concept to evaluate quality of care based on complexity. Curr Opin Pediatr. 2005;17(3):412–7.
19. Axt-Fliedner R, Tenzer A, Kawecki A, Degenhardt J, Schranz D, Valeske K, Vogel M, Kohl T, Enzensberger C. Prenatal assessment of ventriculocoronary connections and ventricular endocardial fibroelastosis in hypoplastic left heart. Ultraschall Med. 2014;35(4):357–63.
20. Edwards A, Veldman A, MD, Nitsos I, Chan Y, Brew N, Teoh M, Menahem S, Schranz D, Wong F. Percutaneous fetal cardiac catheterization technique for stenting the foramen ovale in a midgestation lamb model. Circ Cardiovasc Interv. 2015;8(3):e001967.

21. Latus H, Gummel K, Diederichs T, Bauer A, Rupp S, Kerst G, Jux C, Akintuerk H, Schranz D, Apitz C. Aortopulmonary collateral flow is related to pulmonary artery size and affects ventricular dimensions in patients after the Fontan procedure. PLoS One. 2013;8(11):e81684
22. Rupp S, Michel-Behnke I, Valeske K, Akintürk H, Schranz D. Implantation of stents to ensure an adequate interatrial communication in patients with hypoplastic left heart syndrome. Cardiol Young. 2007;17(5):535–40.
23. Schranz D, Jux C, Akintuerk H. Novel catheter-interventional strategy for intracardiac connecting of total anomalous pulmonary venous return (TAPVR) in newborns with hypoplastic left heart-syndrome (HLHS) prior to hybrid approach. Catheter Cardiovasc Interv. 2013;82(4):564–8.
24. Schranz D, Michel-Behnke I. Advances in interventional and hybrid therapy in neonatal congenital heart disease. Semin Fetal Neonatal Med. 2013;18(5):311–21.
25. Schranz D. Chapter 25. Patent ductus arteriosus stenting in duct-dependent systemic circulation. In: Butera G, Chessa M, Eicken A, Thompson J. Cardiac catheterization for congenital heart disease. Milan: Springer; 2015. p. 401–20.
26. Schranz D. Chapter 38. Hybrid approach in hypoplastic left heart syndrome (HLHS). In: Butera G, Chessa M, Eicken A, Thompson J. Cardiac catheterization for congenital heart disease. Milan: Springer; 2015. p. 649–66.
27. Rupp S, Schieke C, Kerst G, Mazhari N, Moysich A, Latus H, Michel-Behnke I, Akintuerk H, Schranz D. Creation of a transcatheter fenestration in children with failure of fontan circulation: Focus on extracardiac conduit connection. Catheter Cardiovasc Interv. 2015;86(7):1189–94.
28. Dapper F, Bauer J, Kroll J, Zickmann B, Bohle RM, Hagel KJ, Schranz D. Clinical experience with heart transplantation in infants. Eur J Cardiothorac Surg. 1998;14(1):1–5.
29. Gibbs JL, Wren C, Watterson KG, Hunter S, Hamilton JRL. Stenting of the arterial duct combined with banding of the pulmonary arteries and atrial septectomy or septostomy: a new approach to palliation for the hypoplastic left heart syndrome. Br Heart J. 1993;69:551–5.
30. Schranz D. Hybrid approach in hypoplastic left heart syndrome. Heart. 2014;100(10):750–1.
31. Bacha EAM, Hijazi ZM. Hybrid procedures in pediatric cardiac surgery. Semin Thorac Cardiovasc Surg Pediatr Card Surg Annu. 2005;8:78–85.

Hybrid Approach: The Columbus Way 29

John P. Cheatham

The neurodevelopmental outcomes after surgical repair of hypoplastic left heart syndrome (HLHS) are the worst of any congenital heart disease (CHD). In addition, the mortality for the conventional stage I surgical approach, the Norwood/Sano procedure, remains high in many institutions across the globe. Although our institution mortality was acceptably low, we wondered whether there could be a more "gentle" approach to stage I palliation that might lead to both lower mortality/morbidity risks and perhaps to improve neurodevelopmental outcomes. Our strategy was to perform an initial hybrid approach using simple surgical and transcatheter techniques of cardiopulmonary bypass, followed by a more robust comprehensive stage II repair at 4–6 months, followed by a transcatheter Fontan completion.

For the initial hybrid approach, we went through four phases. Phase 1 was a total percutaneous palliation by placing Amplatzer pulmonary artery flow restrictors (PAFR) (St. Jude Medical, Minneapolis, MN) in both pulmonary arteries, along with a balloon-expandable patent ductus arteriosus (PDA) stent, and finally a balloon atrial septostomy (BAS) (Fig 29.1). Unfortunately, the delivery system to implant the PAFR was too large and rigid causing significant tricuspid and pulmonary regurgitation and low cardiac output during the procedure that required inotropic support. So, we went to phase 2. The PDA stent and balloon atrial septostomy were performed in the traditional cath lab first, and the patient was transferred to the operating room (OR) for Gore-Tex pulmonary artery (PA) bands bilaterally. Unfortunately, placing the left pulmonary artery (LPA) band was too difficult because of the adjacent rigid balloon-expandable PDA stent. Next came phase 3. The surgical PA bands were placed in a traditional operating room first, and then the baby was transferred to the cath lab where PDA stenting and balloon atrial septostomy were performed. This method of performing the stage I palliation was going

J.P. Cheatham, MD, FAAP, FACC, MSCAI
The Heart Center, Nationwide Children's Hospital, Pediatrics & Internal Medicine, Cardiology, The Ohio State University, Columbus, OH, USA
e-mail: John.Cheatham@nationwidechildrens.org

G. Butera et al. (eds.), *Fetal and Hybrid Procedures in Congenital Heart Diseases*, DOI 10.1007/978-3-319-40088-4_29

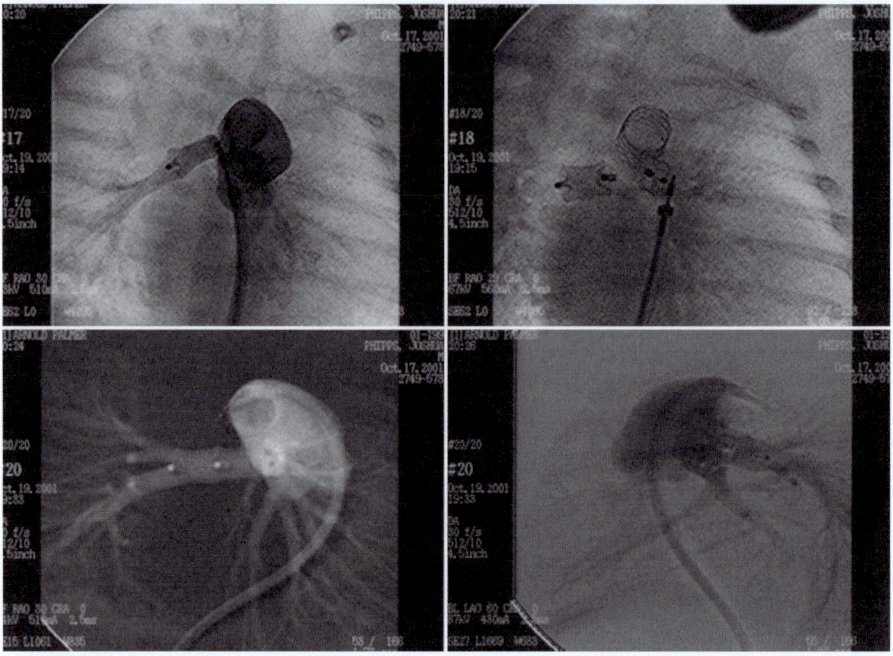

Fig 29.1 During phase 1 of our initial attempt at developing a hybrid strategy for stage I palliation of HLHS, we placed a balloon expandable stent (BES) PDA stent and then Amplatzer PAFR in both pulmonary branches with a BAS to follow. This was an all percutaneous palliation

very well and is the same technique currently used in many institutions. However, Dr. Galantowicz called me to the operating room one day while placing the PA bands and said "Here's the PDA. If I can give you direct access through a purse-string above the pulmonary valve leaflets, why can't you just put the stent through a sheath directly into the PDA?" We then explored imaging possibilities to perform this procedure, and portable fluoroscopy was the answer. The true "hybrid" approach was now a reality and could be performed in any traditional operating room (Fig 29.2a, b). The timing of the balloon atrial septostomy was deferred and performed prior to the patient's discharge, when using a 2 mL (13.5 mm) septostomy catheter (B. Braun Medical, USA) was possible and usually would maintain an adequate atrial septal defect (ASD) until Comprehensive Stage II repair.

Soon after the true "hybrid stage I palliation" was developed, we designed and built Hybrid Cardiac Catheterization and Operative Suites (Fig 29.3). This allowed hybrid stage I palliation, as well as other hybrid procedures, to be performed in a more accommodating setting. Since all of the hybrid suites were designed to meet "OR standards," we could perform the procedures in any of the suites. We discovered that there were few, if any, contraindications in performing hybrid stage I palliation, unlike that for the Norwood/Sano procedure. Size, prematurity, ventricular dysfunction, high morbidity, genetic abnormalities, etc.... were not contraindications to performing this palliation. We have successfully performed this procedure

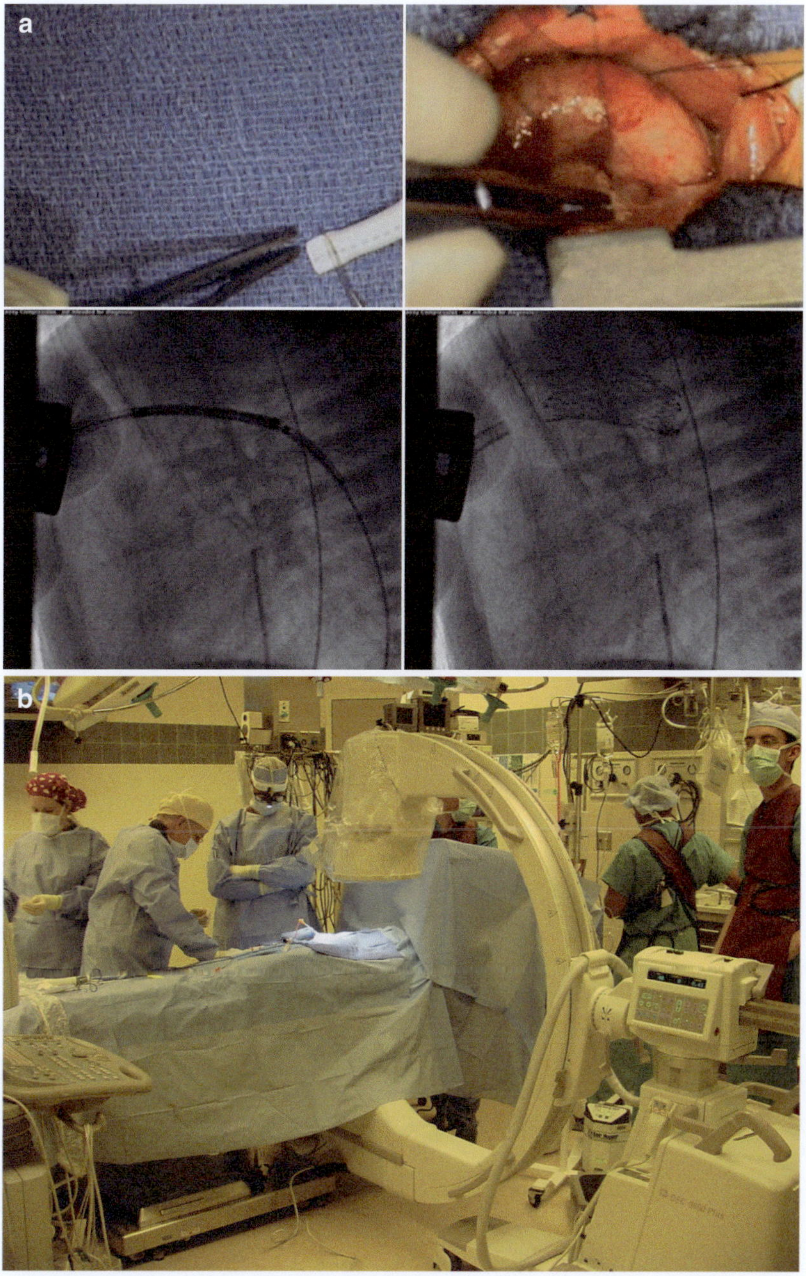

Fig 29.2 In (**a**), the Gore-Tex PA bands are cut to be placed around the left pulmonary artery (LPA) and right pulmonary artery (RPA), while the patent ductus arteriosus (PDA) stent is delivered directly though the main pulmonary artery (MPA) via a purse-string suture. In (**b**), this procedure could be performed in a conventional OR with portable fluoroscopy

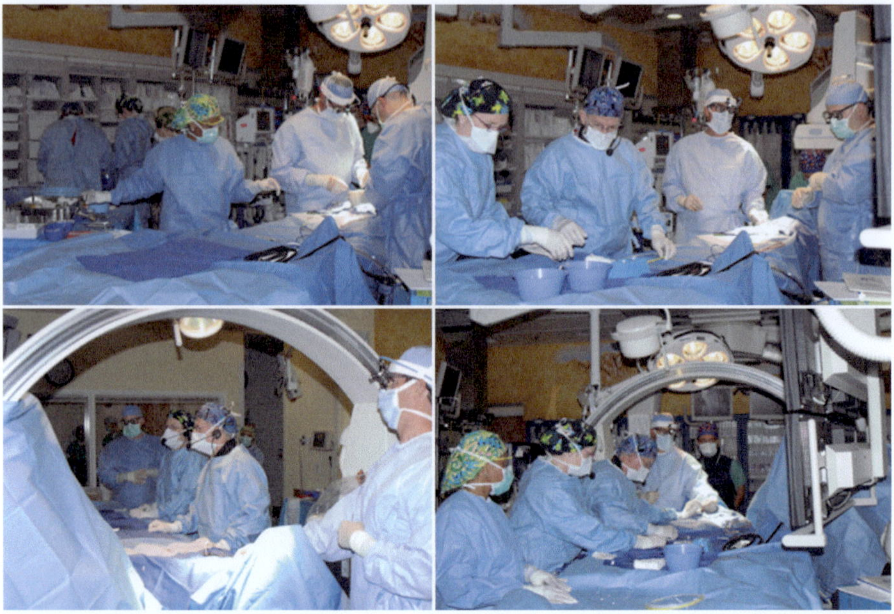

Fig 29.3 After specialized hybrid suites were constructed at Nationwide Children's Hospital (NCH), it was much easier for all of the teams to perform the hybrid stage I palliation. Typically, the entire procedure lasted only 1 h

in premature babies weighing only 1 kg and in others that were already several months old (Fig 29.4). We also found that blood transfusion was seldom necessary, leading to many families of Jehovah Witness faith to be referred to our heart center. In addition, inotropic support was seldom required. In our own institution, only native retrograde aortic arch obstruction was a contraindication. However, in some institutions, a "reverse Blalock-Taussig (BT) shunt" was suggested in these patients.

The patients, after hybrid stage I palliation, were followed closely in the outpatient by the single ventricle team that was formed by the initiative in our heart center named LAUNCH. The patients were followed every 1–2 weeks with physical exam, oximetry, and echocardiography. Our home monitoring nurses also call the family on a regular basis with a defined protocol that would result in the patient being seen earlier if a "breach" is detected. The goal was to allow growth of the baby until 4–6 months of age or approximately 6 kg. At this time, comprehensive stage II repair is performed, which is the first procedure to require cardiopulmonary bypass. During this surgery, the pulmonary artery bands and the PDA stent are removed, patch LPA plasty performed, the aortic arch is reconstructed with a modified Damus-Kaye-Stansel operation, atrial septectomy is performed, and a bidirectional Glenn is performed, initially with markers to "set up" a transcatheter Fontan completion in patients around 2 years of age. Once we built our hybrid suites, we routinely performed exit angiography at the end of the comprehensive stage II repair and, if necessary, performed any surgical or transcatheter interventions before returning to the cardiothoracic intensive care unit (CTICU).

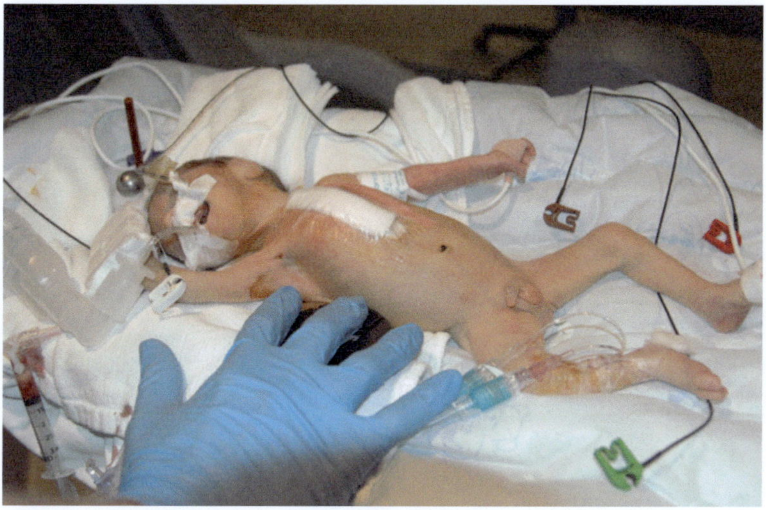

Fig 29.4 Because size is not a contraindication to the hybrid stage I palliation for HLHS, even this 1 kg baby was no different than a term baby, technically speaking

The final goal of our hybrid approach to HLHS was to be able to complete the Fontan procedure in the cath lab. Between 2000 and 2002, we performed 5 out of 5 successful transcatheter Fontan completions in patients averaging 2 years of age and weigh 11 kg. The NuMED covered CP stent (CCPS) (NuMED Inc. Hopkinton, NY) was used as a "customized" device with the distal and proximal rows of zigs left uncovered to allow flow into the pulmonary arteries and hepatic veins, respectively (Fig 29.5a, b). Unfortunately, with issues from the regulatory agencies and NuMED Inc., the covered CP stent was unavailable in the USA for many years, and transcatheter Fontan completion was discontinued. Instead, an extracardiac pericardial baffle is created surgically to complete the Fontan circuit.

The results of hybrid stage I palliation have been reported by our institution, as well as the experience of the center from Giessen, Germany, and have demonstrated this palliation as a preferred approach or at least at equipoise to the Norwood/Sano procedure [1–4]. However, these two institutions have committed to this approach and have become "experts" in performing the procedures, as well as following these patients as outpatients. The main criticism of the hybrid stage I palliation has been the reliance of maintaining the fetal circulation for retrograde aortic arch and coronary perfusion through the stented PDA. We have adapted a strategy of stent therapy in those patients demonstrating retrograde aortic arch obstruction, which can be seen in up to 25–28 % of patients.

The real question and one of the main reasons to endorse hybrid stage I palliation is to assess if the ultimate neurodevelopmental outcomes are different from the poor outcomes published after the Norwood/Sano repair. The report by Cheatham, SL. et al. describes neurodevelopmental testing using tissue inhibitor of metalloproteinase (TIMP), Bayley-III, and transcranial Doppler in infants undergoing hybrid stage

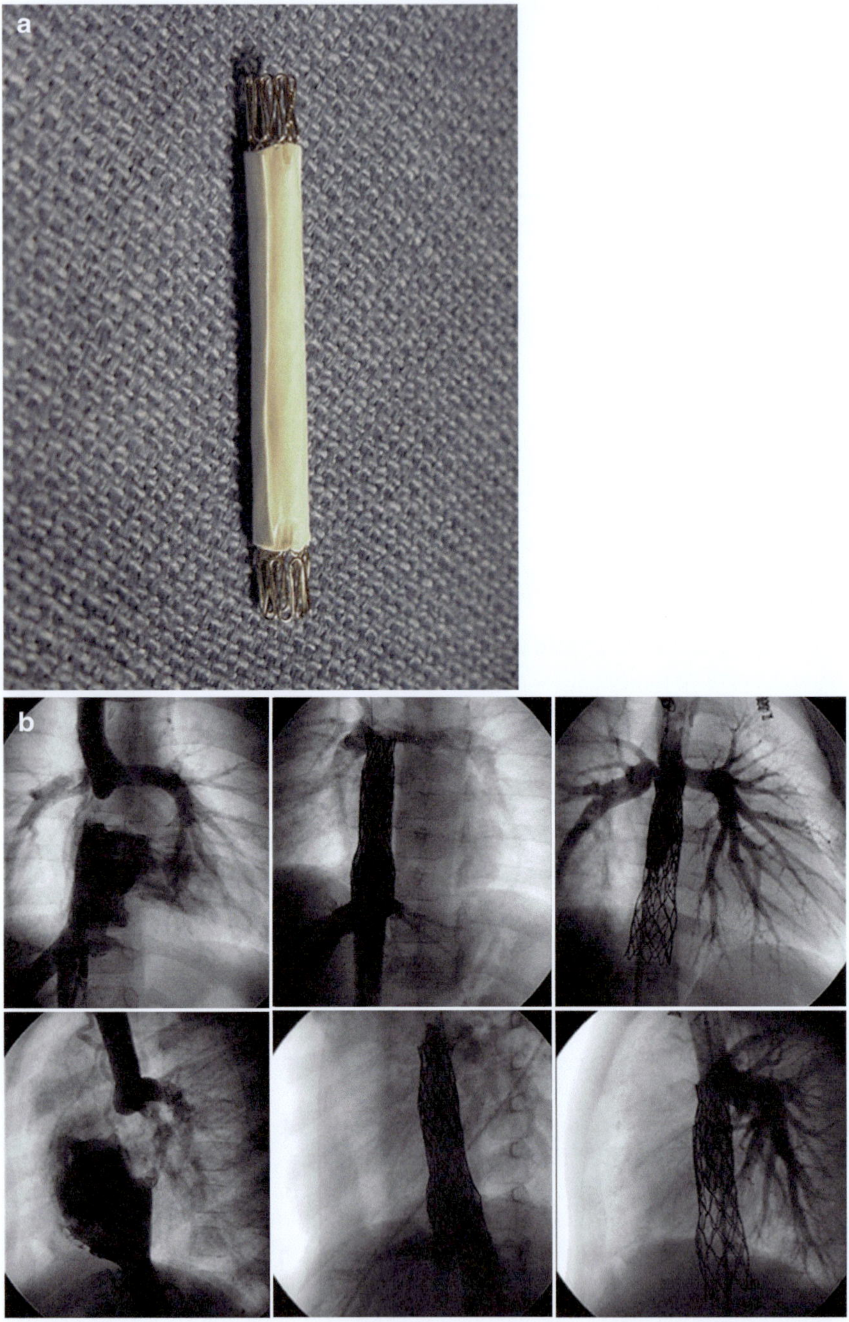

Fig 29.5 In (**a**), the custom-ordered NuMED CCPS was left uncovered at each row of zigs to allow flow into the PAs and the hepatic veins after transcatheter Fontan completion, which is shown in (**b**)

I palliation [5]. While the motor skills remained low compared with age-matched normal infants, they were similar to those patients after Norwood/Sano procedure [6]. In addition, there was no instance in which the infants after hybrid palliation scored lower than those of the Norwood/Sano operation, which dispelled some of the beliefs that continuing retroaortic flow through the PDA for an additional 4–6 months would be deleterious to brain function. Unfortunately, we did not see a significant improvement in the neurodevelopmental scores after the hybrid stage I palliation.

So in summary, the real values of the hybrid stage I palliation in babies with hypoplastic left heart syndrome are:

1. No size, age, or morbidity limitation
2. High procedural success with a short "learning curve" in most institutions
3. Can even be performed in "high-risk" infants in the Norwood/Sano institutions
4. Act as a bridge to heart transplant or even to repair complex two-ventricle neonates that have unacceptable risk for complete repair as a newborn
5. But most importantly, it brings the cardiothoracic (CT) surgical and interventional cardiology teams closer in collaboration so that new and innovative management strategies can be developed for these babies, as well as others with complex heart disease.

References

1. Galantowicz M, Cheatham JP, Phillips A, Cua CL, Hoffman TM, Hill SL, et al. Hybrid approach for hypoplastic left heart syndrome: intermediate results after the learning curve. Ann Thorac Surg. 2008;85(6):2063–70; discussion 2070–1.
2. Akinturk H, Michel-Behnke I, Valeske K, Mueller M, Thul J, Bauer J, et al. Hybrid transcatheter-surgical palliation: basis for univentricular or biventricular repair: the Giessen experience. Pediatr Cardiol. 2007;28(2):79–87.
3. Schranz D, Bauer A, Reich B, Steinbrenner B, Recla S, Schmidt D, et al. Fifteen-year single center experience with the "Giessen Hybrid" approach for hypoplastic left heart and variants: current strategies and outcomes. Pediatr Cardiol. 2015;36(2):365–73.
4. Ohye RG et al. Comparison of shunt types in the Norwood procedure for single-ventricle lesions. N Engl J Med. 2010;362(21):1980–92.
5. Cheatham SL, Carey H, Chisolm JL, Heathcock JC, Steward D. Early results of neurodevelopment following hybrid stage I for hypoplastic left heart syndrome. Pediatr Cardiol. 2015;36(3):685–91.
6. Newburger JW et al. Early developmental outcome in children with hypoplastic left heart syndrome and related anomalies: the single ventricle reconstruction trial. Circulation. 2012;125(17):2081–91.

30 The Brazilian Hybrid Approach for Hypoplastic Left Heart Syndrome

Carlos A.C. Pedra, Simone Fontes Pedra, and Marcelo B. Jatene

30.1 Introduction and Historical Aspects

Until the adoption of the hybrid approach, the management of neonates with hypoplastic left heart syndrome (HLHS) had always been frustrating in our hands. The classical Norwood or the Norwood-Sano operation had had prohibitive in-hospital mortality rates. Therefore, when the concept and the technique of the hybrid approach were introduced to our group in the mid-2000s by Drs. Cheatham, Galantowicz [1], and Schranz [2], the decision to embark on this strategy was made on necessity grounds. Nevertheless, our initial results with stage I were disappointing [3], which prompted the writing of two editorials [4, 5] in a scientific journal addressing the need to improve the whole infrastructure surrounding this procedure. Our learning curve was somewhat slow in the first 5 years due to a myriad of reasons including cultural resistance to changes, lack of trained human resources (both in the medical and nursing fields), use of limited X-ray equipment (C-arm), unavailability of a dedicated hybrid room, inappropriate follow-up, among others. Since our first case done in January 2005, our technique and, more importantly, the perioperative and interstage care evolved significantly resulting in better and reasonable in-hospital and follow-up outcomes. This chapter reports our current results with this approach emphasizing the modifications that occurred over years of practice and probably had a beneficial effect on overall results.

C.A.C. Pedra, MD, PhD, FSCAI, FACC (✉) • S.F. Pedra, MD, PhD • M.B. Jatene, MD, PhD
Hospital do Coração da Associação Sanatório Sírio, São Paulo, Brazil
e-mail: cacpedra@uol.com.br

G. Butera et al. (eds.), *Fetal and Hybrid Procedures in Congenital Heart Diseases*, DOI 10.1007/978-3-319-40088-4_30

30.2 Technique and Indications (Stage I and II)

Most of our patients with HLHS are now diagnosed in utero. They are born in our institution within a strong fetal program supported by the Brazilian Ministry of Health. Hospital do Coração (HCor) is a referral cardiology center (not a maternity hospital) and had to undergo some internal adaptations to push forward this project. Mothers undergo an elective C-section at 38–39 weeks of gestation to better plan the procedure for the neonate. Although this is medically debatable for both the mother and the baby, we now have over 50 C-section deliveries with babies born with HLHS with no complications in the delivery room for the neonate and no complications for the mother during their hospital stay. Same results are observed after 280 deliveries at HCor taking into account other fetal heart diseases.

After delivery, the umbilical vein and artery are catheterized in the intensive care unit (ICU) for monitoring purposes and intravenous (IV) fluids and prostaglandin infusion. Neonates are kept NPO and under spontaneous ventilation. The use of vasopressors, bladder catheterization, and frequent blood samples for labs are avoided. If there are signs of overcirculation, patients are placed in a hood with a hypoxic mixture (FiO2 17–19 %). Carbon dioxide administration is not used. The initial stage I procedure is usually performed between 24 and 72 h of life in a dedicated hybrid suite that was built in early 2012. From 2005 to 2012, all cases were performed in the operating room (OR) using a C-arm machine, which had had significant imaging limitations until 2008 when it was changed for a better portable X-ray piece of equipment. If the atrial septal defect (ASD) or patent foramen ovale (PFO) is absent or highly restrictive during fetal life, the baby is rapidly transferred from the delivery room in the OR to the catheterization laboratory, and atrial septostomy is performed in an urgent basis. It is our impression that in-hospital delivery allowed for a smoother preoperative course in our 10-year experience. Occasionally, we still receive neonates born at community hospitals, which may put them at risk due to the need of transport and excessive manipulation resulting in an unbalanced circulation before the procedure.

The hybrid approach is offered to all neonates with HLHS at our institution, regardless of clinical and anatomical associated risk factors such as prematurity, low weight, comorbidities and malformations, size of the aorta, and right ventricular (RV) dysfunction. If there is significant narrowing of the isthmus or a sub-atretic coarctation of the aorta (CoA), a 4–5 mm reversed shunt is placed between the main pulmonary artery (MPA) and the innominate artery as suggested by Carderone and colleagues in Toronto [6]. Less than 5 % of patients needed this modification.

Prostaglandin infusion is stopped while the neonate is prepped in the hybrid suite. Although the anesthetic strategy varies a bit among different professionals, we have employed the Columbus protocol [7] in most of our patients. A sternotomy is performed, and the chest opened in the usual fashion and the pulmonary arteries are dissected out carefully. Bilateral pulmonary artery banding is performed before ductal stenting using 3.0 mm (for smaller babies) or a 3.5 mm (for babies >2.5 kgs) ePTFE bands based on the Galantowicz guidelines [2]. Fine adjustment is highly surgeon dependent and requires experience!

We use balloon-expandable stents (Cordis, Boston, or Biotronik) implanted through 6–7 F sheaths placed within a purse-string suture in the MPA. At the beginning of our experience (first 5–10 patients), the delivery sheaths were secured in the right ventricular outflow tract (RVOT) due to the longer shoulders of the available balloons at that time, which might have had a negative impact on RV function. The whole ductal tissue should be covered by the stent, from just before the takeoff of the pulmonary arteries until the initial portion of the descending aorta, usually marked by the esophageal thermostat on fluoroscopy. The usual final diameter of the stent is 8 or 9 mm. Occasionally 6–7 mm stents are implanted in smaller babies. Lengths vary between 15 and 25 mm. Nowadays we would rather use a longer stent with some proximal and distal protrusion than run the risk of leaving uncovered ductal tissue. Careful measurements are made in lateral view after 2–3 ml of low-osmolality contrast agent is injected through the side arm of the sheath positioned in the MPA. A regular wire is parked in the abdominal descending aorta for support. A single inflation is usually necessary to deliver the stent appropriately. Although there is some hypotension during inflation, this is generally well tolerated with rapid recovery, and no signs of ischemia and hemodynamic compromise. After the stent is deployed, another contrast injection is performed to assess the immediate results. The whole system (balloon and wire) is withdrawn under fluoroscopic guidance. Although we have avoided the use of vasopressors during the hybrid procedure, approximately 70 % of our patients needed some epinephrine infusion to maintain acceptable blood pressure levels. The chest is closed in the usual fashion, and a drain is left in the mediastinum. The neonate is finally transferred to the ICU for routine post-op care.

An elective atrial septostomy is typically performed between 1 and 3 weeks after the initial hybrid approach (Fig. 30.1). The use of the Z5 atrioseptostomy balloon (NuMED, Cornwall, ON, Canada) has significantly diminished the need for alternative techniques such as radiofrequency perforation of the interatrial septum and septal stenting. Because of the complexity of the anatomy of the interatrial septum (malalignment ASDs are common) in HLHS patients, frailty of such patients, and the limited steerability and pushability of the Z5, we perform septostomies in the catheterization laboratory with the aid of a 23 cm long sheath placed across or at the mouth of the ASD/PFO. The 6 F Z5 is used for term or big neonates and the 5 F for the premies, neonates under 2.5 kgs or with smaller left atria (LAs).

Interstage monitoring is of paramount importance. Although we cannot provide home visits due to financial constraints, parents or guardians are encouraged to come to HCor or to a reliable health facility every other week. Weight gain and systemic saturation are important markers of the overall infant well-being. Low weight gain, low or high sats, and irritability should prompt in-hospital investigations. Echocardiographic monitoring is performed in every clinical visit to check for ASD size, RV function, band tightness adequacy, stent obstruction, and retrograde flow through the arch.

The Norwood-Glenn operation is generally performed at around 6 months of age and/or when the patient is around 6 kgs. Although we have not performed a diagnostic catheterization routinely before this big operation, our threshold to cath these

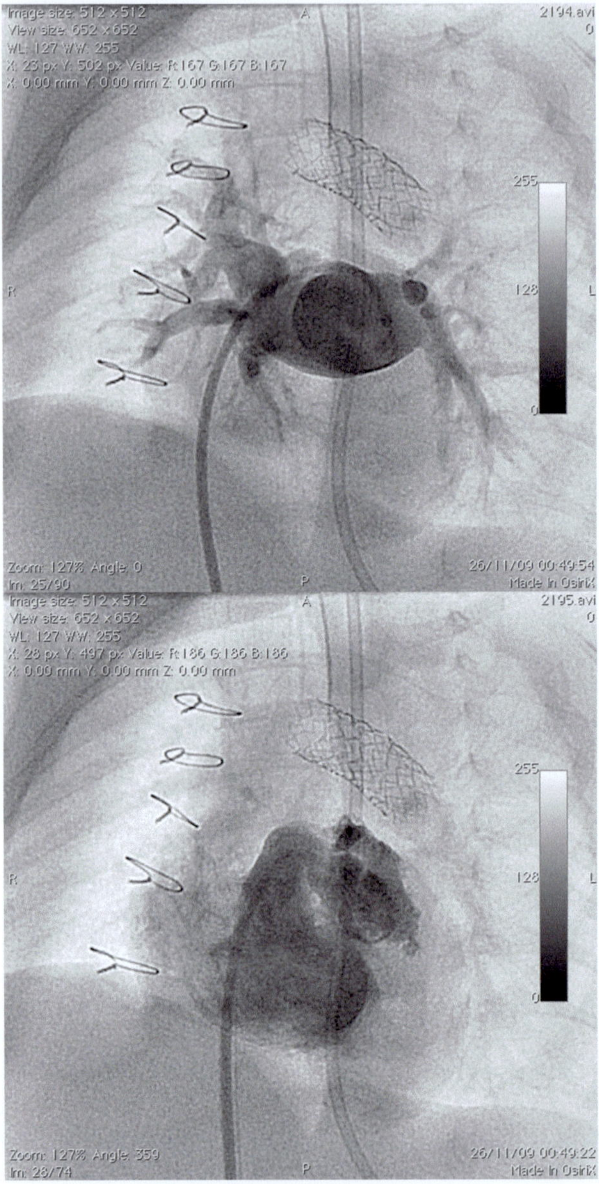

Fig. 30.1 Atrial septostomy 3 weeks after the initial hybrid procedure in the catheterization laboratory using a Z5 atrioseptostomy balloon. (**a**) Left atrial angiogram in left anterior oblique view showing a very dilated left atrium with a tiny atrial septal defect located superiorly within the interatrial septum. (**b**) After the septostomy was performed, the left atrium diminished in size, and a wide-open unobstructed atrial septal defect is seen shunting left-to-right

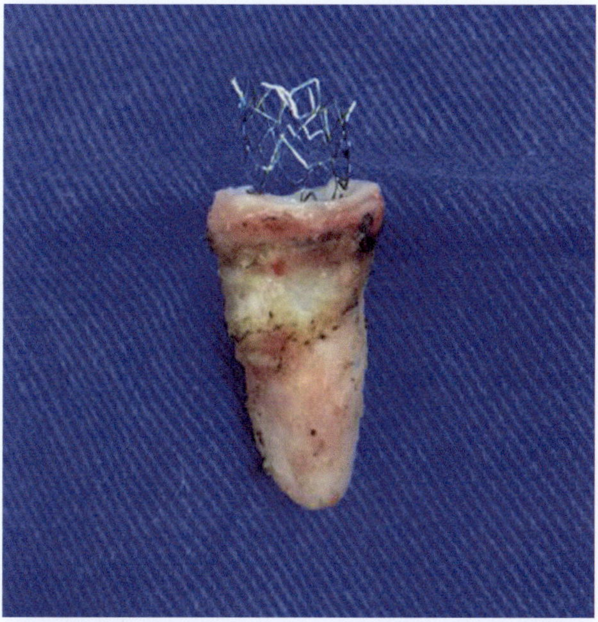

Fig. 30.2 Anatomical specimen obtained after the Norwood-Glenn operation. The stent was taken out of the duct and descending aorta as a unit along with the vessel wall. No attempts at finding a plane of dissection were performed

patients diminished over time. Some patients require new catheter interventions in the interstage period anyways. Some patients are screened with angio-computed tomography depending on the clinical and echo findings (see below in "Results" section). In the Norwood-Glenn operation, the stent is removed entirely as a single block (not dissected out from the aorta finding a plane of dissection) (Fig. 30.2), and the arch is reconstructed using a homograft. If the ascending aorta is tiny (<2.5 mm) and long, we now transfer it to the right aspect of the MPA (neo-aorta) using a terminal to side anastomosis to minimize possible myocardial ischemia (Fig. 30.3). The bands are removed, and the confluence of the pulmonary arteries is reconstructed eliminating the redundant tissue remnant of the MPA. Until early 2012, the surgeon used to patch the left pulmonary artery (LPA) if there was local stenosis or distortion because the operation was conducted in a regular OR without the means to perform an exit angiography. We now take a different approach. The right pulmonary artery (RPA) can and should be repaired by the surgeon while the Glenn anastomosis is performed. When the patient comes off cardiopulmonary bypass, an exit angiography is now performed in the dedicated hybrid suite (Fig. 30.4). A 7 F sheath is secured through a purse-string suture in the high superior vena cava (SVC) near the entrance of the innominate vein, and some contrast is injected through the side

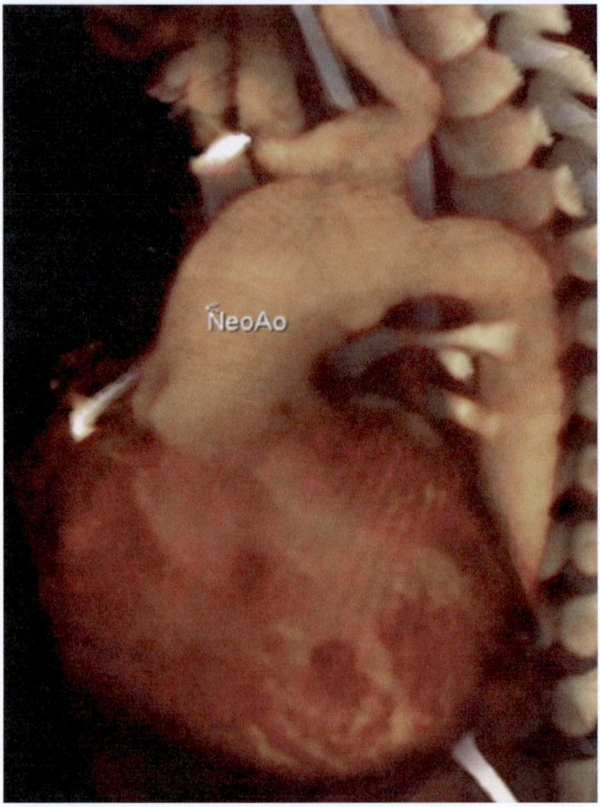

Fig. 30.3 Angio-computed tomography performed after the Norwood-Glenn operation to assess the pulmonary arteries (not shown here) and the ascending aorta. (**a**) The arch has excellent size after surgical reconstruction with a homograft. (**b**) A tiny and long ascending aorta (*marked by small arrows*) is seen on the right side of the former main pulmonary artery. Because of intermittent ischemia and mild right ventricular dysfunction, a decision was made to reimplant the ascending aorta in a more proximal position close to the neo-aortic valve. Abbreviations: *NeoAo* neo-aorta, *Ao asc* ascending aorta

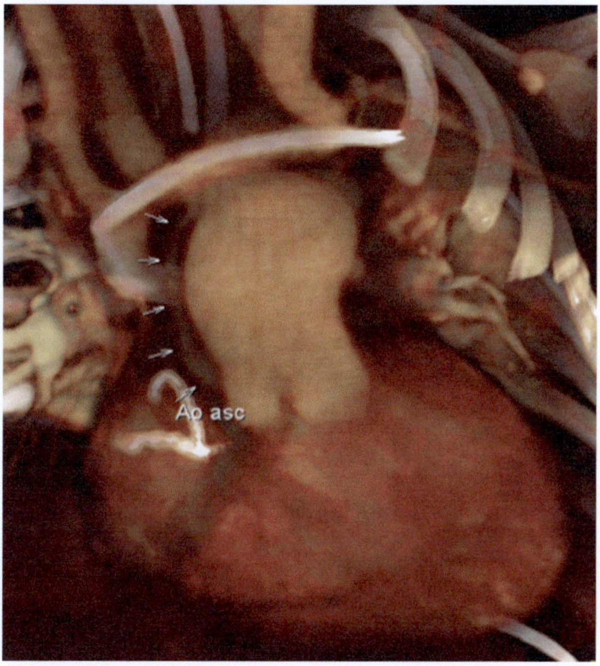

Fig. 30.3 (continued)

arm. If there is stenosis, twisting or distortion of the vessel, the LPA is now under the interventionist domain, and a stent is immediately placed in the OR (Fig. 30.4). If the RPA or the Glenn anastomosis does not look good, the surgeon can fix whatever problem off or on a new run of pump. Using this strategy we significantly reduced the need of early post-op catheter interventions.

The Fontan operation is performed around 3 years of age. Before the operation, all patients undergo a diagnostic catheterization to assess pulmonary anatomy, pressures, and resistance. An extra-cardiac conduit is placed between the inferior vena cava (IVC) and the inferior aspect of the confluence of the pulmonary arteries. A 4 mm fenestration is now left in the conduit to decrease the incidence and length of effusions.

30.3 Results

We have 117 patients who underwent the hybrid approach for HLHS and variants, with 98 performed for HLHS exclusively. Mean age and weight were 3.9 ± 1.5 days and 2.9 ± 0.9 kgs, respectively. Our current mortality rate for stage I is 25 %. Morbidity is still high with median time of mechanical ventilation of 10 days, ICU stay of 15 days, and hospital stay of 27 days. Almost all patients required some kind

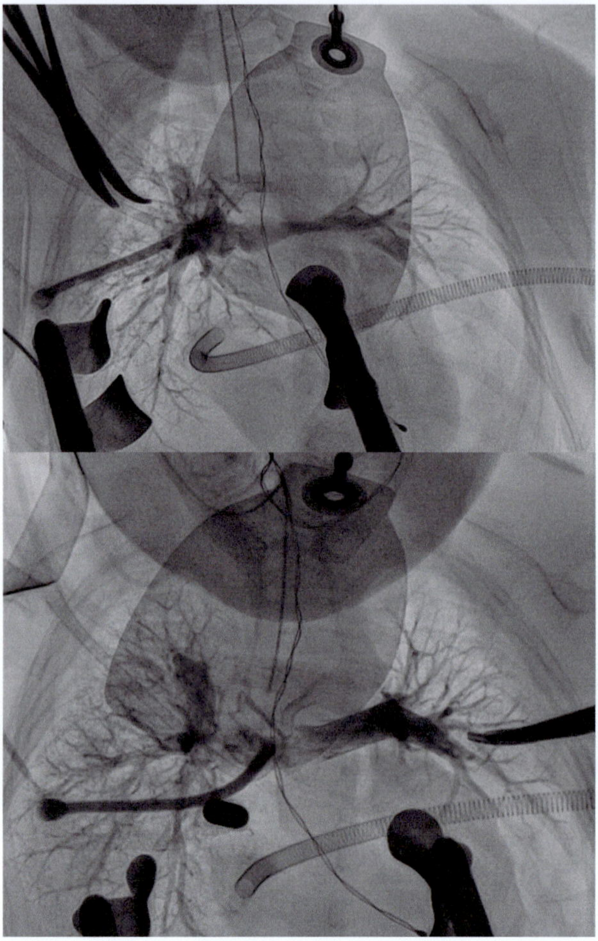

Fig. 30.4 Exit angiography after completion of cardiopulmonary bypass on left anterior oblique with cranial angulation projection. (**a**) The left pulmonary artery is distorted after the band was removed. (**b**) Normalization of the vessel diameter is seen after intraoperative stent implantation

of inotropic support in the ICU. Despite this initial struggle, 50 % of our patients who are discharged home are breast-fed!

Interstage need for cath reinterventions is common in our experience. A third of our patients underwent some kind of reintervention, mainly due to retrograde aortic obstruction (Fig. 30.5). Although we initially performed standard balloon dilatation of the cells of the PDA stent, we now tend to put a coronary stent through the struts of the PDA stent in a retrograde fashion using the distal arch as the reference diameter (usually a 4–4.5 mm stent) and a 4 Fr long sheath. New PDA stenting to cover uncovered ductal tissue may also be occasionally required. Hemodynamic instability is common in this procedure because the pulmonary and tricuspid valves are

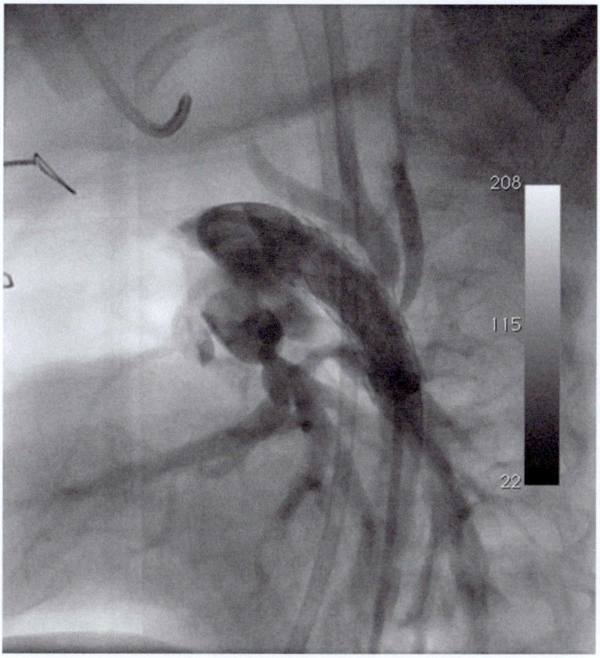

Fig. 30.5 Stent implantation to the arch due to retrograde aortic obstruction. (**a**) Aortic angiography in the lateral projection showing stenosis within the struts of the previously implanted ductal stent causing retrograde aortic obstruction, ischemia, and right ventricular dysfunction. (**b**) Significant improvement in the diameter within the stent cell with optimization of retrograde flow

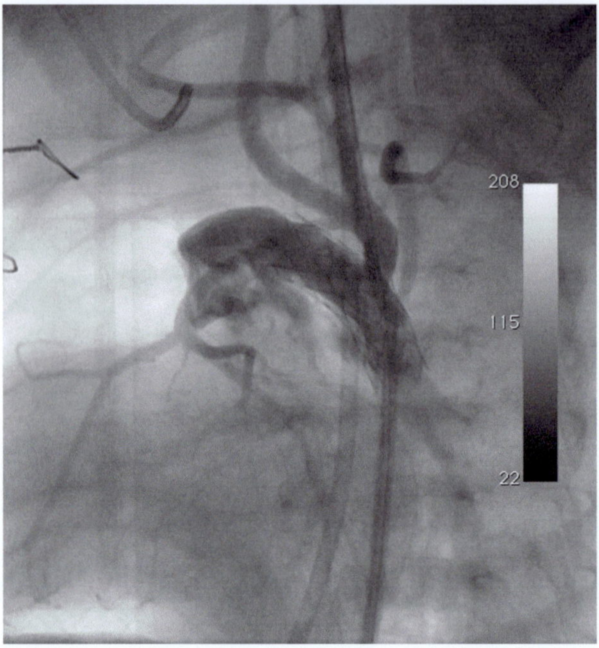

Fig. 30.5 (continued)

propped open during the delivery system progression. Use of longer stents at stage I usually avoids this complication. Significant in-stent proliferation was not observed in our experience. Whether this is due to the use of balloon-expandable stent is debatable. In 5–10 % of patients, one or both of the bands became tighter over time resulting in low sats and/or hypoperfusion of the ipsilateral lung and were successfully dilated using 3.5 mm coronary balloons (Fig. 30.6). Occasionally loosen bands requires tightening in the OR. Interstage mortality is now rare because these patients are followed more closely.

We have 32 patients who had a Norwood-Glenn operation with 22 % mortality mainly due to RV dysfunction. Early on in our experience, most patients needed some kind of pulmonary artery stenting in the early post-op period. This is now unusual because we started to perform exit angios in a dedicated hybrid room. Currently, patients who have less than optimal intra-op PA results are either stented (LPA) or redo (RPA) before going to the ICU. Unfortunately, morbidity after Norwood-Glenn is also common with prolonged ICU stay (median 17 days), use of inotropes in all patients, and 20 % need for diaphragmatic plication.

However, such infants do remarkably well after they are discharged home after this big operation. Arch obstruction is rare (Fig. 30.3). Weight gain is acceptable. We have 17 patients who underwent Fontan completion with no

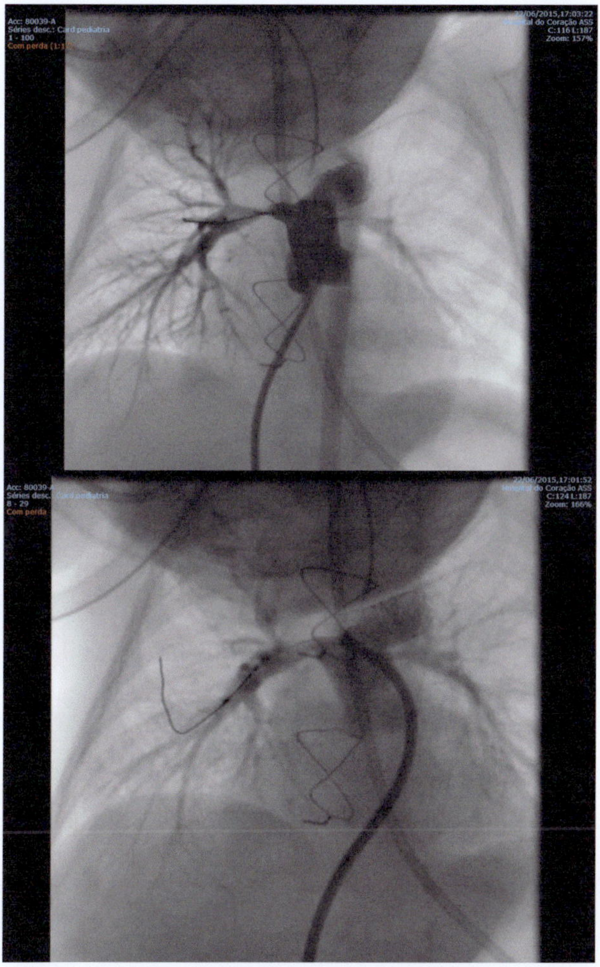

Fig. 30.6 Balloon angioplasty of a tight right pulmonary artery band. (**a**) Right pulmonary artery angiogram in right anterior oblique view with cranial angulation showing a very tight band with the minimum diameter measuring less than 1 mm. A coronary wire was passed through it. (**b**) After an angioplasty was performed with a compliant 3.5 × 15 mm coronary balloon, the minimal diameter increased to ~2 mm with improvement of the patient systemic saturation. The left pulmonary artery (not shown herein) was also dilated in the same procedure

mortality. The 10 more recent patients in whom a fenestrated conduit was used had shorter length of stay due to less days of effusions and need for drainage. All patients are well after Fontan, except for a single one who developed protein-losing enteropathy (PLE). Longer follow-up is needed to better assess our overall results, including neurologic outcomes.

30.4 Final Considerations

We have presented an evolving experience with the hybrid approach for HLHS in a Latin American country with reasonable outcomes. Our results are not comparable as yet with those observed at other institutions that have applied this strategy for a longer period of time such as Giessen and Columbus. Institutions that have good results with the classical or modified Norwood also do significantly better. However, some considerations should be made for those institutions that want to embark on this strategy. Our results started to improve after 10–15 cases (only after our surgeon really embraced the program), and persistence was a must. We simply decided to continue to do what we were doing better. Continuous adjustments in the infrastructure and improvements in the ICU were necessary. Open and frank (sometimes painful) discussions within our team were required to improve. Continuous medical education played a pivotal role in our learning curve with lessons acquired from Columbus, Toronto, and Giessen. A well-established fetal program seemed to have made a difference in our results, which expanded the hybrid concept. A strong interventional team was required to make these patients reach stage II. Nothing was possible without the hospital administration support (including opening the dedicated hybrid suite) and heavy funding from the Ministry of Health. All in all, the above comments can be summarized in a single word: team commitment! The price paid was high in every single way: financial (in a single patient, the final hospital bill came to US 500.000!), scientific, physical, and emotional. But the rewards were high. We got better not only with HLHS. Taking care of these babies had a positive impact on the overall neonatal care of other complex CHD. We got better as a team because the hybrid concept forges interaction. We got better as human beings because we also suffered the burden with these families. Whether this concept could be embraced by other institutions that are willing to treat babies with HLHS, especially those with limited resources, remains to be dealt with individually.

References

1. Galantowicz M, Cheatham JP. Lessons learned from the development of a new hybrid strategy for the management of hypoplastic left heart syndrome. Pediatr Cardiol. 2005;26(3):190–9.
2. Akintuerk H, Michel-Behnke I, Valeske K, Mueller M, Thul J, Bauer J, Hagel KJ, Kreuder J, Vogt P, Schranz D. Stenting of the arterial duct and banding of the pulmonary arteries: basis for combined Norwood stage I and II repair in hypoplastic left heart. Circulation. 2002;105(9):1099–103.
3. Pilla CB, Pedra CA, Nogueira AJ, Jatene M, Souza LC, Pedra SR, Ferreiro C, Ricachinevsky CP, Lucchese FA. Hybrid management for hypoplastic left heart syndrome : an experience from Brazil. Pediatr Cardiol. 2008;29(3):498–506.
4. Hijazi ZM. Hybrid therapy for hypoplastic left heart syndrome: reality check. Pediatr Cardiol. 2008;29(3):477–8.
5. Bacha E. Hybrid therapy for hypoplastic left heart syndrome: system-wide approach is vital. Pediatr Cardiol. 2008;29(3):479–80.

6. Caldarone CA, Benson LN, Holtby H, Van Arsdell GS. Main pulmonary artery to innominate artery shunt during hybrid palliation of hypoplastic left heart syndrome. J Thorac Cardiovasc Surg. 2005;130(4):e1–2.
7. Naguib AN, Winch P, Schwartz L, Isaacs J, Rodeman R, Cheatham JP, Galantowicz M. Anesthetic management of the hybrid stage 1 procedure for hypoplastic left heart syndrome (HLHS). Paediatr Anaesth. 2010;20(1):38–46.

Canadian Approach to Hybrid HLHS

31

Lee Benson

When introduced in to clinical practice, bilateral pulmonary artery banding and stenting of the arterial duct added a further dimension to management strategies for hypoplastic left heart syndrome (HLHS) by allowing a delayed arch reconstruction until the infant was ~4 months of age [1, 2]. The procedure was attractive, as post-operative care after the Norwood procedure was challenging, the infants not infrequently in a low cardiac output state for several days with over-circulation and myocardial ischemia an ever-present concern. Furthermore from a neurological standpoint, it was anticipated that the more mature infant would tolerate bypass with less central nervous system compromise during the so-called comprehensive stage II (arch and pulmonary artery reconstruction, stent removal, bidirectional cavopulmonary connection). Early investigations identified a number of drawbacks to this staged approach (i.e., the primary hybrid procedure), which included the risk of retrograde arch obstruction from the ductal stent [3], loose bands [4], difficulties management of the size of the atrial septum [5], low systemic blood flow immediately after the procedure [6], and problems with left pulmonary artery hypoplasia after comprehensive stage II [7] to name a few. Despite these limitations we enthusiastically embraced this as one of the treatment strategies offered to parents of infants with HLHS. However, our program approach to the infant with HLHS was lacking as not being uniform, i.e., not protocolized, but rather reflected the biases of the parents (having gone to the web) and the referring physicians. As such, questions arose as to where to place the hybrid procedure in the overall treatment algorithm. An interesting analogy to the adoption of a management option (or new innovation) can be seen in the Gartner Hype Cycle [8], which is a graphical representation of the adoption of a new technology (Fig. 31.1a). Under this construct, the innovation, in this case the hybrid procedure, undergoes rapid incorporation into

L. Benson, MD, FRCPC, FACC, FSCAI
The Cardiac Diagnostic and Interventional Unit, The Hospital for Sick Children, University of Toronto School of Medicine, Toronto, Canada
e-mail: lee.benson@sickkids.ca

G. Butera et al. (eds.), *Fetal and Hybrid Procedures in Congenital Heart Diseases*, DOI 10.1007/978-3-319-40088-4_31

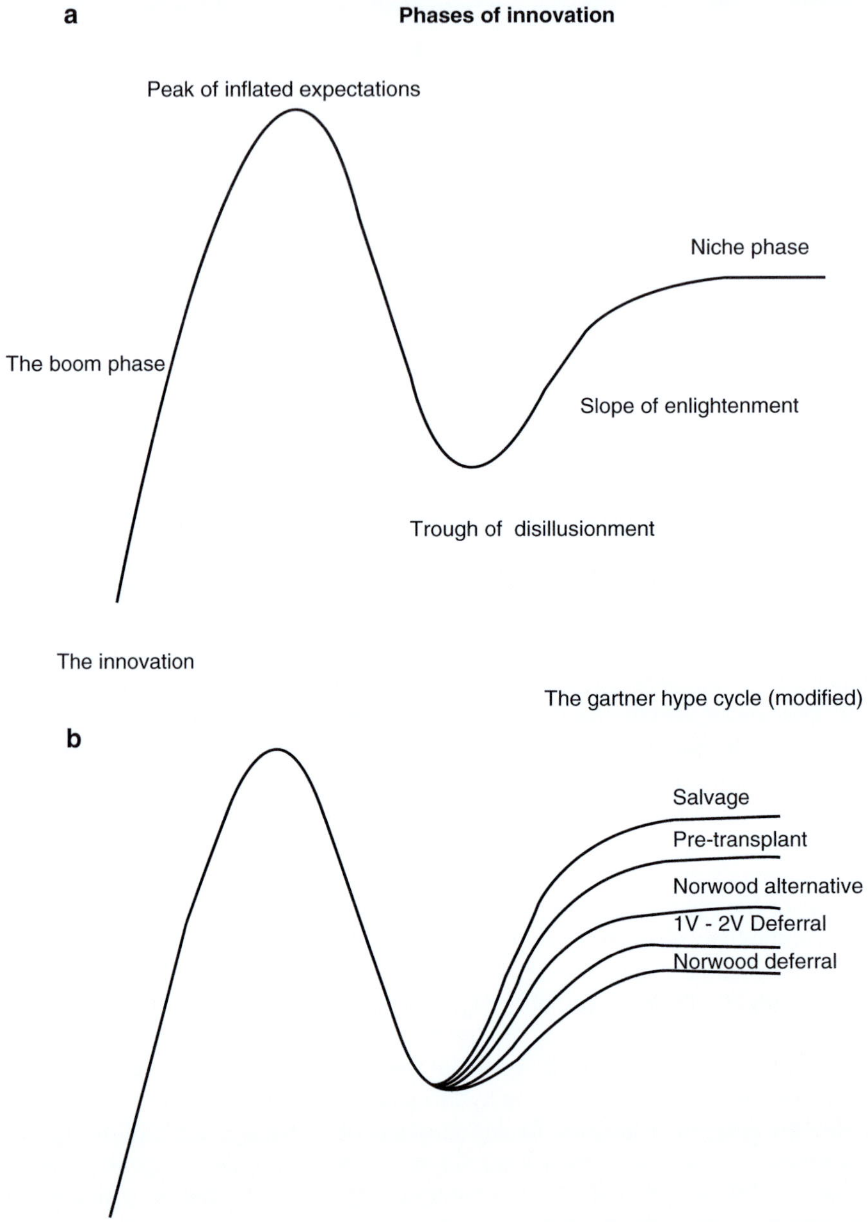

Fig. 31.1 Phases of innovation. Modified Gartner hype cycle panel (**a**). After the application of an innovation (i.e., hybrid procedure), it finds a 'niche' in clinical practice, panel (**b**)

clinical management, the so-called 'boom' phase. After widespread application, weaknesses in the strategy become apparent and centers either abandon the procedure, do not incorporate it into their treatment algorithm, work through the

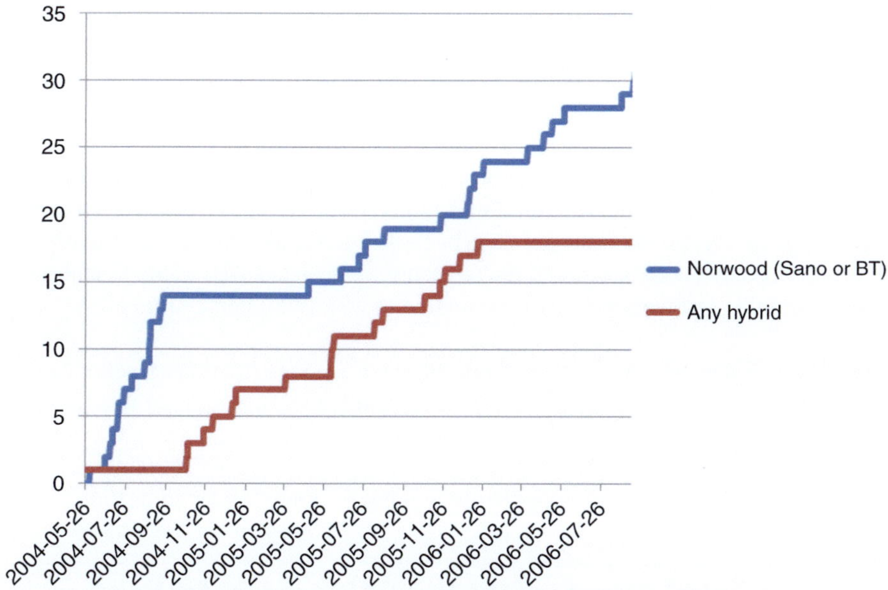

Fig. 31.2 The boom phase, adoption of the hybrid procedure from 2004 to 2006

Table 31.1 Type of surgical palliation for HLHS or its variants

>2.5 kg	Norwood with BT shunt
2–2.5 kg	Norwood-Sano
<2 kg	Hybrid
Bridge to transplant	Hybrid
Potential biventricular repair	Hybrid

identified problems (e.g., impact of an arch coarctation, management of the atrial septum), or identify subgroups where it may be a better alternative to standard therapy (i.e., a primary Norwood) (Fig. 31.1b). The adoption of the hybrid innovation (boom phase) in our unit followed that pathway closely, as can be seen in Fig. 31.2, with rapid introduction of the procedure into clinical practice [9].

31.1 Management of the Infant with HLHS

After a program review and reassessment of treatment approaches in 2012, a focused team was constituted to manage all newborns with HLHS or one of its variants presenting to the hospital to follow a standardized agreed-upon protocol. The choice of surgical palliation was weight based (Table 31.1), with the hybrid procedure for HLHS used for those infants <2 kg. However, it became apparent that there was a subset of infants in whom hybrid physiology would be preferable: those with borderline left ventricular anatomy as a bridge to a biventricular repair, hemodynamic stabilization while awaiting heart transplantation, and as salvage for those infants who present too ill for a Norwood procedure [10, 11]. Furthermore, infants with biventricular hearts, poor ventricular function, and/or significant comorbidities (e.g., infants with truncus arteriosus) could be stabilized over a short period of time, before undergoing definitive surgical repair. A variation on this approach has been the low-birth-weight HLHS infant (or variant) who undergoes a hybrid procedure without ductal stenting and is maintained on prostaglandins until the infant attains a weight where a Norwood procedure can be performed at lower risk [12]. Finally, the hybrid procedure (with or without ductal stenting) has been used as the first component in a rapid (3–4 weeks of age) conversion to a Norwood procedure [13].

Our results Since mid-2012, 13 newborns have undergone a hybrid procedure including five infants as potential biventricular repair candidates, four for poor function, one for prematurity, and three isolated pulmonary artery bands as a bridge to a Norwood, following these guidelines. As can be seen in Fig. 31.3, since 2006, the hybrid procedure has continued to be performed in our unit but for more 'niche' indications.

31.2 Technical Aspects of the Hybrid Procedure for HLHS

The procedure The approach to performing a hybrid procedure in our unit generally follows the recommendations outlined in the early work by Schranz [2], Cheatham [4], and colleagues. There are some features unique to our approach that

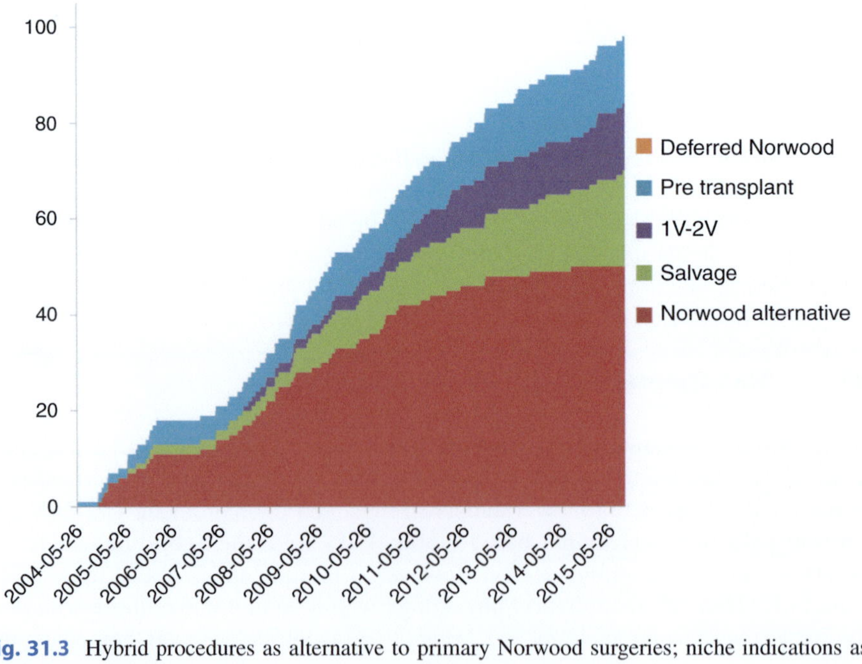

Fig. 31.3 Hybrid procedures as alternative to primary Norwood surgeries; niche indications as applied over the years

will be emphasized. The procedure is performed in one of our hybrid catheterization laboratories using a single AP camera. After the pulmonary artery bands are placed, a radiopaque marker is positioned on left pulmonary artery band, and a 6 Fr short sheath with a sidearm for injection placed with pledgeted sutures just above the pulmonary valve annulus. With the flat panel in a left anterior oblique (LAO), steep cranial projection an angiogram is performed to detail the diameter of the arterial duct and its extent in relationship to the origin of the left pulmonary artery. A 0.035″ exchange guidewire is maneuvered into the descending aorta through the sheath over which a Protégé® GPS® self-expanding stent (eV3, Plymouth, MN) is positioned to traverse the length of the duct. The diameter is chosen to be 1–2 mm greater than the ductal diameter. Care is taken to assure that it is proximal enough toward the pulmonary artery ostium to assure that there is full ductal coverage. Distally, it is ideal to extend up to but not beyond the retrograde aortic ostium, but in our experience, such placement is difficult, and often the stent goes beyond the ostium. Care is also taken not to deliver the stent too distal as that makes subsequent surgical manipulation difficult during later stages. As this stent is a hybrid (closed/open cell) design, the risk of clinically significant retrograde arch obstruction is reduced. If there is aortic atresia, a 'reverse' Blalock-Taussig (BT) shunt is placed (prior to ductal stenting) originating from the main pulmonary artery to the right subclavian artery [14]. If retrograde arch flow is compromised, cerebral and coronary perfusion can be maintained through this connection. If we have not appropriately covered the full length of ductal tissue, there is no hesitancy to implant a second stent.

Post hybrid care The infants are transferred to the cardiac intensive care unit. Initial therapy is goal directed with the mean blood pressure target 45–50 mmHg, SaO_2>70 %, Hgb 140 g/l, NIRS (flanks) >45 %, and a MVO_2>45 %. We use peripheral vasodilation to promote cardiac output with phentolamine, switching to clonidine ± with or without captopril (target 3 mg/kg/day/q8h, but less if low systemic pressure). Attention is paid to evaluation of over-circulation (too loose bands), low saturations (tight bands/restrictive atrial defect), development of tricuspid regurgitation (ductal restriction), or coronary/cerebral ischemia (retrograde arch obstruction). Echocardiographic evaluation is critical, and the decision to perform a cardiac catheterization made early in the child's course as warranted. Management of the atrial septum is the most challenging aspect of care. If the band gradients trend down or saturations fall, we assess the adequacy of the atrial defect and perform a balloon septoplasty/septostomy as required. Although attractive and allowable for a reliable defect, we avoid using an atrial stent as it can become incorporated into the atrial wall and result in pulmonary vein obstruction. Unfortunately, we have found intervening on a fixed atrial defect gradient at times misleading, as repeated measures frequently give conflicting results. If the clinical course is otherwise uncomplicated, in general, we like to perform an elective balloon septostomy just before discharge, particularly if the transatrial gradient is ≥6 mmHg. We have a fixed protocol for transition to the open ward, occurring only between Monday to Thursday before noon, when off any respiratory support for 48 h and without hemodynamic/drug changes for 24 h. The child must be off inotropes for 24 h (except milrinone) with NIRS flank monitoring continuing on the ward. Transition home occurs only if the saturations are 75–85 %; if <75 % or >90 %, they stay on the ward. Function must be better than moderately reduced by echocardiogram. Nutrition is at a minimum 100/kg/day, tolerating 100 kcal/kg/day, and gaining 20 g/day for at least three consecutive days. If a G-tube is required, it must be at a maximum four weeks from initial extubation. Lasix dosage is usually ≤2 mg/kg/day, and the child is on aspirin and Plavix antiplatelet therapy. They also receive clonidine to keep the AVO_2 difference 20–30 based on the NIRS. Finally there must be a minimum 24-h care by parent prior to discharge. If these criteria are not met, the child will remain in hospital during the interstage period. All infants with right or left atrial isomerism are investigated for malrotation; and if so, get a LADDS procedure when stab from the initial procedure. Out of hospital monitoring: Parents are contacted daily for the first week, then weekly by our single ventricle service nurse practitioners. A full-study echocardiogram is obtained every two weeks. We let the child outgrow the clonidine dose if doing well. Immunizations (relative to stage I-II intervals) are performed as standard. The first two clinical visits from discharge are with a single ventricle team physician and nurse practitioner once a week, then every 2 weeks in the single ventricle clinic. There is a weekly conference to review all single ventricle patients including nutrition/feeding and psychological state (monthly)

Conclusion

Innovations go through various stages once introduced into general use. Parallels are found in clinical medicine as exemplified by the introduction of the hybrid procedure for HLHS. Ultimately, no single innovation can fulfill the promise of the “silver bullet,” and with time, experience, and application, what initially was thought of as applicable to all finds a ‘niche’ where the innovation often outperforms its initial expectations.

References

1. Gibbs JL, Wren C, Watterson KG, Hunter S, Hamilton JR. Stenting of the arterial duct combined with banding of the pulmonary arteries and atrial septectomy or septostomy: a new approach to palliation for the hypoplastic left heart syndrome. Br Heart J. 1993;69(6):551–5.
2. Akintürk H, Michel-Behnke I, Valeske K, Mueller M, Thul J, Bauer J, Hagel KJ, Schranz D. Hybrid transcatheter-surgical palliation: basis for univentricular or biventricular repair: the Giessen experience. Pediatr Cardiol. 2007;28(2):79–87.
3. Egan MJ, Hill SL, Boettner BL, Holzer RJ, Phillips AB, Galantowicz M, Cheatham JP, Kovalchin JP. Predictors of retrograde aortic arch obstruction after hybrid palliation of hypoplastic left heart syndrome. Pediatr Cardiol. 2011;32(1):67–75.
4. Galantowicz M, Cheatham JP, Phillips A, Cua CL, Hoffman TM, Hill SL, Rodeman R. Hybrid approach for hypoplastic left heart syndrome: intermediate results after the learning curve. Ann Thorac Surg. 2008;85(6):2063–70; discussion 2070–1.
5. Holzer RJ, Wood A, Chisolm JL, Hill SL, Phillips A, Galantowicz M, Cheatham JP. Atrial septal interventions in patients with hypoplastic left heart syndrome. Catheter Cardiovasc Interv. 2008;72(5):696–704.

6. Li J, Zhang G, Benson L, Holtby H, Cai S, Humpl T, Van Arsdell GS, Redington AN, Caldarone CA. Comparison of the profiles of postoperative systemic hemodynamics and oxygen transport in neonates after the hybrid or the Norwood procedure: a pilot study. Circulation. 2007;116(11 Suppl):I179–87.
7. Rahkonen O, Chaturvedi RR, Benson L, Honjo O, Caldarone CA, Lee KJ. Pulmonary artery stenosis in hybrid single-ventricle palliation: high incidence of left pulmonary artery intervention. J Thorac Cardiovasc Surg. 2015;149(4):1102–10.
8. http://www.gartner.com/technology/research/methodologies/hype-cycle.jsp
9. Caldarone CA, Benson L, Holtby H, Li J, Redington AN, Van Arsdell GS. Initial experience with hybrid palliation for neonates with single-ventricle physiology. Ann Thorac Surg. 2007;84(4):1294–300.
10. Yerebakan C, Murray J, Valeske K, Thul J, Elmontaser H, Mueller M, Mann V, Ostermayer S, Latus H, Apitz C, Schranz D, Akintuerk H. Long-term results of biventricular repair after initial Giessen hybrid approach for hypoplastic left heart variants. J Thorac Cardiovasc Surg. 2015;149(4):1112–20.
11. Guleserian KJ, Barker GM, Sharma MS, Macaluso J, Huang R, Nugent AW, Forbess JM. Bilateral pulmonary artery banding for resuscitation in high-risk, single-ventricle neonates and infants: a single-center experience. J Thorac Cardiovasc Surg. 2013;145(1):206–13; discussion 213–4.
12. Gomide M, Furci B, Mimic B, Brown KL, Hsia TY, Yates R, Kostolny M, de Leval MR, Tsang VT. Rapid 2-stage Norwood I for high-risk hypoplastic left heart syndrome and variants. J Thorac Cardiovasc Surg. 2013;146(5):1146–51; discussion 1151–2.
13. Ota N, Murata M, Tosaka Y, Ide Y, Tachi M, Ito H, Sugimoto A, Sakamoto K. Is routine rapid-staged bilateral pulmonary artery banding before stage 1 Norwood a viable strategy? J Thorac Cardiovasc Surg. 2014;148(4):1519–25.
14. Baba K, Honjo O, Chaturvedi R, Lee KJ, Van Arsdell G, Caldarone CA, Benson LN. "Reverse Blalock-Taussig shunt": application in single ventricle hybrid palliation. J Thorac Cardiovasc Surg. 2013;146(2):352–7.

Prolonged Right-Ventricle-to-Left-Ventricle Support (Hybrid or Surgical) to Delay Decision-Making in Borderline Left Ventricles

32

Stephen C. Brown, Benedicte Eyskens, Bjorn Cools, Filip Rega, Ruth Heing, Derize Boshoff, Bart Meyns, and Marc Gewillig

32.1 Introduction

The management of neonates with hypoplastic left heart syndrome (HLHS) has markedly evolved since the 1950s [1]. Treatment strategies have developed to the extent that now the majority of these children survive until adulthood and beyond. Development of hybrid palliation avoided early circulatory arrest and cardiopulmonary bypass in a neonate, was even possible in low birth weight infants, and combined all the physiological goals requiring only a single surgical sternotomy [2].

Two ends of a spectrum can now clearly be distinguished and managed accordingly. At the one end are neonates with obvious hypoplastic left ventricles (LV) that cannot support the systemic circulation now or later, qualifying only for univentricular repair (UR). At the other end are newborns with a relatively small left heart and a coarctation of the aorta (CoA) that will clearly be able to maintain a biventricular circulation. In between these two extremes are a group at the lower limits of LV functional ability that may or may not sustain a systemic circulation early after birth with a decreasing pulmonary vascular resistance. This ill-defined group, which consists of an LV that is neither rudimentary nor near normal, is generally referred to as "borderline" left ventricles. It includes a heterogeneous group of anatomical and functional LV impairment combined with varying degrees of aortic stenosis

S.C. Brown
Pediatric Cardiology, University of the Free State, Bloemfontein, South Africa

Pediatric Cardiology, University Hospitals Leuven, Leuven, Belgium

B. Eyskens • B. Cools • R. Heing • D. Boshoff • M. Gewillig, MD (✉)
Pediatric Cardiology, University Hospitals Leuven, Leuven, Belgium
e-mail: marc.gewillig@uzleuven.be

F. Rega • B. Meyns
Congenital Cardiac Surgery, University Hospitals Leuven, Leuven, Belgium

G. Butera et al. (eds.), *Fetal and Hybrid Procedures in Congenital Heart Diseases*, DOI 10.1007/978-3-319-40088-4_32

(AS), coarctation of the aorta (CoA), and other forms of the hypoplastic left heart complex such as aortic arch hypoplasia and mitral valve and left ventricle abnormalities alone or in combination. This nebulous group lies in a gray area where no clear definitions or guidelines exist; the clinician is frequently left undecided as to what constitutes the best management. Even more challenging, the decision has to be made soon after birth in patients who might have the potential of catch-up growth. Delaying the decision at this stage will allow some ventricles to develop and expose small LVs which will never cope with a biventricular circulation.

32.2 Hemodynamic Considerations

32.2.1 Fetal Circulation

Normal physiology During fetal life, the right ventricle is responsible for two-thirds of the combined cardiac output allowing parallel development of the fragile pulmonary vascular bed and the complex structured left ventricle. For the left ventricle, 30 % of the preload comes from left-to-right shunting via the foramen ovale (FO) and about 8 % from the pulmonary veins. The main stimulus for growth appears to be the shear stresses as a result of blood flow over the vascular endothelium [3].

Small left hearts If the FO is restrictive, a decrease down to 25 % of normal LV preload may occur. This will decrease LV growth due to a decrease in flow-related shear stresses. In the case of left ventricular outflow and/or aortic obstruction, pressure rises in the developing left ventricle. This pressure overload leads to myocardial hypertrophy resulting in reduction of left heart volume and compliance and, in extreme cases, endocardial fibroelastosis. Mitral valve abnormalities may also compromise LV flows and impact on LV growth. Fetal somatic development is rarely affected because of compensatory increased right heart output.

Fetal intervention Fetal intervention by means of balloon angioplasty may assist in LV growth in antenatally diagnosed borderline left ventricles [4].

32.2.2 Newborn

As long as the ductus arteriosus remains patent, the majority of infants with a borderline left heart will not immediately become severely symptomatic. Other postnatal circulatory changes will also benefit these hearts.

Normal physiology Preload to the left ventricle will increase immediately after birth due to a significant increase in pulmonary flow to the lungs and thus increase pulmonary venous return; this will lead to the so-called unfolding of the left ventricle. This phenomenon can also be observed in infants where the interventricular septum was pushed to the left due to increased right heart pressures or flow antenatally. This unfolding on the LV was also been seen by clinicians within hours and days following prostaglandin administration. Adequate or sufficient catch-up development of the left ventricle may, however, take weeks to months to occur.

Small left hearts Afterload reduction by means of aortic balloon angioplasty in the case of aortic stenosis (AS) will decrease pressure overload on the ventricle resulting in reduction of hypertrophy with resultant improvement in LV filling, compliance, and growth. Left ventricular outflow tract obstruction (LVOTO) and the majority of mitral valve abnormalities are not amenable to percutaneous treatment and will be discussed in the next chapter.

Growth potential The summation of all of the physiological and treatment effects may lead to catch-up growth of the small LV over weeks to months analogous to LV growth observed in severely hypertrophied ventricles of infants of diabetic mothers [5] .

32.3 Criteria for the Diagnosis of Borderline Left Ventricle

A closer look at current decision-making algorithms is validated. These were developed in the previous era where limited options were available and any decision needed to be made within days: Norwood for HLHS or biventricular repair for critical CoA to be performed within days after birth. A biventricular circulation is clearly the preferred option if this can be obtained in a safe and predictable manner. Several parameters have to be taken into account including anatomic (e.g., aortic valve, outflow tract, mitral valve and left ventricular dimensions, and volume) and functional (e.g., ejection fraction, diastolic function, etc.) evaluations using echocardiographic and radiological information:

- Rhodes score (1991) [6] includes variables of indexed aortic root and mitral valve dimensions as well as left ventricle dimensions. Mainly applicable to infants with aortic stenosis.
- Colan score (2006) [7] uses body surface area and valve z-score. Mainly applicable to infants with aortic stenosis.
- Congenital Heart Surgeons Society score (2007) [8]: Apart from the above measurements, it also includes variables of the aortic arch. It can be accessed at www.chs.org.

Several publications have shown these scoring systems not to be universally applicable to all infants with borderline left hearts, still leave a large gray zone, and have shown that different scores predict different outcomes of strategies if calculated for the same patient [9–11]. As a result different calculations, including LV volume assessments, have been used, and newer echocardiographic scoring systems are being developed which combine anatomical and flow characteristics of the left heart or risk of mortality scores [12, 13] . However, to date, no single measurement or combination of measurements is able to unequivocally predict best treatment option for an individual patient. The reason why predictors differ reflects the true nature of a borderline left heart and the shortcomings of current predictors [14].

No clear consensus exists regarding which selection criteria should be used to decide on a UR of BV strategy in infants with a borderline LV. Essentially the question that needs answer is what constitutes the absolute minimum dimensions to allow for BV repair. Even more important some patients clearly show the potential for significant catch-up growth, if sufficient time is allowed. This is important, since going down the wrong pathway can lead to avoidable early and late mortality and morbidity [9, 15–17].

Hybrid strategies (Fig. 32.2) The development of hybrid palliation in recent years and the technical simplicity of this option opened up new avenues of treatment. In the scenario of borderline left hearts, it becomes an attractive option for the following reasons:

- Provide support of the LV by using the RV as temporary assistance
- Can be performed without cardiopulmonary bypass
- Give weeks to months for LV catch-up growth
- Give time and opportunity to treat reversible lesions, e.g., AS, CoA, and left ventricular hypertrophy (LVH)

This could potentially allow for a more weighted decision regarding a univentricular or biventricular strategy and convert more patients safely to a biventricular circulation.

32.4 Right Ventricle-Left Ventricle Assist Strategy

32.4.1 Overview

Our current preferred strategy for infants with borderline left hearts is termed right ventricle-left ventricle assist (RLa) and is demonstrated in Fig. 32.1.

32.4.2 Therapeutic Options

Prostaglandin The immediate decision regarding what to do can initially be delayed by the intravenous administration of prostaglandins (Alprostadil) to maintain ductal patency. This will allow the clinician 1–2 weeks for thorough serial assessment of the left-sided structures and give time for the left ventricle to "unfold" and grow as a result of the augmented preload.

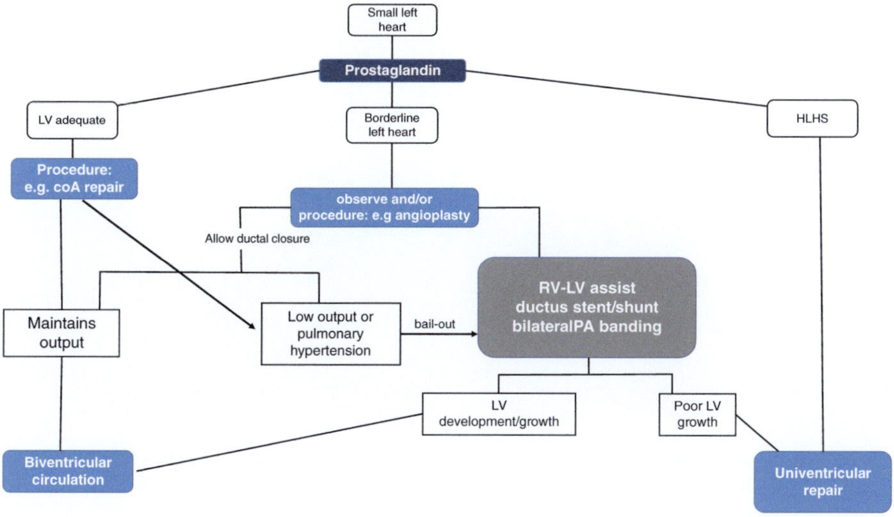

Fig. 32.1 Management strategy

In the latter case, we typically follow with a procedure to unburden the left ventricle. In the case of aortic stenosis, this will consist of aortic valve balloon angioplasty or in the case of aortic arch obstruction coarctectomy or stenting. If the left heart is able to maintain the systemic output, biventricular circulation is aggressively supported.

Right ventricle-left ventricle assist (RLa) This usually consists of bilateral pulmonary artery banding and ductal stenting [18, 19] (Fig. 32.2). Although an elective combined surgical-interventional approach is preferred, a similar result can be accomplished as bail-out procedure by surgery only after an adequate coarctectomy but circulatory failure (see later).

Growth potential If after initial prostaglandin administration after some days the left ventricle remains small but has growth potential (no mitral stenosis, endocardial fibroelastosis) or we are undecided, a hybrid palliation remains our treatment of choice. If the left ventricle after weeks to months shows evidence of development, this option of RV-LV circulatory assist can serve as a bridge to future biventricular circulation [20–22].

No growth potential In the absence of demonstrable or expected left ventricular catch-up growth, the univentricular route with Norwood procedure or hybrid procedure can be chosen.

Surgical RLa In rare cases where the neonatal evaluation and scoring system suggest a good biventricular outcome, but where the postoperative course shows the left heart is not (yet) able to maintain cardiac output, a surgical RLa may be a life saving

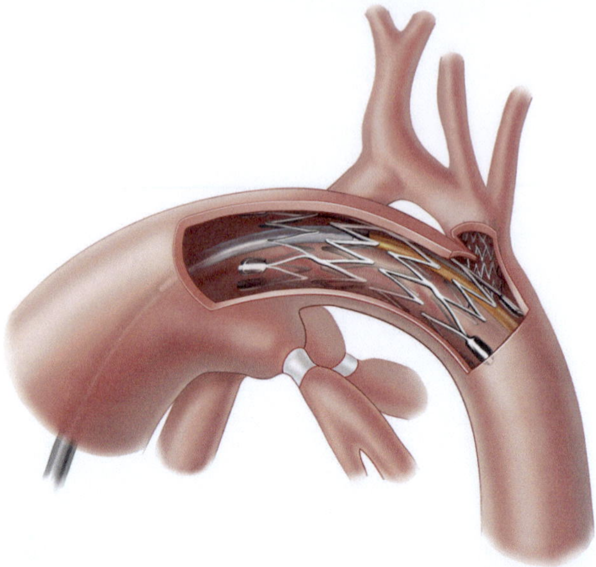

Fig. 32.2 Hybrid right ventricle-left ventricle assist: bilateral pulmonary artery bands and stent in ductus arteriosus also demonstrated. Note: a small stent in aortic isthmus – coarctation; if indicated, the coarctation stent is easier implanted prior to the ductal stent

bail-out procedure. Circulation failure is usually not due to inability of the LV to generate forward flow but as a result of backward failure with the development of retrograde pulmonary hypertension. Pulmonary hypertension may develop early or late, and the resulting interventricular septal shift impinges on the small LV. The surgeon performs bilateral pulmonary artery bandings and a Gore-Tex tube from the pulmonary trunk to thoracic aorta (Fig. 32.3, "reversed" shunt) [23, 24].

32.4.3 Outcomes

32.4.3.1 Results of Strategy

We have performed 18 RV-LV circulatory assist (RLa) procedures for borderline left hearts since 2005. Eleven infants had RLa as the initial procedure as a bridge to biventricular circulation, and two of these proceeded to a univentricular circulation. The majority of these infants (9/11) evolved to a biventricular circulation with a median of 4.4 months (range: 1.5 – 45.8) after the RLa procedure. In the other group ($n=7$) where an initial attempt to relieve LV obstruction was carried out, three ($n=3$) infants of whom one demised evolved to a univentricular circulation. Fifty seven percent ($n=4$) returned to a biventricular circulation with a median of 4 months (range 3.0 – 6.1) after RLa procedure, and one is currently still in follow-up. Characteristics of the groups can be viewed in Table 32.1.

Patients 10 and 11 both initially had a coarctectomy and transection of the ductus arteriosus. After initial stable hemodynamics, they both developed within hours

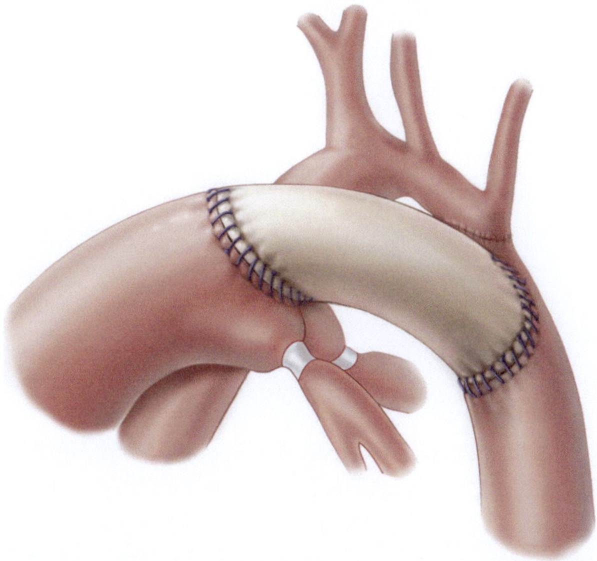

Fig. 32.3 Surgical right ventricular-left ventricular assist procedure "reversed shunt." Bilateral pulmonary artery bands and Gore-Tex pulmonary artery to systemic shunt. Note also that aortic arch was previously reconstructed

suprasystemic retrograde acute pulmonary hypertension with severe RV dilation and compression of the LV. As a result, the small left ventricle could not sustain the systemic output. A "reversed shunt" RLa procedure was performed: a 6 mm Gore-Tex® graft was constructed between the main pulmonary artery and thoracic aorta together with 3.5 mm bilateral pulmonary artery bands (Fig. 32.3). One patient evolved to biventricular repair 4 months later, the other patient to Fontan circulation; both children are doing well.

Patient 13, with a hypoplastic aortic arch complex, proceeded to early RLa. Extensive arch reconstruction (Fig. 32.4b) was carried out 6 months later together with creation of a restrictive interatrial communication to partially decompress the left atrium.

Patient 16 was diagnosed after 6 weeks with Kabuki syndrome, and after consultation with the parents, it was decided that the RLa procedure would be the final palliation. At the last follow-up, the child was 5.5 years old and doing well. This case highlights the fact that RLa procedures can provide long-term palliation with reasonable quality of life in selected cases.

32.4.3.2 Treating Associated Conditions

We have a low tolerance for intervention in these infants following RLa procedures since associated conditions may impede development of the left heart. Aortic valvular stenosis can be safely managed by simple balloon angioplasty. Residual coarctation should be detected early, and balloon angioplasty has been successfully carried out during follow-up.

Table 32.1 Patient characteristics

No	Main lesion	Initial procedure	Age at RLa (day)	Technique	Final procedure	Age (year)
1	AS		9	Percutaneous surgery	Ross	6.5
2	AS		6	Percutaneous surgery	Fontan	
3	AS	BA	28	Percutaneous surgery	PDA closed, bands dilated percutaneously	0.9
4	AS	BA	15	Percutaneous surgery	Arch reconstruction	0.3
5	AS	BA	13	Percutaneous surgery	Fontan	
6	AS	BA	15	Percutaneous surgery	BDG, demise	
7	CoA		8	Percutaneous surgery	Arch reconstruction, subAS resection	1.4
8	CoA		11	Percutaneous surgery	Coarctectomy	0.5
9	CoA		7	Percutaneous surgery	Follow-up	
10	CoA	Coarctectomy	14	Surgical	Arch reconstruction	4
11	CoA	Coarctectomy	14	Surgical	Fontan	
12	CoA-ha		7	Percutaneous surgery	Ventricular septal defect (VSD) closure, debanding	1.6
13	CoA-ha		3	Percutaneous surgery	Arch reconstruction, restrictive fenestration IAS	0.6
14	CoA-ha		3	Percutaneous surgery	Arch reconstruction	0.3
15	CoA-ha	stent CoA	15	Percutaneous surgery	Arch reconstruction	0.6
16	HLHC		8	Percutaneous surgery	Palliative (5.1 year)	
17	HLHC		8	Percutaneous surgery	Kawashima	
18	HLHC		27	Percutaneous surgery	BDG	

AS aortic valve stenosis, *BA* balloon angioplasty, *CoA* coarctation of the aorta, *CoA-ha* coarctation-hypoplastic arch, *HLHC* hypoplastic left heart complex, *BA* balloon valve angioplasty, percutaneous, percutaneous ductus arteriosus stent, and bilateral pulmonary artery banding; surgical, surgical systemic to pulmonary artery shunt and bilateral pulmonary artery banding, *PDA* patent ductus arteriosus, *IAS* interatrial septum, *BDG* bidirectional Glenn

Since ductal stents may show peal or ductal ingrowth over time, these can be balloon dilated or re-stented. Using dilatable bands for the left and right pulmonary arteries is advisable since these can be tailored to adjust flow in relation to somatic growth by balloon angioplasty [25].

Patient 3, with severe AS, had aortic balloon valvuloplasty. The left ventricle was borderline, and an RLa was performed three weeks later. The LV showed continuous improvement in structure and function. The ductus arteriosus stent was later closed by a duct occluder and pulmonary artery bands dilated (Fig 32.4a). This patient was completely rehabilitated by percutaneous means [26].

32.4.3.3 Options for Repair

Fontan Patients proceeding to univentricular circulation typically had extensive aortic arch repair and a Damus-Kaye-Stansel procedure. We often had to treat residual stenosis especially of the left pulmonary artery as a result of banding by means of balloon angioplasty and stenting.

Biventricular circulation This could be accomplished using surgery or by means of percutaneous intervention (see above). Surgery usually consisted of extensive aortic arch reconstruction, clipping the ductus arteriosus, and debanding the pulmonary arteries (Fig 32.4b). Some children required patch plasty at the site of

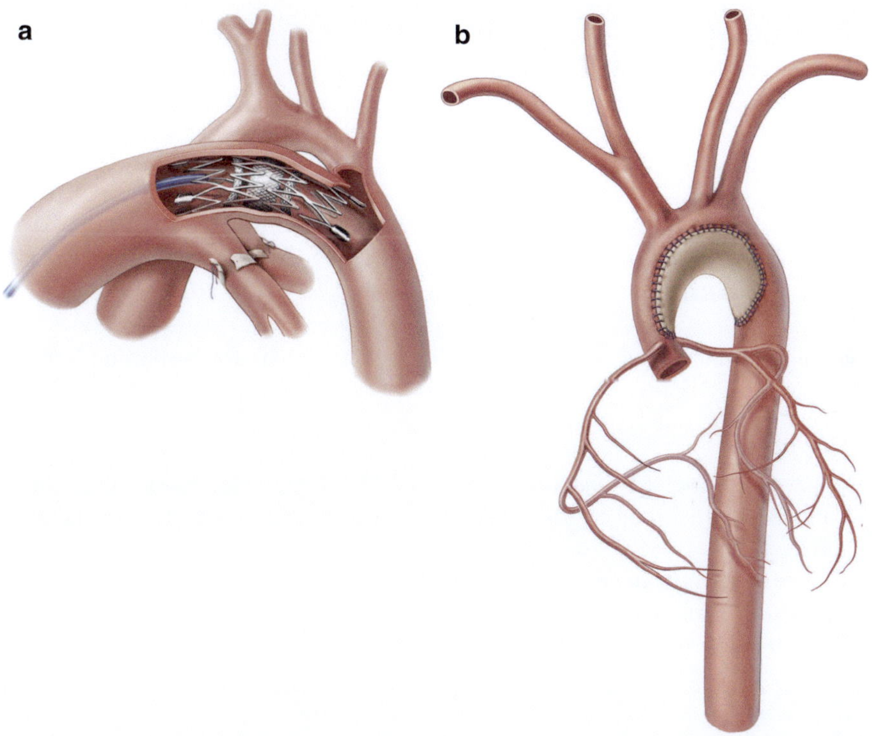

Fig. 32.4 Abolishment of RLa: (**a**) if the aortic arch has sufficiently grown and does not contain a circular stent, the RLa can be occluded percutaneously after balloon release of the PA strips. (**b**) If the aortic arch still shows significant hypoplasia or a circular stent, surgical aortic arch reconstruction is performed

pulmonary artery banding. Several studies have documented good biventricular outcomes in infants with small left hearts [27–31].

32.4.3.4 Impediments to Left Ventricular Growth After RLa Procedures

Mitral Valve

In our experience, certain congenital abnormalities of the mitral valve are an important limiting factor for left ventricular growth in infants with borderline left hearts. Similar to the experience of Del Nido et al., annular hypoplasia, thickened leaflets, commissural fusion, and chordal and papillary muscle abnormalities are common morphological abnormalities seen in these infants and should carefully be assessed and addressed if possible [32].

Endocardial fibroelastosis (EFE) EFE hampers both systolic and diastolic functions of the small left ventricle, and high grades of EFE have been demonstrated to be risk factors for mortality after biventricular repair [33, 34]. Both of our patients with EFE required univentricular circulation.

Atrial septal defect A mildly restrictive shunt through the atrial septal defect (ASD) still allows LV development and further catch-up growth but avoids left atrial hypertension. In selected patients with a small left heart, a mild left-to-right shunt with limited LA hypertension is better tolerated than no shunt but severe retrograde pulmonary hypertension.

32.5 Advantages of Right Ventricle-Left Ventricle Assist Procedure

The main advantages of following this "hybrid approach" for borderline left ventricles are:

- Buy time.
- Allows potential for catch-up growth of LV if possible; most successful in patients where a fetal restrictive foramen ovale was the root cause of the small left heart.
- Can be performed in small and low birthweight infants.
- Allows time for ventricular and somatic growth.
- This strategy can be used as medium term palliation.

Conclusion

The management of infants with borderline left hearts remains a challenge. Current algorithms lacks in ability to discriminate whether biventricular circulation is possible in time if catch-up growth occurs. Right ventricle assist of left ventricle (hybrid) procedures offer the clinician the ability to buy some time to better discriminate which ventricles have adequate growth potential.

Acknowledgement Figures by Medical-illustration: s_philippaerts@hotmail.com

References

1. Lev ML. Pathologic anatomy and interrelationship of hypoplasia of the aortic tract complexes. Lab Invest. 1952;1:61–70.
2. Galantowicz M, Cheatam JP. Lessons learned from the development of a new hybrid strategy for the management of hypoplastic left heart syndrome. Pediatr Cardiol. 2005;26:190–9.
3. Hickey EJ, Caldarone CA, McCrindle BW. Left ventricular hypoplasia: a spectrum of disease involving the left ventricular outflow tract, aortic valve, and aorta. J Am Coll Cardiol. 2012;59(1 Suppl):S43–54.
4. Jantzen DW, Gelehrter SK, Yu S, et al. Echocardiographic factors discriminating biventricular versus univentricular approach in the foetus with borderline left ventricle. Cardiol Young. 2015;25:941–50.
5. Hayati AR, Cheah FC, Yong JF, et al. The role of serum insulin-like growth factor I (IGF-I) in neonatal outcome. J Clin Pathol. 2004;57:1299–301.
6. Rhodes LA, Colan SD, Perry SB, et al. Predictors of survival in neonates with critical aortic stenosis. Circulation. 1991;84(6):2325–35.
7. Colan SD, McElhinney DB, Crawford EC, et al. Validation and re-evaluation of a discriminant model predicting anatomic suitability for biventricular repair in neonates with aortic stenosis. J Am Coll Cardiol. 2006;47(9):1858–65.
8. Hickey EJ, Caldarone CA, Blackstone EH, et al. Critical left ventricular outflow tract obstruction: the disproportionate impact of biventricular repair in borderline cases. J Thorac Cardiovasc Surg. 2007;134(6):1429–36.
9. Tani LY, Minich LL, Pagotto LT, et al. Left heart hypoplasia and neonatal aortic arch obstruction: is the Rhodes left ventricular adequacy score applicable? J Thorac Cardiovasc Surg. 1999;118(1):81–6.
10. Davis CK, Pastuszko P, Lamberti J, et al. The hybrid procedure for the borderline left ventricle. Circulation. 2001;104(6):682–7.
11. Tuo G, Khambadkone S, Tann O, et al. Obstructive left heart disease in neonates with a "borderline" left ventricle: diagnostic challenges to choosing the best outcome. Pediatr Cardiol. 2013;34(7):1567–76.
12. Checchia PA, McGuire JK, Morrow S, et al. A risk assessment scoring system predicts survival following the Norwood procedure. Pediatr Cardiol. 2006;27(1):62–6.
13. Mart CR, Eckhauser AW. Development of an echocardiographic scoring system to predict biventricular repair in neonatal hypoplastic left heart complex. Pediatr Cardiol. 2014;35(8):1456–66.
14. den Dekker MH, Slieker MG, Blank AC, et al. Comparability of Z-score equations of cardiac structures in hypoplastic left heart complex. J Am Soc Echocardiogr. 2013;26(11):1314–21.
15. Hickey EJ, Caldarone CA, Blackstone EH. Biventricular strategies for neonatal critical aortic stenosis: high mortality associated with early reintervention. J Thorac Cardiovasc Surg. 2012;144(2):409–17.
16. Tuo G, Khambadkone S, Tann O, et al. Obstructive left heart disease in neonates with a "borderline" left ventricle: diagnostic challenges to choosing the best outcome. Pediatr Cardiol. 2013;34(7):1567–76.
17. Emani SM, del Nido PJ. Strategies to maintain biventricular circulation in patients with high-risk anatomy. Semin Thorac Cardiovasc Surg Pediatr Card Surg Annu. 2013;16(1):37–42.
18. Galantowicz M, Cheatam JP. Lessons learned from the development of a new hybrid strategy for the management of hypoplastic left heart syndrome. Pediatr Cardiol. 2005;26:190–9.
19. Ringewald JM, Stapleton Elsa G, Suh J. The hybrid approach – current knowns and unknowns: the perspective of cardiology. Cardiol Young. 2011;21:47–52.
20. Brown SC, Boshoff D, Eyskens B, Gewillig M. Hybrid approach as bridge to biventricular repair in a neonate with critical aortic stenosis and borderline left ventricle. Eur J Cardiothorac Surg. 2009;35(6):1080–2.

21. Davis CK, Pastuszko P, Lamberti J, et al. The hybrid procedure for the borderline left ventricle. Circulation. 2001;104(6):682–7.
22. Ballard G, Tibby S, Miller O. Growth of left heart structures following the hybrid procedure for borderline hypoplastic left heart. Eur J Echocardiogr. 2010;11(10):870–4.
23. Brown SC, Boshoff DE, Heying R, et al. Stent expansion of stretch Gore-Tex grafts in children with congenital heart lesions. Catheter Cardiovasc Interv. 2010;75(6):843–8.
24. Brown S, Boshoff D, Rega F, et al. Dilatable pulmonary artery banding in infants with low birth weight or complex congenital heart disease allows avoidance or postponement of subsequent surgery. Eur J Cardiothorac Surg. 2010;37(2):296–301.
25. Brown S, Boshoff D, Rega F, et al. Dilatable pulmonary artery banding in infants with low birth weight or complex congenital heart disease allows avoidance or postponement of subsequent surgery. Eur J Cardiothorac Surg. 2010;37(2):296–301.
26. Brown SC, Boshoff D, Eyskens B, Gewillig M. Hybrid approach as bridge to biventricular repair in an infant with borderline hypoplastic left ventricle. Eur J Cardiothorac Surg. 2009;35:1080–2.
27. Kalish BT, Banka P, Lafranchi T, et al. Biventricular conversion after single ventricle palliation in patients with small left heart structures: short-term outcomes. Ann Thorac Surg. 2013;96(4):1406–12.
28. Han RK, Gurofsky RC, Dipchand AI, et al. Outcome and growth potential of left heart structures after neonatal intervention for aortic valve stenosis. JACC. 2007;50:18–25.
29. Emani SM, Bacha EA, McElhinney DB, et al. Primary left ventricular rehabilitation is effective in maintaining two-ventricle physiology in the borderline left heart. J Thorac Cardiovasc Surg. 2009;138:1276–82.
30. Freund JE, den Dekker MH, Blank AC, et al. Midterm follow-Up after biventricular repair of the hypoplastic left heart complex. Ann Thorac Surg. 2015;99(6):2150–6.
31. Davis CK, Pastuszko P, Lamberti J, et al. The hybrid procedure for the borderline left ventricle. Cardiol Young. 2011;21(1):26–30.
32. Emani SM, Bacha EA, McElhinney DB, et al. Primary left ventricular rehabilitation is effective in maintaining two-ventricle physiology in the borderline left heart. J Thorac Cardivasc Surg. 2009;138:1276–82.
33. Lofland GK, McCrindle BW, Williams WG, et al. Critical aortic stenosis in the neonate: a multi-institutional study of management, outcomes, and risk factors. J Thorac Cardiovasc Surg. 2001;121:10–27.
34. Khambadkone TG, Tann O, Kostolny M, et al. Obstructive left heart disease in neonates with a borderline left ventricle: diagnostic challenges to choosing the best outcome. Pediatr Cardiol. 2013;34:1567–76.

The Anatomical or Functional Borderline Left Ventricle and Strategies for Staged Rehabilitation

33

Pedro J. del Nido

33.1 Introduction

The concept of the "borderline left heart" was introduced following the experience with fetal catheter interventions that aimed to change the natural history of critical aortic stenosis in the fetus. Early attempts to rescue the severely obstructed left ventricle during mid-gestation by transuterine, balloon aortic valvotomy yielded encouraging results in some, with progressive recovery of left ventricle (LV) contractile function in the fetus and associated continued growth of the LV cavity as gestation progressed [1, 2]. However, in about 60 % of these patients, LV growth was inadequate, and at birth, the LV was deemed incapable of supporting the systemic circulation. The constellation of anatomic features varied from that seen in young infants with Shone's syndrome with mitral and aortic valve stenosis and coarctation to that of hypoplastic left heart syndrome. These features included mitral valve stenosis and hypoplasia, aortic valve stenosis, and varying degrees of endocardial fibroelastosis. The latter appeared to develop in utero and we theorized that its presence restricted LV growth in utero and postnatally.

A postnatal program was therefore started to aggressively recruit the left heart structures in infants with borderline left heart by addressing each of the components that were found to be abnormal. The rationale for this approach was based on previous observations that appropriate left heart growth occurred in infants undergoing balloon aortic valvotomy with adjunctive surgical repair of coarctation and mitral stenosis [3, 4]. Also, resection of endocardial fibroelastosis at the time of mitral valvuloplasty for congenital mitral stenosis was found to be feasible and appeared to be associated with improved LV compliance. Staged LV recruitment was utilized in patients where the LV was deemed inadequate because of size and was combined

P.J. del Nido, MD
Department of Cardiac Surgery, Boston Children's Hospital, Harvard Medical School, Bader 275, 300 Longwood Ave, Boston, MA 02115, USA
e-mail: Pedro.delnido@childrens.harvard.edu

G. Butera et al. (eds.), *Fetal and Hybrid Procedures in Congenital Heart Diseases*, DOI 10.1007/978-3-319-40088-4_33

with palliative procedures including the Norwood operation to permit LV recruitment without compromising systemic perfusion. Many lessons were learned in this process, and this concept has now been expanded to other forms of borderline left heart including unbalanced complete atrioventricular (AV) canal defects and complex valve anatomy such as straddling AV valve or common AV valve with inlet VSD and conotruncal anomalies as seen in forms of heterotaxy syndrome.

33.1.1 The Borderline Left Heart

The anatomic and physiologic features that define a borderline left heart have evolved significantly as we have gained a better understanding of the conditions required to maintain adequate systemic circulation under physiologic filling pressures and afterload. Anatomic criteria rely on valve diameter normalized to body surface area, z-score. For ventricular chambers, this criteria applied to cavity volume has been less predictive of ventricular performance under physiologic loads as the interventricular septum can shift with right ventricle (RV) unloading, resulting in a substantial increase in LV volume. Instead, we rely more on the extent to which the LV cavity reaches the apex of the heart as viewed by a standard four-chamber view on echocardiography. LV length along with LV volume are used together to decide whether the chamber size is adequate as we have successfully performed two-ventricle conversion procedures with LV volumes of about 35 ml/m^2 and greater.

33.1.1.1 Anatomic Features

Significant hypoplasia of the inlet and outlet valves, as defined by a z-score between −5 and −2, is frequently found in borderline left hearts. The valves are most often not only hypoplastic but also abnormal in structure. Abnormalities of the mitral valve can include thickened leaflets with fibroelastic tissue on the atrial surface often causing commissural fusion. Fused and shortened chords with basally displaced papillary muscles are a very frequent feature. Abnormal tethering of the leaflets, particularly the mural leaflet by secondary chords, is common. Bicuspid and unicuspid aortic valves are an invariable feature which functionally results in stenosis of varying degrees. After balloon aortic valvotomy, mixed disease with stenosis and regurgitation often is seen and the regurgitation tends to progress.

Endocardial fibroelastosis (EFE) is one of the most variable findings and can range from minimal small patches to extensive covering of the entire endocardial surface including papillary muscles. In the most extreme cases, the fibroelastic layer can reach several millimeters in thickness and is very inelastic. Histologic analysis of EFE tissue has shown a well-organized elastin layer along with collagen, similar to that seen in the walls of great vessels. Unlike the fibroelastic tissue that forms in the sub-aortic region in older infants and young children, the EFE in the borderline left heart is highly cellular. The etiology of the EFE has been studied and appears to arise from endocardial cells that transform into fibroblasts by a process termed endothelial-to-mesenchymal transformation [6].

33.1.2 Physiologic Assessment

Functional assessment of the borderline left heart can be done, in large part, with echocardiography to asses LV cavity dimensions and calculate LV volume and assess systolic function and regional wall motion as well as valve leaflet morphology and movement. With the Doppler interrogation, the degree of valve stenosis and regurgitation can be estimated, and indirect measures of LV chamber compliance can be obtained. For a qualitative assessment of blood flow through heart chamber, color flow Doppler is most helpful. Echo bright endocardium is suggestive of EFE; however, more accurate and quantitative assessment requires magnetic resonance imaging (MRI) with contrast looking for delayed enhancement of the endocardial layer [7]. Cardiac catheterization is reserved for direct pressure measurements of atrial and ventricular pressures, which is most important for assessing LV compliance when deciding whether the LV diastolic function is acceptable for two-ventricle conversion.

33.2 Surgical Strategy

LV growth depends on blood flow through the ventricle and on the fluid forces in diastole that promote chamber growth. Surgical strategies, therefore, aim to promote blood flow into and out of the LV chamber in the borderline heart and to eliminate the fluid force dampening effect of a thick endocardial layer. We hypothesized that EFE, when extensive, can prevent LV growth by serving as an internal dampener of fluid forces and potentially a physical restraint on chamber distention. Therefore, EFE resection is an integral part of the strategy to elicit "catch-up" growth of the left ventricle. To further promote LV growth, the restriction of the interatrial communication was found to be necessary to create a physiologic gradient between the left and right atrium.

33.2.1 Mitral Valve

Mitral valvuloplasty aims to improve valve orifice size, leaflet mobility, and subvalvar restrictions to leaflet movement. The fibroelastic layer commonly found on the atrial surface of the valve leaflets can be peeled away as it forms a layer of inelastic tissue on the leaflet surface, with relatively normal leaflet underneath. This layer covers the commissures and often extends on to the chords and papillaries. Careful removal of the layer frequently leads to opening of the commissures, enlarging the effective orifice of the valve, and improving leaflet mobility. Similarly, the subvalvar structures can be mobilized by removal of the fibroelastic layer. Rarely is leaflet augmentation with pericardium necessary early in infancy. The exception is when there is mitral regurgitation present in association with stenosis.

33.2.2 Aortic Valve

There is often aortic annular hypoplasia in addition to leaflet abnormalities in the borderline left heart. Techniques aim to enlarge the effective orifice and repair torn leaflets in case of regurgitation following balloon dilation. Commissurotomy, leaflet thinning, and resection of any subvalvar tissue often result in substantial reduction in the flow gradient across the valve, even moderately hypoplastic valves. If regurgitation is present following balloon dilation, the disruption is most often on the anterior leaflet and requires leaflet augmentation with pericardium to repair. Reapproximation of a torn leaflet will recreate the obstruction and is rarely effective in reducing or eliminating regurgitation without stenosis. In young infants, the goal is to reduce the outflow obstruction but to preserve the valve if at all possible. Valve replacement is rarely necessary and complicates the procedure and long-term management. Options for replacement are limited in infants and most surgeons will use the Ross procedure with a pulmonary autograft. While effective, the Ross operation is best reserved for when two-ventricle physiology can be achieved. In procedures aiming to recruit the LV, aortic valve repair, sometimes with pericardial augmentation of deficient leaflets, is the best approach.

33.2.3 Endocardial Fibroelastosis

Resection of EFE is a key component of LV rehabilitation [8]. The thick endocardial layer severely restricts LV growth when the extent of endocardium covered by EFE is large and particularly when it involves the posterior free wall and apex of the ventricle. Visualization to remove EFE from the posterior LV wall, papillary muscles, and apex is best achieved through the mitral valve. This is greatly facilitated by the mitral valvotomy. The LV outflow and the outflow part of the septum can be visualized through the mitral valve, but a transaortic approach, particularly at the time of the Ross procedure, is preferred. Sharp dissection is required to remove the EFE tissue as it is densely adherent to the myocardium underneath. The sharp demarcation between the whitish EFE tissue and myocardium guides the extent and depth of resection. All visible EFE should be removed to effectively improve LV compliance and diastolic function.

33.2.4 Restriction of Atrial Septal Defect

Due to the compliance mismatch between the LV and RV in the borderline left heart, an unrestrictive interatrial communication will result in only a small fraction of pulmonary venous return to enter the LV. Thus, in conjunction with measures to improve LV compliance, a restriction must be placed in the atrial septum with a goal of creating a pressure gradient between the atria. We have found that a gradient of 4–6 mmHg is ideal as this will maintain left atrial pressures within a range that will not interfere with pulmonary blood flow, a critical factor in infants and children with single ventricle physiology [9]. As many of these patients will have had single ventricle palliation performed in infancy while LV recruitment is undertaken, adjusting the size and therefore interatrial pressure gradient is important. This is best done with a patch on the septum with a calibrated fenestration. In our experience, a 4 mm fenestration is effective in infants, and 6 mm is ideal in children between 1 and 2 years of age. Further enlargement of the fenestration can be done by catheter balloon dilation and stenting if the septum is thick.

33.2.5 Two-Ventricle Conversion

Conversion from single ventricle palliated physiology to two-ventricle physiology should be done after careful assessment of LV volume and estimate of LV compliance, extent of aortopulmonary collateral blood flow, and mitral and aortic valve function. Of all these factors, LV compliance or diastolic function is the hardest to quantify. Cardiac catheterization is required to measure left atrial and LV end diastolic pressure, but this must be done in the absence of a large left to right shunt at atrial level. Balloon occlusion of the atrial septal fenestration can be a useful maneuver; however, if this communication is large, balloon occlusion is not possible without interfering with mitral inflow. MRI measurements of LV volume, ejection fraction, extent of residual EFE, and, importantly, LV blood flow are critical to assess the ability of the left ventricle to assume systemic circulation under physiologic preload and afterload. Combining MRI measures of LV volume (>35 ml/m^2), with left atrial or LV end-diastolic pressure <20 mmHg and an LV flow of >2.5 L/m^2, usually predicts a good outcome following two-ventricle conversion.

Elimination of as much aortopulmonary collateral blood flow as possible in the catheterization laboratory as well as in surgery will reduce the risk of having significantly elevated left atrial pressures after two-ventricle conversion.

Valvar dysfunction must be addressed at this procedure and often requires aortic valve repair or replacement, commonly done with a Ross operation. Since the takedown of a Stansel connection is usually required, combining this with a Ross procedure is generally the best approach to address LV outflow hypoplasia or residual aortic valve dysfunction. Similarly, the mitral valve must be repaired at least to a level of mild regurgitation or stenosis.

Reconnection of the superior vena cava to the right atrium is part of the two-ventricle conversion procedure in almost all the patients who have had a bidirectional Glenn operation as an interim step for palliation. In almost all cases, the superior vena cava can be connected directly to the right atrium at the appendage; however, this procedure does require that both the cava and the appendage be extensively mobilized so that they can be connected directly with minimal tension.

Anterior patch augmentation and the cavo-atrial connection is a helpful maneuver to prevent stenosis [10].

33.2.6 Unbalanced AV Canal Defects

Children with a common AV valve and an inlet septal defect where the inlet valve is primarily over one ventricle most often have varying degrees of hypoplasia of one ventricular chamber. This subgroup of borderline left heart patients very rarely have endocardial fibroelastosis and, in our experience, have the most predictable response to LV recruitment. LV growth can be achieved by partitioning the AV valve and fenestrated closure of the interatrial communication. In children with heterotaxy syndrome, systemic venous and pulmonary venous abnormalities are common and require baffle diversion to the appropriate atrium at the time of atrial partitioning. We have found that it is not necessary to close or restrict the ventricular septal defect to achieve LV growth and augmenting LV inflow by atrial and AV valve partitioning is sufficient in most.

The decision to convert to two-ventricle physiology involves the same assessment as described for more conventional borderline left heart patients, except that we have found that LV volumes as low as 25 ml/m^2 are sufficient for conversion in this group as shift of the interventricular septum immediately after conversion add significant cavity volume.

33.3 Outcomes and Future Work

Our initial experience with LV recruitment spanned 9 years from 2001 to 2010 [9]. During that time, the techniques for mitral valve and aortic valve reconstruction were developed and combined with resection of EFE. In that period, restriction of the interatrial septum was demonstrated to be a key factor in recruiting the LV. A cohort of 34 patients was compared to a case-matched group of 34 infants with hypoplastic left heart that underwent conventional staged single ventricle palliation [9]. Overall mortality was not different between the two groups and 12 of the initial 34 patients who underwent staged LV recruitment achieved two-ventricle circulation. LV growth was achieved in nearly all the experimental group as shown in Fig. 33.1. The impact of restricting the interatrial communication is shown in Fig. 33.2. The resection of EFE and the restriction of the atrial septum were done at the time of the Glenn procedure in most patients. Gain in LV volume occurred within a year after the Glenn and most patients who ultimately underwent biventricular conversion had gained sufficient LV volume to be considered for two-ventricle conversion within that period of time (Fig. 33.3). Currently, our practice is to begin LV recruitment in early infancy but defer extensive EFE resection and restriction of the interatrial septum to the time of the Glenn, which is typically done between 4 and 6 months of age. The exception is in patients with unbalanced AV

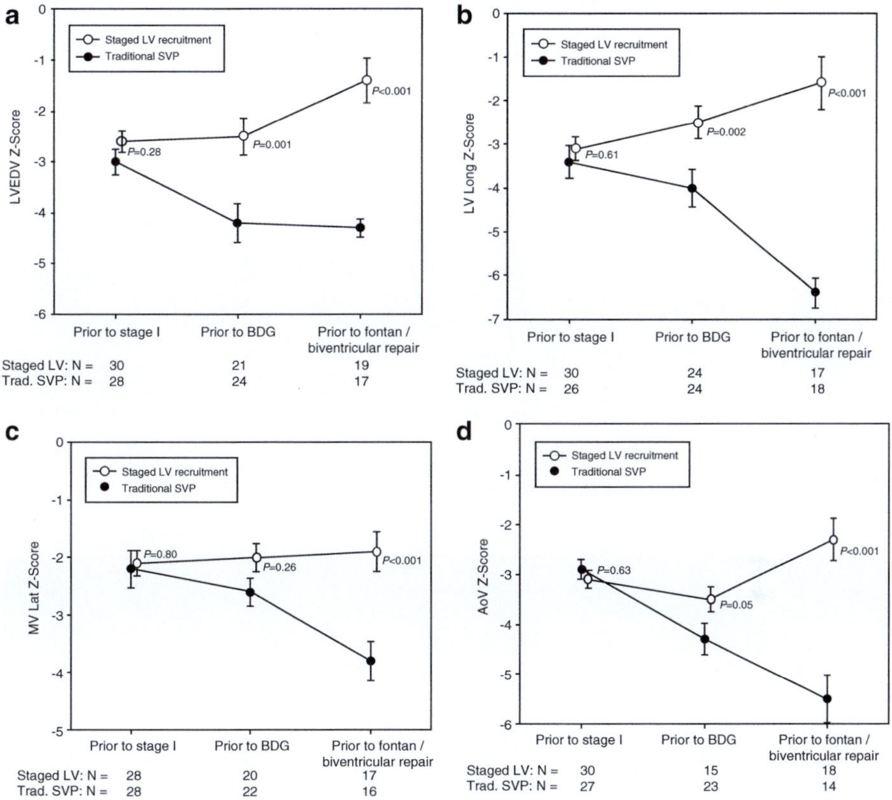

Fig. 33.1 Left heart dimensions at various palliative stages in patients undergoing staged LV recruitment (From Emani et al. [9])

canal defect group where atrial and AV valve partitioning can be done in early infancy.

Age is an important factor with respect to LV growth as we have found that young infants respond much more rapidly to LV recruitment than older children. Our oldest patient to undergo successful staged two-ventricle conversion was 14 years of age at the time of conversion and had Fontan physiology from the age of 3 years. LV volume growth required 2 years of recruitment and even after two-ventricle conversion LV compliance as measured by left ventricular end-diastolic pressure remained abnormal for several years. Thus, we restrict our efforts for two-ventricle recruitment to younger children, typically less than 7–8 years of age.

Late results following two-ventricle conversion indicate that most patients survive the procedure (Fig. 33.4). Reoperation, particularly for mitral and/or aortic valve repair or replacement, is common on late follow-up (Fig. 33.5). By 5 years after the conversion procedure, half of the patients required reinterventions with most of these procedures occurring in the first 2 years. Currently, we prefer to

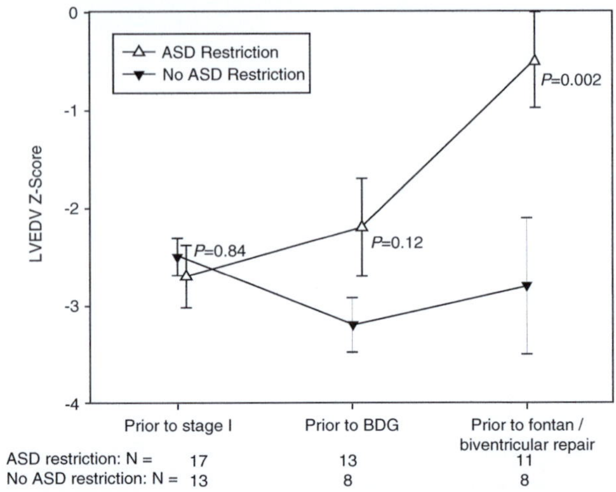

Fig. 33.2 Comparison of left heart dimension between unrestricted atrial septal defect group (*No ASD*), and restricted atrial septal defect group (*ASD restriction*) (From Emani et al. [9])

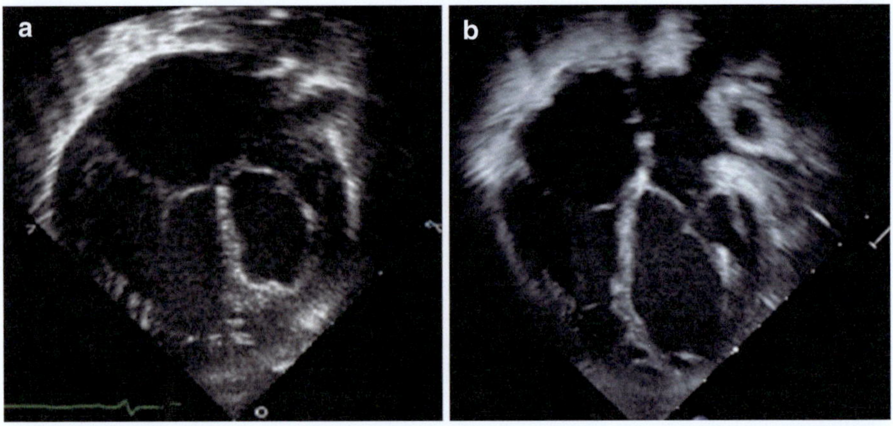

Fig. 33.3 Echocardiogram of representative patient who underwent staged LV recruitment. The LV is endocardial fibroelastosis-bound and non-apex forming (**a**) before stage 1, but apex forming and normal in size (**b**) before biventricular conversion. (From Emani et al. [9])

address the valve defects with more definitive procedures such as a Ross pulmonary autograft at the time of two-ventricle conversion rather than aortic valvuloplasty as this tends to be a longer-term solution for aortic valve dysfunction in these patients. Mitral valvuloplasty in young infants is still our preferred approach as prosthetic replacement carries a high reoperation rate in children less than 5 years of age. In very young infants, we have used a stent-mounted bioprosthetic valve that can be dilated as the child grows [11, 12]. While this experience is limited, we have found

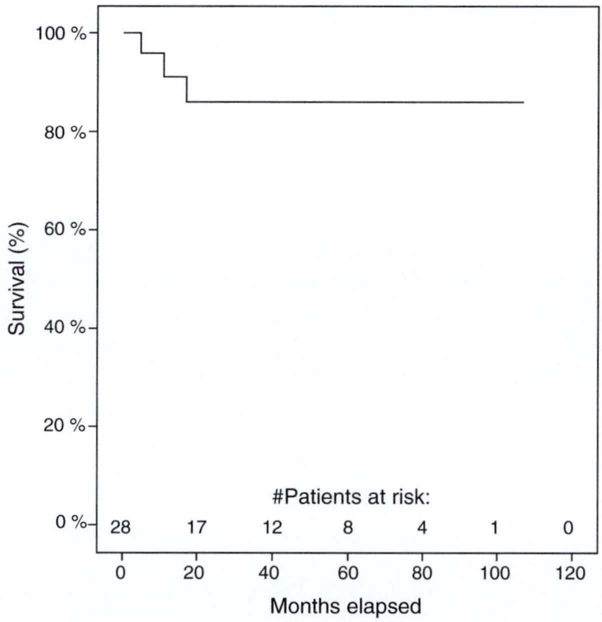

Fig. 33.4 Kaplan-Meier curve of survival after biventricular conversion (From Kalish et al. [5])

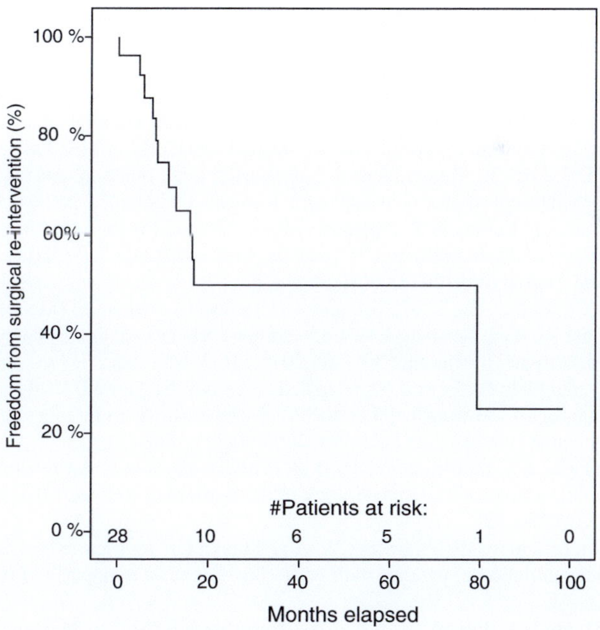

Fig. 33.5 Kaplan-Meier curve of freedom from surgical re-intervention after biventricular conversion (From Kalish et al. [5])

that balloon redilation can be effective in enlarging the prosthetic valve and still maintains valve competence in most [12].

Conclusions

Staged LV recruitment is a viable strategy to achieve two-ventricle physiology in children with a borderline left heart. The specific steps required are dictated by the anatomic features that are present at birth and can include EFE resection, mitral and aortic valvuloplasty, and restriction of interatrial communication. Patients with unbalanced AV canal defects represent a subgroup that rarely if ever have EFE and staging is best achieved by partitioning the common AV valve and restricting the atrial septum. Initial palliative procedures are almost always required as attempts at neonatal biventricular repair often carry a prohibitive risk. In patients with EFE, resection and recruitment of the LV is best started at the time of the Glenn procedure as the larger heart structures in this age group permit a more effective resection as compared to the neonatal period. Late results with this strategy are encouraging in that most children survive late. However, mitral and aortic valve repair or replacement procedures are common following biventricular conversion.

References

1. McElhinney DB, Marshall AC, Wilkins-Haug LE, et al. Predictors of technical success and postnatal biventricular outcome after in utero aortic valvuloplasty for aortic stenosis with evolving hypoplastic left heart syndrome. Circulation. 2009;120:1482–90.
2. Freud LR, McElhinney DB, Marshall AC, et al. Fetal aortic valvuloplasty for evolving hypoplastic left heart syndrome postnatal outcomes of the first 100 patients. Prenat Diagn. 2014;31:695–8.
3. Han RK, Gurofsky RC, Lee KJ, et al. Outcome and growth potential of left heart structures after neonatal intervention for aortic valve stenosis. J Am Coll Cardiol. 2007;50:2406–14.
4. McElhinney DB, Lock JE, Keane JF, et al. Left heart growth, function, and reintervention after balloon aortic valvuloplasty for neonatal aortic stenosis. Circulation. 2005;111:451–8.
5. Kalish BT, Banka P, Lafranchi T, Tworetzky W, del Nido P, Emani SM. Biventricular conversion after single ventricle palliation in patients with small left heart structures: short-term outcomes. Ann Thorac Surg. 2013;96(4):1406–12.
6. Xu X, Friehs I, Zhong Hu T, Melnychenko I, Tampe B, Alnour F, Iascone M, Kalluri R, Zeisberg M, del Nido PJ, Zeisberg EM. Endocardial fibroelastosis is caused by aberrant endothelial to mesenchymal transition. Circ Res. 2015;116(5):857–66.
7. Tworetzky W, del Nido PJ, Powell AJ, Marshall AC, Lock JE, Geva T. Usefulness of magnetic resonance imaging of left ventricular endocardial fibroelastosis in infants after fetal intervention for aortic valve stenosis. Am J Cardiol. 2005;96(11):1568–70.
8. Emani SM, Bacha EA, McElhinney DB, et al. Primary left ventricular rehabilitation is effective in maintaining two-ventricle physiology in the borderline left heart. J Thorac Cardiovasc Surg. 2009;138:1276–82.
9. Emani SM, McElhinney DB, Tworetzky W, et al. Staged left ventricular recruitment following single ventricle palliation in patients with borderline left heart hypoplasia. J Am Coll Cardiol. 2012;60:1966–74.
10. Baird CW, Myers PO, Borisuk M, Kalish B, Hofferberth S, Nathan M, Emani SM, del Nido PJ. Takedown of cavopulmonary shunt at biventricular repair. J Thorac Cardiovasc Surg. 2014;148(4):1506–11.

11. Abdullah I, Ramirez FB, McElhinney DB, Lock JE, del Nido PJ, Emani S. Modification of a stented bovine jugular vein conduit (melody valve) for surgical mitral valve replacement. Ann Thorac Surg. 2012;94(4):e97–8.
12. Quiñonez LG, Breitbart R, Tworetsky W, Lock JE, Marshall AC, Emani SM. Stented bovine jugular vein graft (Melody valve) for surgical mitral valve replacement in infants and children. J Thorac Cardiovasc Surg. 2014;148(4):1443–9.

Part VIII

Pulmonary Arteries

Pulmonary Arteries: Surgical Point of View

34

Matteo Trezzi and Adriano Carotti

Surgical repair of the pulmonary artery (PA) branches encompasses many different clinical scenarios and technical challenges. Branch PA stenosis can occur either primarily or following a previous attempt at surgical repair. In cases of complex congenital heart disease (CHD) requiring reoperations or staged palliation, surgical patch angioplasty is often needed and may prove challenging. Aside from elective indications, surgical PA plasty is necessary following complications of percutaneous stent implantation such as PA dissection or rupture, stent migration, suboptimal stent expansion, stent thrombosis, stent restenosis, airway compression, and inhibition of PA growth. The main challenge in PA surgery is to obtain a spatially pleasing reconstruction in three dimensions.

Exposure can be suboptimal secondary to adhesions, scarring with concomitant calcification, bleeding, excessive collateral flow and previous stent implantations. In addition, extensive dissection around the PA branches can lead to thinning and rupture of the vessel and injury to the phrenic nerve, lymphatics and other vascular structures. The repair is routinely carried out anteriorly, through a midline sternotomy, generally on bypass, as access to the distal branches compromises the pulmonary blood flow. The usual approach includes extensive PA dissection with control of peripheral branches, which are temporarily occluded using neurovascular clips. The pulmonary vessel is opened longitudinally, overcoming the area of stenosis or hypoplasia both proximally and distally, trying to keep the incision line far from secondary branch takeoff. Patch reconstruction is achieved using subtle running sutures. When adhesions do not allow for external control of the vessel or its peripheral branching, the principle of endovascular clamping can be applied using small sized Pruitt or Fogarty catheters. Although a wide variety of materials have been proposed for PA reconstruction, we give our preference to untreated autologous pericardium, pulmonary homograft tissue, and, more recently, commercially

M. Trezzi (✉) • A. Carotti
Unit of Pediatric Cardiac Surgery, Bambino Gesù Children's Hospital IRCCS, Rome, Italy
e-mail: matteo.trezzi@opbg.net

G. Butera et al. (eds.), *Fetal and Hybrid Procedures in Congenital Heart Diseases*, DOI 10.1007/978-3-319-40088-4_34

available bio-scaffolds. In this chapter, we present a focused description of our experience with surgical PA plasty in relation to few specific conditions.

34.1 PA Plasty Following Pulmonary Atresia/Ventricular Septal Defect/Major Aortopulmonary Collaterals Repair

The condition of pulmonary atresia, ventricular septal defect (VSD), and major aortopulmonary collaterals (MAPCAs) can have an extremely variable pulmonary blood supply. Surgical repair can be very challenging though it has been carried out with increasing frequency and success, creating a new population of patients who require a specific and complementary surgical and interventional strategy in order to address residual distal PA stenosis. Between September 1994 and July 2015, 94 patients underwent one-stage repair of pulmonary atresia with MAPCAs at our institution. Median age and weight at operation were 1.09 years and 7.9 kg (range, 2.5–68), respectively, whereas median number of MAPCAs unifocalized was 3.5 (range, 1–7). Forty-eight patients (65.5 %) underwent either surgical or interventional procedure during the follow-up. Freedom from reintervention was 25 % at 12.5 years after initial surgery. Actuarial analysis showed that reintervention rate was progressive during the entire follow-up interval. While right ventricular to PA conduit reinterventions are routinely performed to bridge the patient to the next surgery, we do not recommend PA stenting (unless in patients who have almost reached complete body development) but only PA balloon angioplasty in order to promote PA growth and allow comfortable subsequent stage reconstructive surgery.

34.2 PA Plasty Following Hybrid Palliation for Hypoplastic Left Heart Syndrome

PA hypoplasia and stenosis often complicates the second stage palliation after a Norwood procedure. Mechanisms contributing to PAs compromise are multiple and include narrowing at the ductal remnant site, extrinsic compression by the neoaorta or the ductal stump, and distortion by the modified Blalock-Taussig shunt insertion. Particularly at risk for these influences is the retroaortic segment of the common PA and the proximal and mid segments of the left PA. Compromised flow may contribute to PA hypoplasia over time, which can increase morbidity of the subsequent bidirectional cavopulmonary anastomosis and Fontan procedures. Higher rates of PA intervention (particularly the left) and less developed PA structures have also been reported with hybrid-based palliation when compared with Norwood palliation [1, 2]. Reinterventions are primarily related to the PA bands placed at the time of the hybrid procedure. In addition, smaller PA band diameter and PA band duration longer than 90 days are both thought to be detrimental to the branch PAs [3]. We recently moved to a four-stage approach to hypoplastic left heart syndrome, performing the Norwood procedure 40–50 days after the initial hybrid palliation, thus avoiding neonatal cardiopulmonary bypass. A few weeks after hybrid palliation, fibrosis around the PAs has not yet developed, allowing for simple PA debanding without the need for surgical patch plasty (Fig. 34.1). If surgical reconstruction of the PAs is needed, we utilize autologous tissue excised from the exuberant pulmonary confluence. We elect is to resect the redundant pulmonary confluence, reestablish it by direct suture, and use the resected tissue to create an extended reconstruction of the neopulmonary arterial confluence (Fig. 34.2). The long-term

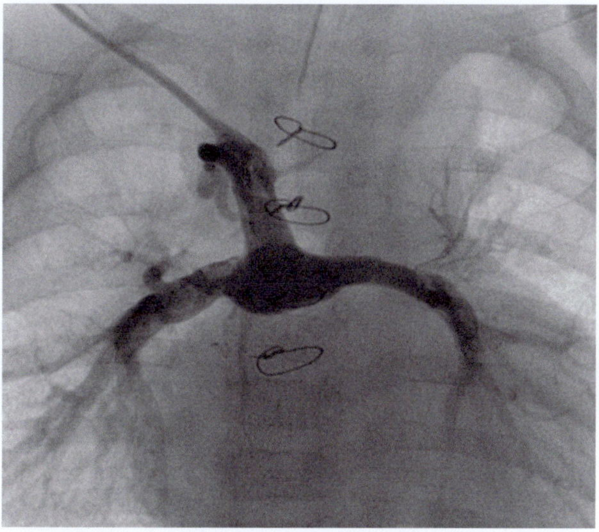

Fig. 34.1 Post-operative angiography following bidirectional Glenn shunt

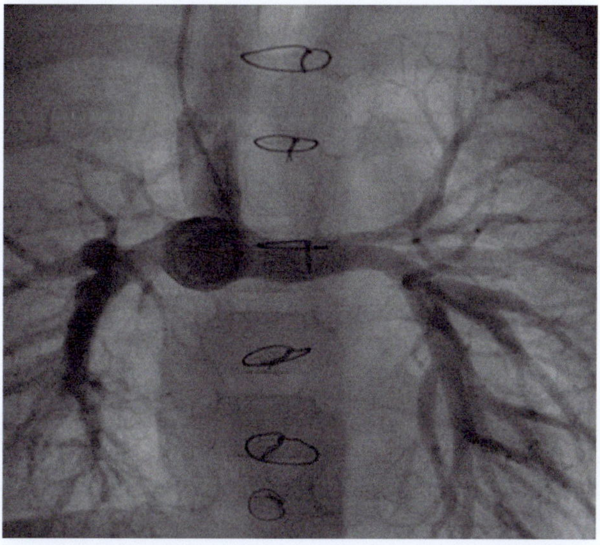

Fig. 34.2 Postoperative angiography following bidirectional Glenn anastomosis and central PA reconstruction

impact of multiple reinterventions on pulmonary arterial growth (both central and peripheral) is not clear. It remains to be seen whether long-term Fontan circuit pressures and ultimately clinical failure rates will be affected by the multiple pulmonary arterial interventions required to bring them to Fontan.

34.3 PA Plasty in Case of Previously Delivered Stents

Surgical reconstruction of PAs in case of previously delivered stents can be a difficult undertaking, due to the stiffness of the tissue to be incised and sutured to, especially in long-standing conditions. The usual approach, when possible, is to remove either the stent itself or together with the pulmonary arterial tissue merged with it. In case of recent stent deployment, up to 3 months, in our experience, under direct vision the stent can be carefully crumpled up and removed, producing minimal damage to the vessel intima. Subsequent vessel reconstruction is carried out in the usual manner. When the stent is strongly merged into its wall, we try to achieve an extended vessel mobilization, resect the stented PA segment, and perform a posterior end-to-end anastomosis with anterior patch enlargement (Fig. 34.3). This latter approach, however, is feasible only when the distal end of the stent is sufficiently

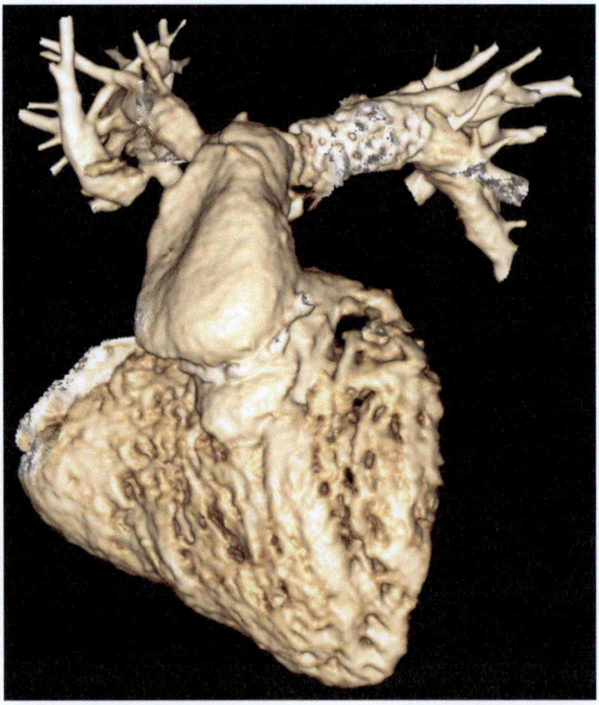

Fig. 34.3 Postoperative 3D CTA rendering

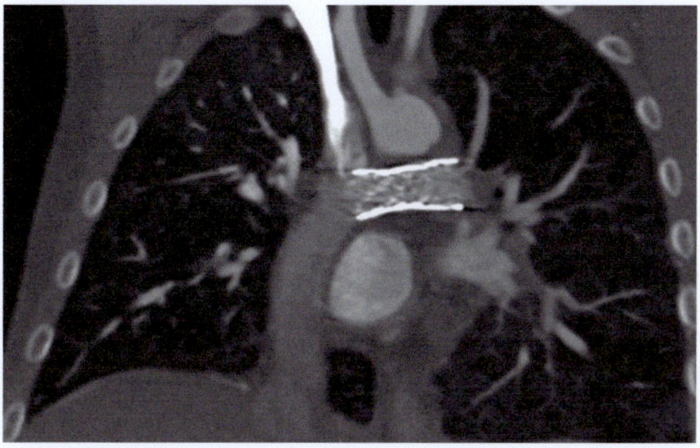

Fig. 34.4 Stent placed at the level of the pulmonary confluence

far from secondary branching of the pulmonary artery. When the stent either approximates or includes secondary branching of PAs, it is safer to leave the stent in place, open it longitudinally including into the incision both proximal and distal PA's native tissue, and perform the patch reconstruction of the pulmonary artery in the usual manner. The interrupted struts of the stent enhance the risk of bleeding along with patch or suture damage.

34.4 PA Plasty at the Time of Fontan Completion in Patients with Hypoplastic Left Heart Syndrome

Pulmonary artery growth is an important determinant of outcome in single-ventricle strategies. Flow dynamic models of Fontan pathways point to the importance of PA geometry as a determinant of pulmonary flow efficiency in relation to early and late outcomes [4]. In addition, when a failing Fontan patient undergoes heart transplantation, surgery may be challenging at the site of previous PA stenting (Fig. 34.4).

34.5 Conclusive Surgical Considerations

PAs stenosis/hypoplasia constitutes a challenge which may negatively affect both early and late outcomes in patients with CHD. Whenever percutaneous balloon dilation proves either unfeasible or ineffective, surgical reconstruction should be considered the treatment of choice, both for native and post-surgical PA lesions, especially in pediatric patients who have not reached their full body development. Stent placement into the PAs may reduce the potential for vessel growth and make subsequent surgery difficult and risky. For this reason, it should be reserved for rescue situations, in case of very difficult surgical approach or in any case in patients with almost completed body development.

References

1. Baba K, Kotani Y, Chetan D, Chaturvedi RR, Lee KJ, Benson LN, Grosse-Wortmann L, Van Arsdell GS, Caldarone CA, Honjo O. Hybrid versus Norwood strategies for single-ventricle palliation. Circulation. 2012;126(11 Suppl 1):S123–31.
2. Rahkonen O, Chaturvedi RR, Benson L, Honjo O, Caldarone CA, Lee KJ. Pulmonary artery stenosis in hybrid single-ventricle palliation: high incidence of left pulmonary artery intervention. J Thorac Cardiovasc Surg. 2015;149(4):1102–10.
3. Davies RR, Radtke WA, Klenk D, Pizarro C. Bilateral pulmonary arterial banding results in an increased need for subsequent pulmonary artery interventions. J Thorac Cardiovasc Surg. 2014;147(2):706–12.
4. Hsia TY, Migliavacca F, Pittaccio S, Radaelli A, Dubini G, Pennati G, de Leval M. Computational fluid dynamic study of flow optimization in realistic models of the total cavopulmonary connections. J Surg Res. 2004;116(2):305–13.

Exit Angiography

35

Ralf J. Holzer

35.1 Introduction

Very few physicians would disagree that it is in the best interest of a patient to leave the operating room with a good surgical result. Significant residual pathology complicates postoperative recovery, and the outcome of patients requiring cardiac catheterization after cardiac surgery prior to hospital discharge is poor. Asoh and colleagues reported on the outcome of 49 children who underwent 62 cardiac catheterization procedures after cardiothoracic surgery prior to hospital discharge and found a need for catheter interventions in 56 % and surgical reoperation in 37 %, with an overall mortality of 43 % [1]. With this data, identifying and preemptively treating residual structural pathology reduces postoperative hemodynamic compromise and is clearly preferable to rescue interventions. Yet, despite those very convincing arguments for completion (exit) angiography after cardiothoracic surgery, the technique is only selectively used in most centers. While there are many reports of using exit angiography in peripheral vascular interventions, coronary artery bypass grafting, as well as carotid thromboendarterectomy (TEA) [2–5], only very few reports exist on the findings and clinical implications of exit angiography [6, 7]. This is in sharp contrast to transesophageal echocardiography which has become a standard intraoperative diagnostic tool with data having documented a significant impact through the use of routine perioperative transesophageal echocardiography [8]. However, while transesophageal echocardiography is an excellent tool for assessing intracardiac anatomy and ventricular function, its use is much more limited for the evaluation of extra cardiac vascular structure. This is where completion angiography has distinct advantages, and this chapter will outline some of the technical considerations as well as discussing patient selection and outcomes of completion angiography.

R.J. Holzer, MD, MSc, FSCAI
Division Chief Cardiology (Acting), Sidra Cardiovascular Center of Excellence, Sidra Medical and Research Center, PO Box 26999, Doha, Qatar
e-mail: rholzer@sidra.org

G. Butera et al. (eds.), *Fetal and Hybrid Procedures in Congenital Heart Diseases*, DOI 10.1007/978-3-319-40088-4_35

35.2 Patient Selection

Given the limited data available on exit angiographies after cardiothoracic surgery for congenital hart disease, selecting the appropriate patients for completion angiography can be somewhat subjective. In the data reported by Holzer and colleagues, the most common lesions that resulted in interventions after exit angiography included patients undergoing a bidirectional Glenn, comprehensive stage II, Fontan completion, or other vascular interventions such as tetralogy of Fallot repair [6].

Many additional questions remain unanswered given the lack of data presently available. For example, it is unclear whether exit angiography should be limited to patients with specific surgical concerns or whether angiographies should be performed in all patients with a specific surgical diagnosis. This dilemma is not unique to congenital heart disease. For example, exit angiography after carotid TEA has been performed since the 1980s [9]. A study published in 2006 found no significant difference in neurological complications or a 30-day stroke and death rate when comparing a group that routinely underwent completion angiography to a group that only performed completion angiography selectively at the surgeon's discretion [5]. Despite this data, controversies on when completion angiography should be performed after carotid TEA are still ongoing [10, 11]. All those concerns apply equally to completion angiographies performed after congenital cardiothoracic surgery.

Furthermore, once an anomaly is identified, it is also unclear which finding would require surgical or transcatheter intervention and which findings can be left alone. Imaging appearance immediately after surgical correction with the patient still on cardiopulmonary bypass and an open chest may be different from what we would expect in the catheterization laboratory. This may lead to some patients undergoing unnecessary re-explorations with potential associated complications. Whether prospective studies will ultimately be able to provide a definitive answer to these questions is unclear, given that in order to identify which lesion would need to be corrected, it would require to have a group of patients in whom residual pathology would be left uncorrected, which clearly poses an ethical dilemma.

For the time being and with the lack of data, careful patient selection is required and the surgical as well as the interventional team should review the scheduled surgical procedures and decide in advance if a "routine" completion angiography should be performed. In addition to preoperative selection, there will always be patients where a surgical concern arises during the procedure, thereby requiring an unplanned exit angiography. Given the data reported by Holzer and colleagues, it would be beneficial to select all patients that undergo a Glenn or comprehensive stage II procedure, as well as most patients with complex pulmonary artery, aortic, or coronary reconstructions for a routine exit angiography.

35.3 Technique

Completion angiography does not require any unusual equipment, and while a dedicated hybrid suite has some advantages in the setup, it is not required, and a simple portable c-arm combined with a power injector (especially for larger patients) is all that is needed. However, careful planning is of utmost importance. It is beneficial to review the surgical schedule well in advance to identify those patients most likely benefitting from a completion angiography. If a dedicated hybrid operating room is available at an institution, those procedures should then be scheduled within that room. If this is not the case, then arrangements need to be made to have a portable c-arm and power injector readily available within the time frame of the surgery. The exact timing can be difficult to predict and therefore it is important that the equipment is available for the entire procedure, and not suddenly being removed by other departments. In addition, it is important to be sure to have the necessary expertise in operating the portable c-arm, especially as it relates to available image storage and calibrating options. Identifying a problem or lack of "know-how" during a procedure should be avoided and problems solved in advance. Furthermore, arrangements need to be made to have the necessary supplies (angiographic catheters, adapters for the power injector, contrast, sterile covers for c-arm, etc.) available within the operating room, so that no time is wasted by having to retrieve the items from the catheterization laboratory.

Radiation protection is very important when performing completion angiographies. While lead aprons should be readily available and are suitable for staff not scrubbed in during the procedure, this is clearly not a feasible option for the surgeon and surgical assistant(s) who are scrubbed in for a longer period. However, Sawdy and colleagues have documented the usefulness of sterile bismuth-based radiation protection drapes during hybrid procedures, which have very similar radiation protection qualities than a standard lead apron [12]. The drapes can easily be attached with clamps to the surgical gown and disposed after the angiography is performed. In addition, it is advisable that staff not immediately required near the operating table move away from the c-arm, preferably in a shielded area if available.

Education and training of operating room staff is crucial and should include not only radiation protection, but also an overview of the catheters and equipment used for completion angiographies, so that these procedures can be performed with the aid of staff working in the operating room.

The completion angiography also requires some advanced coordination with the cath lab staff as well as an interventional cardiologist or nurse practitioner. This is crucial to aid in performing the angiography and the associated setup, as well as providing the necessary expertise to choose the appropriate camera angles and injection parameters. There is no point performing a completion angiography if the area of interest is not profiled appropriately.

Advancing the c-arm into position, whether ceiling mounted or portable, can be challenging. However, the more frequently these procedures are performed, the more expertise is gained by all members of staff working in the operating room, which usually leads to a significant improvement in the time required for setup. A variety of equipment has to be navigated, which includes the anesthesia setup, the cardiopulmonary bypass, as well as any portable surgical trays and tables. For these reasons, the angles that can be achieved in the OR are somewhat limited, but higher degrees of right anterior oblique (RAO) or left anterior oblique (LAO) angulation can be achieved by carefully tilting the operating room table. The injection site is usually determined by the vascular structure that needs to be visualized, and the chosen angiographic catheter is advanced through either a surgical suture line or a purse string. Care has to be taken when choosing the appropriate angiographic settings, as a freshly operated vessel – in particular a fresh suture line – is more susceptible to staining and vascular injury (Fig. 35.1), especially if the injection site is in close proximity to a fresh suture line. Therefore it is advisable to choose lower power injections with a higher rate of rise to limit those problems. The angiographic image quality can be improved by temporarily coming off cardiopulmonary bypass, which should be considered in each patient whenever feasible.

The angiographic setup for performing a rotational angiography in the operating room is even more complex. While this technique can add invaluable information in selected patients, the setup can be time consuming and to some degree disrupts the surgical procedural flow (Fig. 35.2). Therefore patient selection is crucial when considering a rotational technique in the operating room.

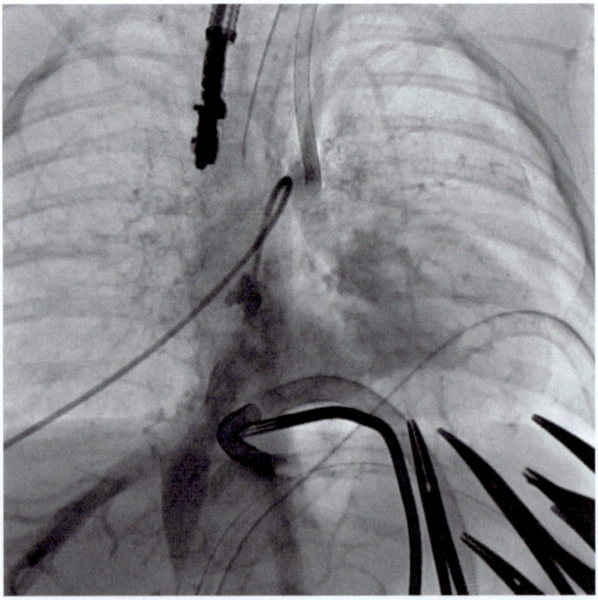

Fig. 35.1 Staining after exit angiography. A 2-year-old patient undergoing Fontan completion. The angiographic catheter was inserted in close proximity to the suture line, leading to vascular injury/staining

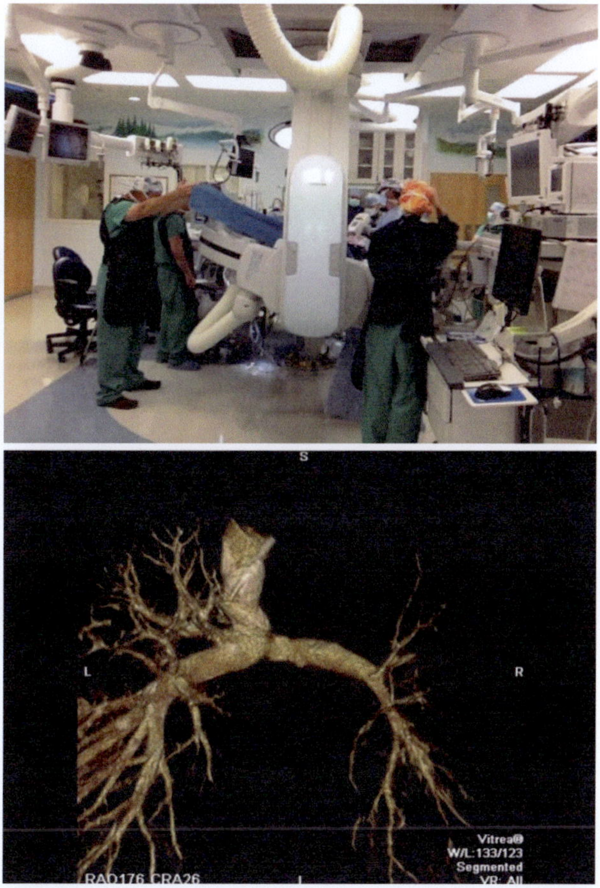

Fig. 35.2 Rotational exit angiography. An 8-month-old infant undergoing a bidirectional Glenn procedure. A rotational angiography was performed. *Top image*: setup prior to performing a rotational angiography in the hybrid operating room. *Bottom image*: 3D reconstruction of the rotational angiography documenting a mild left pulonary artery (LPA) stenosis

35.4 Outcomes

Outcome data on completion angiographies is limited [6]. Data reported by Holzer and colleagues documented an unexpected pathology in 56 % of exit angiographies, with a change in patient management occurring in as much as 28 % of exit angiographies [6]. Updated data on exit angiographies (not published) was presented at the Pediatric Interventional Cardiac Symposium (PICS) in 2013, documenting an 11 % rate of intraoperative interventions (either transcatheter intervention or surgical revision) resulting from exit angiographies. In general, change in management includes surgical revision on cardiopulmonary bypass (Fig. 35.3), surgical revision of cardiopulmonary bypass (Fig. 35.4), transcatheter intervention such as a pulmonary artery stent placement (Fig. 35.5), change in medical management (such as change in anticoagulation), or early recatheterization. While for many of the identified abnormalities there would be very little disagreement in whether to intervene or

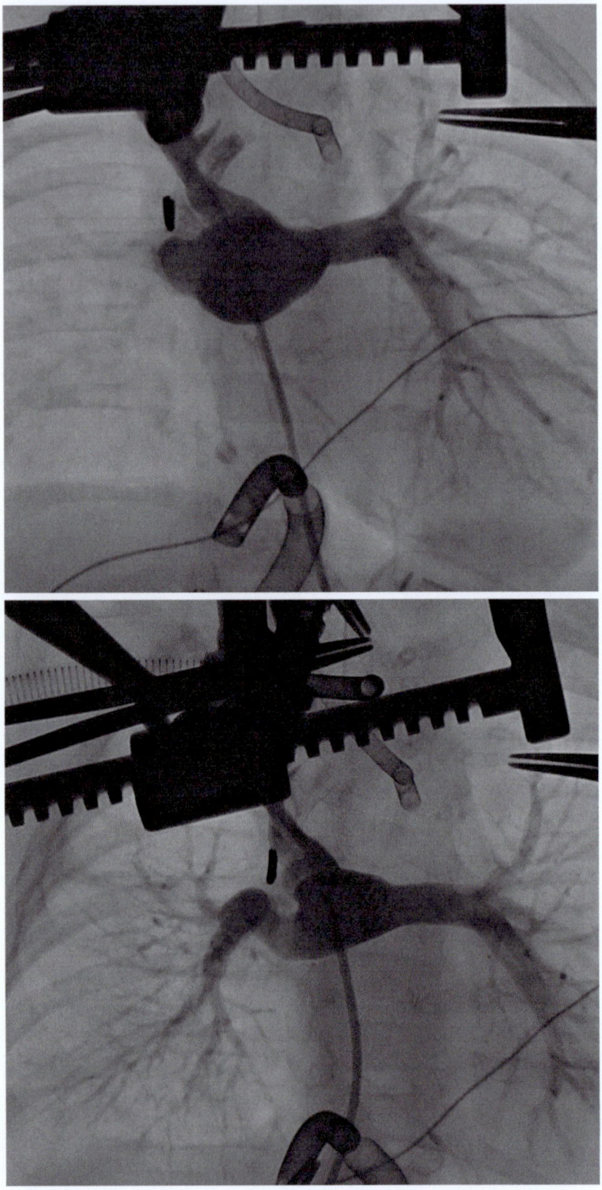

Fig. 35.3 Revision on CPB as a result of exit angiography. A 9-month-old infant undergoing a bidirectional Glenn procedure. Exit angiography documented absent flow to the right pulmonary artery. A revision was performed on cardiopulmonary bypass with an excellent anatomical result

not, this however does not apply to all cases, and therefore when to intervene after an abnormal finding remains an important unanswered question. The updated data on exit angiographies performed at Nationwide Children's Hospital (presented at PICS 2013) identified 9 % of patients with exit angiography that required early recatheterization after surgery, clearly highlighting the difficulty in deciding which lesion to treat or not.

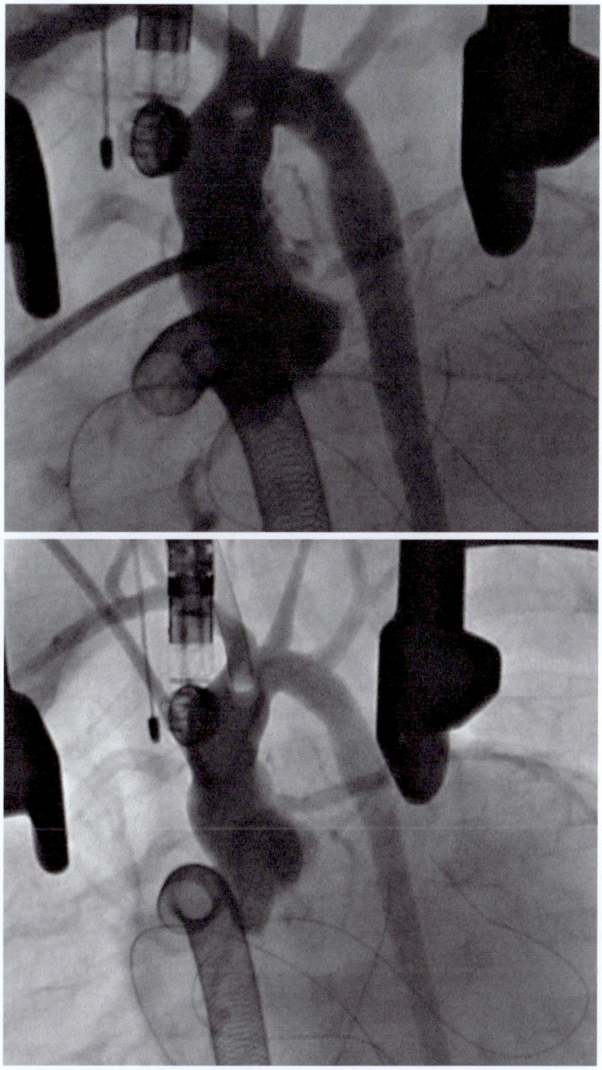

Fig. 35.4 Revision of CPB as a result of exit angiography. A 2-month-old infant with anomalous origin of the left coronary artery from the pulmonary artery. After surgical repair an angiography was performed in the ascending aorta documenting a proximal filling defect of the left coronary artery. Adhesions and external compression were removed without the use of cardiopulmonary bypass and a subsequent angiography documented an appropriate surgical result

35.5 Summary

Exit angiography is an excellent tool to identify postoperative vascular abnormalities. It requires careful planning and a proactive approach to selecting the appropriate patients. While many questions remain unanswered, in particular, relating to patient selection and which lesions require treatment, this should not be a deterrent from using this tool diligently, as it has the ability to identify postoperative abnormalities that would otherwise not be detected by conventional imaging modalities. With careful planning, this tool has the ability to

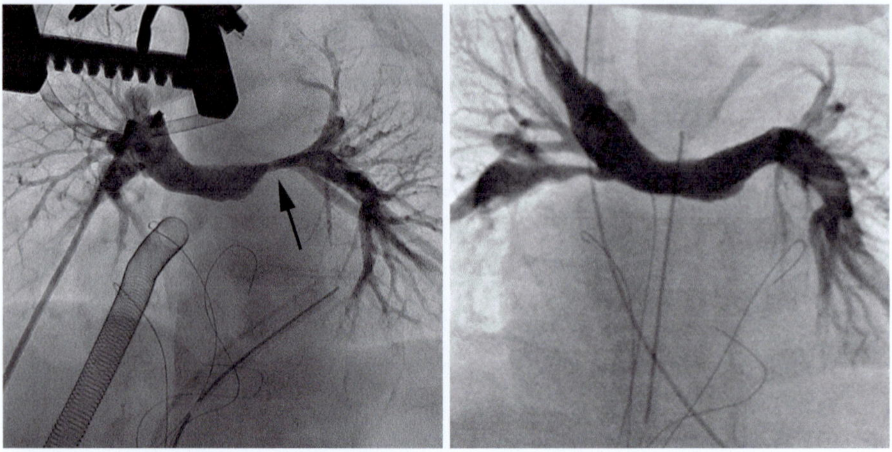

Fig. 35.5 Intraoperative stent placement as a result of exit angiography. A 6-month-old infant undergoing a comprehensive stage II palliation. Exit angiography documented a distal stenosis of the behind left pulmonary artery (*arrow*). A stent was placed intraoperatively

improve postoperative outcomes and should be part of the standard intraoperative imaging techniques used in every center.

References

1. Asoh K, Hickey E, Dorostkar PC, et al. Outcomes of emergent cardiac catheterization following pediatric cardiac surgery. Catheter Cardiovasc Interv. 2009;73(7):933–40.
2. Khilnani NM, Trost D, Jagust MB, Sos TA. Multiple-side-hole catheter technique for selective over-the-wire completion angiography following renal angioplasty. J Vasc Interv Radiol. 1994;5(2):387–9.
3. Helmick RA, Mesh CL. The importance of antegrade completion angiography in aortobifemoral bypass limb revision. J Vasc Surg. 2012;55(4):1141–4.
4. Zhao DX, Leacche M, Balaguer JM, et al. Routine intraoperative completion angiography after coronary artery bypass grafting and 1-stop hybrid revascularization results from a fully integrated hybrid catheterization laboratory/operating room. J Am Coll Cardiol. 2009;53(3):232–41.
5. Pratesi C, Dorigo W, Troisi N, et al. Routine completion angiography during carotid endarterectomy is not mandatory. Eur J Vasc Endovasc Surg. 2006;32(4):369–73; discussion 374.
6. Holzer RJ, Sisk M, Chisolm JL, et al. Completion angiography after cardiac surgery for congenital heart disease: complementing the intraoperative imaging modalities. Pediatr Cardiol. 2009;30(8):1075–82.
7. Shuhaiber JH, Bergersen L, Pigula F, et al. Intraoperative assessment after pediatric cardiac surgical repair: initial experience with C-arm angiography. J Thorac Cardiovasc Surg. 2010;140(1):e1–3.
8. Randolph GR, Hagler DJ, Connolly HM, et al. Intraoperative transesophageal echocardiography during surgery for congenital heart defects. J Thorac Cardiovasc Surg. 2002;124(6):1176–82.
9. Jernigan WR, Fulton RL, Hamman JL, Miller FB, Mani SS. The efficacy of routine completion operative angiography in reducing the incidence of perioperative stroke associated with carotid endarterectomy. Surgery. 1984;96(5):831–8.

10. Ricco JB, Schneider F, Illuminati G. Part one: for the motion. Completion angiography should be used routinely following carotid endarterectomy. Eur J Vasc Endovasc Surg. 2013;45(5):416–9.
11. Samson RH. Part two: against the motion. Completion angiography is unnecessary following carotid endarterectomy. Eur J Vasc Endovasc Surg. 2013;45(5):420–2.
12. Sawdy JM, Gocha MD, Olshove V, et al. Radiation protection during hybrid procedures: innovation creates new challenges. J Invasive Cardiol. 2009;21(9):437–40.

Role of Three-Dimensional Rotational Angiography in Imaging the Pulmonary Arteries

36

Darren P. Berman

36.1 Introduction

Noninvasive imaging modalities such as echocardiography, cardiac MRI, and CT have greatly enhanced our abilities to assess the pulmonary arteries (PAs) in complex forms of congenital heart disease (CHD). These noninvasive modalities have helped reduce the need for diagnostic cardiac catheterization while simultaneously allowed for effective preprocedural planning for either transcatheter or surgical intervention of complex problems, including PA stenosis.

When intervening, biplane angiography in the cardiac catheterization remains the primary method for assessing the pulmonary arterial anatomy. Calibrated measurements from these two-dimensional angiograms serve as the basis for final decision-making when performing catheter-based interventions. Three-dimensional rotational angiography (3DRA) was first described as an emerging technology in the management of CHD by Kapins et al. in 2010 [1]. It has since been utilized as an adjunctive enhanced real-time imaging modality in the catheterization suite to help understand and properly treat complex anatomical problems in CHD [1–3].

This chapter will provide a broad overview of the role and utility of 3DRA in imaging the PAs in the setting of (1) palliated single ventricle (SV), (2) surgically corrected biventricular CHD (i.e., conotruncal defects following repair), and (3) neonates requiring delineation of pulmonary blood flow.

D.P. Berman
The Heart Center, Nationwide Children's Hospital, Columbus, OH, USA
e-mail: Darren.Berman@nationwidechildrens.org

G. Butera et al. (eds.), *Fetal and Hybrid Procedures in Congenital Heart Diseases*, DOI 10.1007/978-3-319-40088-4_36

36.2 3DRA Acquisition

Acquiring high-quality 3DRA images is fundamentally different in comparison to biplane angiography. Our experience with 3DRA is within a Toshiba Infinix-i biplane flat panel catheterization suite (Toshiba, Japan). While each system has slight variations in image acquisition, the following general principles hold true across all systems. Image acquisition is performed with a single flat panel detector with the lateral detector out of the way. After centering the area of interest on the frontal flat panel, and assuring appropriate table height with the frontal flat panel in the lateral position, an automated series of steps prepares the operator for image acquisition. A single 200° high-speed rotation of the frontal detector over 4–5 s while obtaining 100 digital acquisition frames produces the rotational angiogram. The dataset is transferred to a 3D workstation (Vitrea, Vital Solution, Toshiba) where a 3D reconstruction is created, post-processed, and directly linked back to the Toshiba system. Additional CT-like cross-sectional tomographic images are also generated providing adjunctive information. Current systems now have almost immediate 3D overlay capabilities with live fluoroscopy as deemed necessary for the rest of the procedure.

To maximize image quality, a breath-hold is essential to minimize motion artifact. Additionally, the area of interest must remain fully opacified with nonionic contrast media throughout the acquisition. Tips to help achieve this include the following:

1. Position the angiographic catheter proximal to the area of interest (as opposed to directly within).
2. Program the rotational angiogram with a 0.5–1 s delay such that contrast media begins to inject prior to gantry rotation so that contrast media will have already filled the area of interest from the onset of image acquisition.
3. Rapid ventricular pacing throughout image acquisition with the goal of decreasing blood pressure by ~50 % effectively decreases stroke volume. This not only maximizes opacification of the area of interest, but also reduces unwanted opacification of pulmonary venous return, thus minimizing artifact.

36.2.1 Role of 3DRA Following Cavopulmonary Connection Palliation for SV

Patients born with complex single ventricle (SV) forms of CHD undergo a series of surgical palliations to achieve a stable circulation. Once palliated with a bidirectional Glenn (BDG) or total cavopulmonary connection (TCPC), this group of patients relies primarily on residual kinetic energy provided by a single systemic ventricle and the sucking of blood from the left atrial diastole to allow systemic venous return to reach the distal pulmonary vascular bed and ultimately the left atrium. Unobstructed pulmonary circulation is vital for maximizing circulatory efficiency and reducing early and late morbidity [4, 5]. Unfortunately, a significant number of these patients are at risk for hemodynamically important PA stenoses secondary to either congenital abnormalities or as a consequence of prior surgeries.

Catheter-based intervention is an important tool for addressing these PA stenoses. 3DRA performed within the BDG or TCPC provides significant insight into the mechanism(s) of stenosis (and can thus guide appropriate intervention) as well as improve post-intervention assessment with regard to potential negative impact on surrounding structures, i.e., the aorta and airway [2, 6] (Fig. 36.1).

With this patient population, high-quality 3DRA image acquisition is the norm. Modifying cardiac output in the form of rapid ventricular pacing is typically not needed given the lack of pulsatility through the PAs in these patients. However, if planning to perform simultaneous injections in the reconstructed aorta and BDG to further understand the interaction of adjacent structures, rapid pacing would be recommended to improve image quality within the pulsatile systemic arterial system. Additionally, to maximize image quality in the TCPC, simultaneous injection into two identical catheters positioned within different portions of the TCPC, but "Y-ed" back to a single injector, enables the entire TCPC to be imaged with a single 3DRA with reliably good image quality.

36.2.2 Role of 3DRA Following Surgical Correction of Complex Biventricular CHD

Patients born with conotruncal defects including tetralogy of Fallot (TOF), truncus arteriosus, and D-transpositon of the great arteries (D-TGA) undergo complex surgical correction that requires manipulation of the PAs. This can include patch augmentation of a congenitally stenotic PA, unifocalization of aortopulmonary collaterals, mobilization and reimplantation of a PA, and the Lecompte maneuver as part of the arterial switch operation (ASO). It is thus not unexpected that a number of these patients develop recurrent PA stenosis that can be effectively treated with transcatheter options.

As in patients who have undergone TCPC, 3DRA in this subset of patients provides a number of advantages. A single rotational angiogram in the right ventricle or right ventricular outflow tract (RVOT) provides a volume-rendered 3D reconstruction of the entire RVOT and PA architecture that can be viewed in essentially an endless number of virtual angles (Fig. 36.2). This 3D reconstruction can provide a roadmap with the ideal gantry angles to then perform selective biplane angiograms to guide interventions. This should increase efficiency of correctly profiling PA stenoses and therefore may reduce the total number of digital acquisitions required throughout potentially long complex procedures and secondarily may reduce the total amount of contrast media needed.

The subsets of patients who have undergone an ASO with the Lecompte maneuver are also at risk for PA stenosis. 3DRA with simultaneous injections in the RVOT and aorta maximize our ability to understand the intimate relationship between the

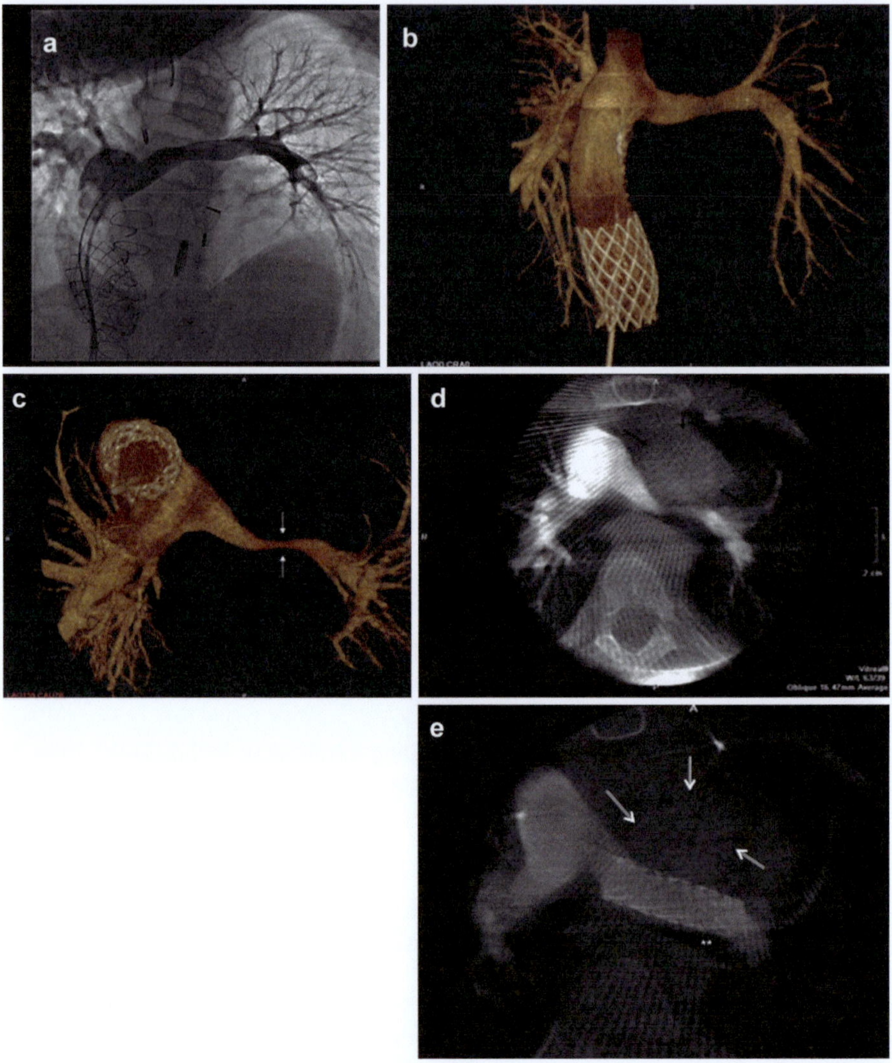

Fig. 36.1 left pulmonary artery (LPA) stenosis secondary to compression from a dilated ascending aorta in a patient following Norwood reconstruction and TCPC with a previously placed IVC stent. A two-dimensional selective LPA arteriogram suggests a diffusely hypoplastic LPA (**a**). A volume-rendered 3D reconstruction in a frontal projection appears similar to the 2D angiogram (**b**). Rotation of the image to a virtual plane (LAO 135, Caudal 78) clearly shows a severe long segment stenosis (**c**), which in a corresponding tomographic image, is shown to be secondary to aortic (*black arrows*) compression (**d**). Following the placement of a large vascular stent, a tomographic slice from a repeat 3DRA clearly demonstrates an expanded LPA and the relationship of the newly stented LPA to the reconstructed aorta (*white arrows*) and left main bronchus (*asterix*) (**e**)

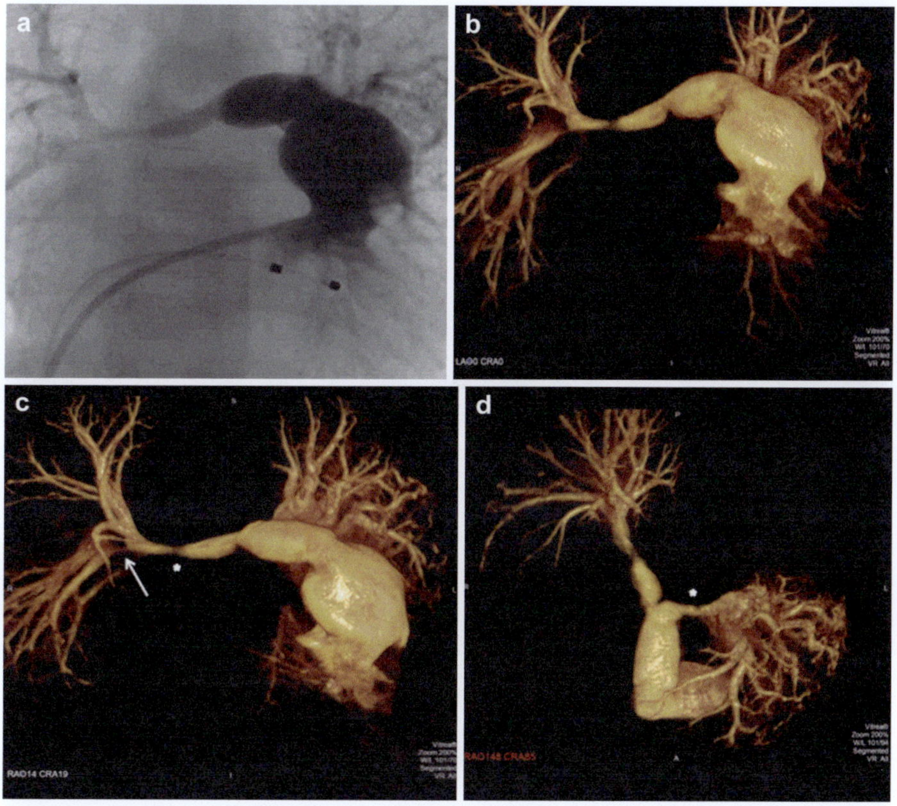

Fig. 36.2 3DRA in a 10-month-old born with TOF and pulmonary atresia who has undergone placement of a conduit to create right ventricle (RV) to PA continuity. The injection was performed with a multi-side-hole catheter positioned in the proximal portion of the RVOT; note the pacing catheter in the body of the RV (**a**). A 3D-reconstructed image of the RVOT and PAs is available within 1–2 min following the angiogram (**b**). The reconstructed image can be used to best profile the right PA and its stenoses (**c**), as well as the more hypoplastic left PA (**d**). Note how the gantry angles correlating with each image is provided in real time as the 3D-reconstructed image is manipulated

stretched PAs and aorta (Fig. 36.3). Further understanding the mechanism of a PA stenosis should help lead to more efficient and effective therapy (i.e., balloon angioplasty versus stent).

36.2.3 Additional Roles of 3DRA in Imaging Pulmonary Arteries

There are several additional scenarios worth mentioning where 3DRA can play a role in effectively imaging the PAs. Patients born with the most complex form

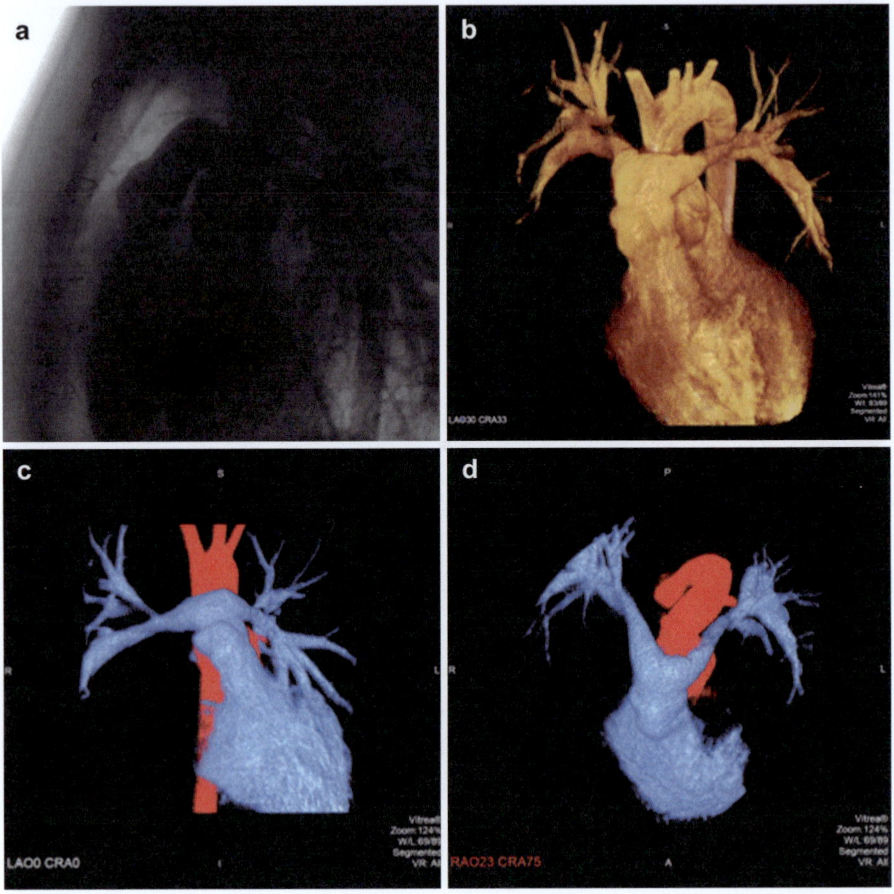

Fig. 36.3 Simultaneous 3DRAs performed in the left and right ventricle in an 18-year-old who has previously undergone an ASO with the Lecompte maneuver for D-TGA (**a**). The 3D reconstruction (**b**) can also be color coded (**c**, **d**) to help show the intimate relationship of the PAs draped over the aorta

of tetralogy of Fallot (TOF) with pulmonary atresia and multiple aortopulmonary collaterals (MAPCAs) require a detailed preoperative assessment of pulmonary blood flow which often includes a cardiac catheterization. 3DRA within the aorta with rapid right ventricular pacing provides a roadmap of pulmonary blood flow (Fig. 36.4).

Additionally, some newborns with ductal-dependent pulmonary blood flow are referred for consideration of arterial duct stenting as a less invasive option for

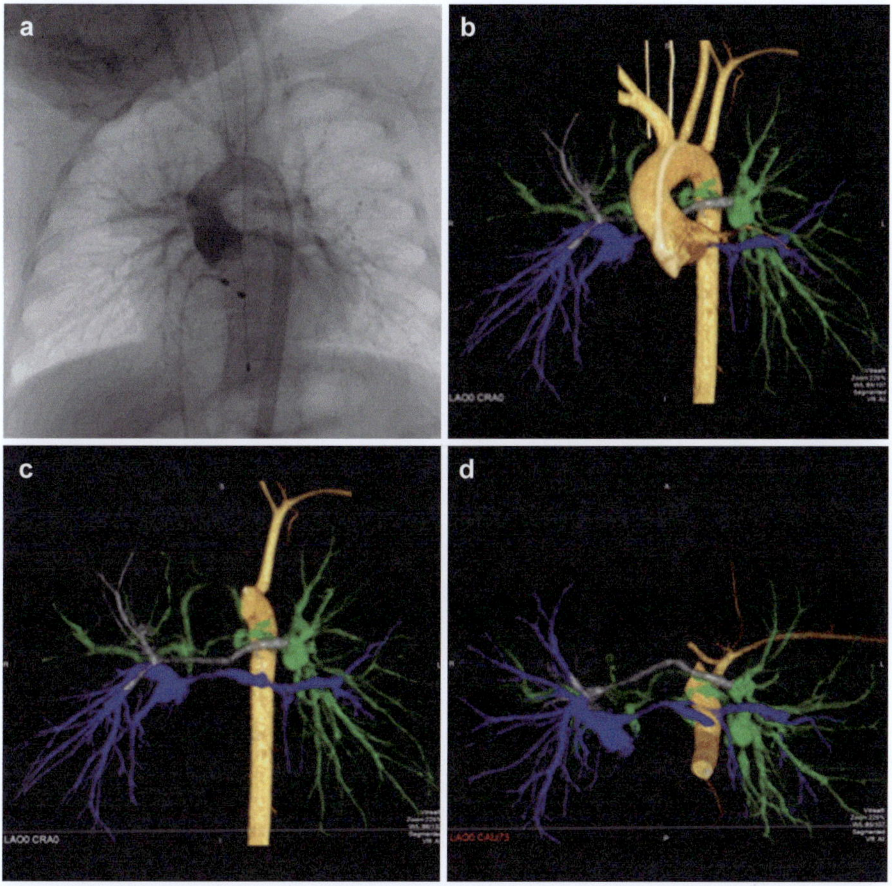

Fig. 36.4 3DRA performed in the aorta with RV pacing (**a**) in this 2-month-old with unrepaired TOF, pulmonary atresia and major aortopulmonary collateral arteries (MAPCAs). This single injection provides a highly informative 3D reconstruction that with additional post-processing (**b–d**) can delineate the diminutive true PAs (*gray*) and the MAPCAs (*blue*, *green*)

securing pulmonary blood flow. The arterial duct itself, as well as its insertion into the proximal PAs, can be tortuous and complex making these procedures challenging. Often, numerous digital acquisitions at various gantry angles are needed in an attempt to best profile the arterial duct and its course as it inserts into the PAs. 3DRA within the aorta with rapid ventricular pacing can help guide these complex procedures (Fig. 36.5).

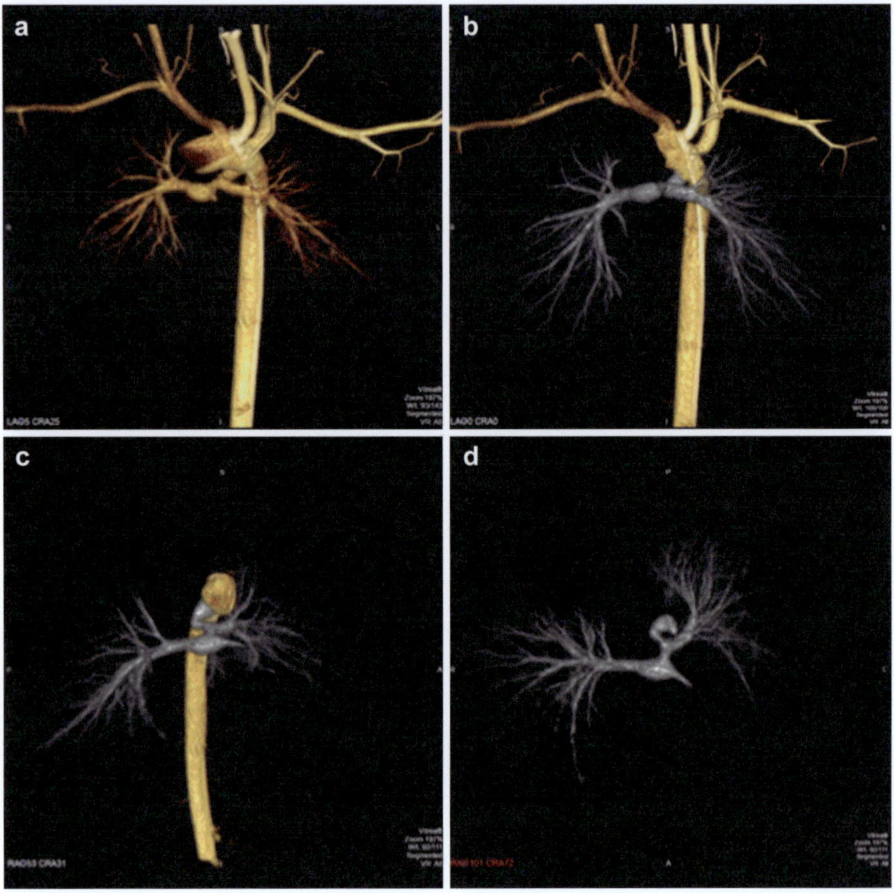

Fig. 36.5 3DRA performed in the aorta with RV pacing in this newborn with TOF and pulmonary atresia adequate sized PAs and ductal-dependent pulmonary blood flow referred for consideration of ductal stenting (**a**). 3D reconstruction nicely demonstrates the origin of the arterial duct, its tortuous course, and its insertion onto the true left PA (**b**, **c**). Further post-processing reveals a significant stenosis to the proximal left PA between the main PA and duct insertion site (**d**). This patient was referred for surgical repair

Conclusion

3DRA is a safe and effective, relatively new technology. It can be used to provide enhanced imaging of the PAs in many of our patients with complex CHD. A single rotational angiogram provides immense data, including a 3D reconstruction that can be viewed in a near endless number of virtual angles, as well as a CT-like tomographic data that can provide insight into the interactions with surrounding structures before and after intervention.

With this immense amount of information gleaned from a single 3DRA, this technology can help reduce the total number of biplane digital acquisitions needed throughout a procedure and, in doing so may reduce total radiation exposure and contrast media needed. Finally, 3DRA allows us to better understand the mechanism(s) of PA stenoses and thus allows us to treat our patients more effectively as well as understand the potential affects our therapies may have.

References

1. Kapins CEB, Coutinho RB, Barbosa FB, Silva CMC, Lima VC, Carvalho AC. Use of rotational 3D (3D-RA) in congenital heart disease patients: experience with 53 cases. Rev Bras Cardiol Invasiva. 2010;18:199–203.
2. Berman DP, Khan DM, Gutierrez Y, Zahn EM. The use of three-dimensional rotational angiography to assess the pulmonary circulation following cavo-pulmonary connection in patients with single ventricle. Catheter Cardiovasc Interv. 2012;80(6):922–30.
3. Glatz AC, Zhu X, Gillespie MJ, Hanna BD, Rome JJ. Use of angiographic CT imaging in the cardiac catheterization laboratory for congenital heart disease. JACC Cardiovasc Imaging. 2010;3:1149–57.
4. Hosein RB, Clarke AJ, McGuirk SP, Griselli M, Stumper O, De Giovanni JV, Barron DJ, Brawn WJ. Factors influencing early and late outcome following the Fontan procedure in the current era. The 'Two Commandments'? Eur J Cardiothorac Surg. 2007;31:344–52.
5. Choussat A, Fontan F, Besse P. Selection criteria for Fontan's procedure. In: Anderson RH, Shinebourne EA, editors. Pediatric cardiology. Edinburgh: Churchill Livingstone; 1978. p. 559–66.
6. Borik S, Volodina S, Chaturvedi R, Lee KJ, Benson LN. Three-dimensional rotational angiography in the assessment of vascular and airway compression in children after a cavopulmonary anastomosis. Pediatr Cardiol. 2015;36(5):1083–9.

Hybrid Approach to Pulmonary Artery Stenosis

37

Evan Zahn

37.1 Introduction

Since its description nearly 25 years ago [1, 2], endovascular stent therapy has become the procedure of choice in many settings involving pulmonary artery stenosis. Early descriptions suggested this therapy was only suitable for larger children and adults; however, advances in technique and technology have allowed pulmonary artery stent therapy to be safely and effectively performed in younger children and infants [3–5]. While improvements in delivery technique, balloon, stent, and sheath technology have made percutaneous stent implantation a more accomplishable procedure, there are numerous clinical scenarios where hybrid stent implantation may be preferable.

37.2 History

Intraoperative pulmonary artery stent implantation was first described by Houde et al. in 1992 [6]. During these early days, stents were placed under direct vision in the operating room with essentially no ability to evaluate the post-implant result. Despite the obvious suboptimal nature of this approach, results reported were good, with improvements in vascular diameter comparable to percutaneous implantation [7–9]. As this therapy was more widely adopted, the technique evolved to include a variety of ways to assess the pertinent anatomy prior to, during, and after stent implantation.

E. Zahn, MD
Guerin Family Congenital Heart Program, Cedars-Sinai Heart Institute, Los Angeles, CA, USA
e-mail: Evan.Zahn@cshs.org

G. Butera et al. (eds.), *Fetal and Hybrid Procedures in Congenital Heart Diseases*, DOI 10.1007/978-3-319-40088-4_37

37.3 Indications and Advantages

There are several important scenarios where hybrid delivery of a PA stent may be advantageous. These include small patient size (e.g., infants and neonates), interventions required in the early postoperative period, limited vascular access, need for concomitant surgical procedures, and as rescue therapy for either a failed percutaneous stent attempt or for a patient unable to separate from cardiopulmonary bypass due to PA stenosis.

Advantages to hybrid PA stent implantation include:

1. The ability to implant a stent with the future capability of achieving an adult diameter regardless of patient size at the time of implant (including young infants)
2. Avoidance of intracardiac catheter manipulation, which may be particularly important for critically ill patients, particularly in the early postoperative period
3. Minimization or avoidance of ionizing radiation
4. Reduction of the total number of invasive procedures by combining several procedures (e.g., conduit replacement and bilateral PA stent placement) into one
5. Improved accuracy of stent placement including the ability to redo the implant if desired and/or flair proximal stents against the PA wall to facilitate future vessel reentry

37.4 Techniques

Two different techniques have evolved for the hybrid delivery of PA stents. The first, stent implantation under direct or endoscopic visualization, is typically a planned procedure performed in the operating room or a hybrid suite. The second, stent implantation via surgically provided vascular access supported with fluoroscopic imaging, can be used to treat not only PA stenoses but several other lesions. This approach can be performed in a standard catheterization suite, surgical operating room (with portable fluoroscopic imaging), or hybrid suite.

37.4.1 Direct or Videoscopic-Guided Stent Implantation

This procedure is typically performed at the time of other required surgical procedures such as right ventricular outflow tract reconstruction, conduit replacement, delayed ventricular septal defect (VSD) closure (in the setting of pulmonary atresia and VSD), bidirectional Glenn, or Fontan palliation. As the availability of fluoroscopy in the operating room and hybrid suites has become more common, this technique has a receding role. A critical component to the success of this technique is a thorough quantitative assessment of all pertinent anatomy *prior to* the actual procedure. Since these implants are done without fluoroscopy/angiography, decisions regarding implant location, stent type/length, and the diameter of the implantation balloon are made prior to the procedure based upon pre-procedural imaging. Typically stents with adult-size potential are chosen, and stent length is determined based on pre-procedural imaging combined with known foreshortened length-diameter relationships, paying special attention to the takeoff of side-branches. The diameter of the implant balloon is chosen to approximate normal vessel diameter adjacent to the stenosis.

Prior to implantation, the target stenosis and surrounding vessel are examined internally and externally using direct visual and/or digital videoscopic examination. A videoscope limits the amount of dissection required to visualize the target lesion, thereby shortening operative and cardiopulmonary bypass times, minimizing trauma to surrounding structures, and preserving supporting tissue as the target stenosis and surrounding vessel are forced to expand with balloon inflation. Landmarks that have been identified on pre-procedural imaging such as side branches are reidentified with the videoscope as final plans for implant are made. Preparation of the stent and balloon differs slightly from normal in several respects. The balloon catheter lumen is flushed, and the balloon itself is inflated and deflated with saline (contrast not needed) prior to mounting the stent to improve stent adherence since no sheath is utilized, and low-profile balloons are preferred for this application. After crimping the stent onto the balloon, stent slippage is assessed by applying gentle traction on the stent. If the stent is loose despite vigorous crimping, the balloon may be inflated slightly to form a "dumbbell" shape, which helps to minimize stent slippage. A slight "hockey stick" curve is placed on the guidewire, which is "preloaded" within the balloon catheter lumen, such that a few centimeters extend beyond the catheter tip. Typically balloons with moderate-burst pressure with low-deflation profiles are used to minimize the chance of pulling back the stent after it has been deployed.

While the surgeon manages the videoscope, the cardiologist places the balloon tip at the orifice of the vessel and advances the tip of the guidewire down the target vessel, directing the wire so as to align the tip with the course of the target vessel (Fig. 37.1). With the wire now advanced several centimeters into a distal branch, the back of the wire is stabilized as the balloon/stent complex is advanced over the wire and across the target lesion. Care should be taken to not damage the balloon or stent if a forceps is being used to advance the complex forward. The videoscope is then advanced down the vessel to confirm and fine-tune positioning prior to inflation. Inflation is typically performed to the manufacturers specified burst pressure, followed by balloon deflation. The balloon catheter is removed over the guidewire in the usual fashion as the surgeon holds gentle pressure on the proximal stent struts to prevent proximal dislodgement. The videoscope is then advanced down the newly stented vessel to assess the end result prior to the removal of the wire. Particular attention is paid to the presence or absence of vascular tears, apposition of the entire stent to the vessel wall, patency of any side branches thought to be at risk, and the integrity of any suture lines that were crossed by the stent. If need be, the stent can be re-dilated with a larger balloon (± higher pressure) if it does not appear fully expanded or apposed to the vessel wall. When satisfied with the end result, the wire is removed, and the surgeon may flare any proximal struts that may be protruding into the main PA, particularly when treating ostial stenoses.

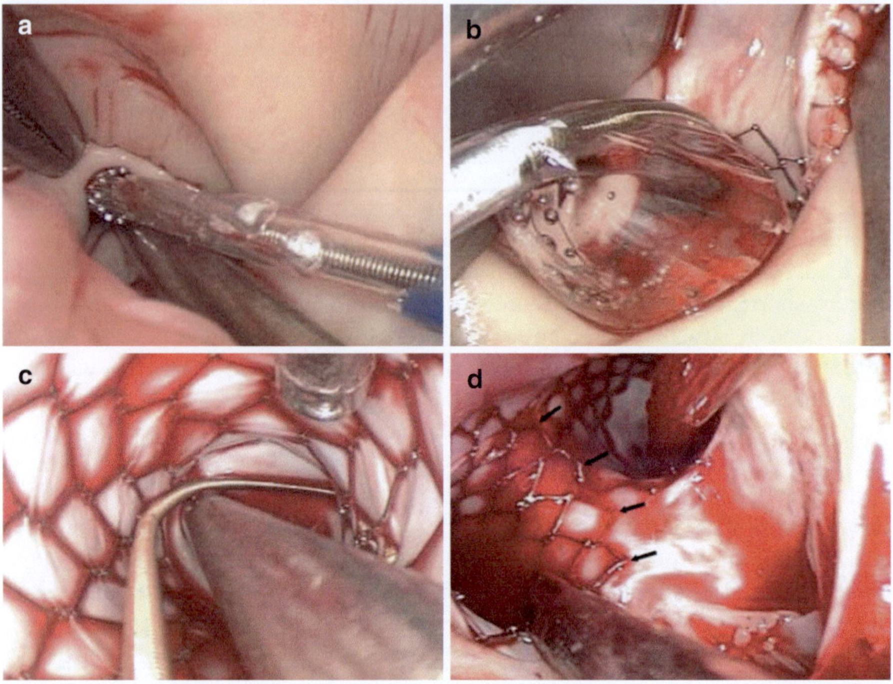

Fig. 37.1 Videoscopic stent implantation procedure to treat central PA stenosis. Pre-implant image used to position stent balloon complex in the right PA (**a**). Note how the proximal stent is brought to the ostium of the vessel. The appearance of the balloon during implantation (**b**). Videoscopic examination of the vessel following stent implantation shows good apposition of the stent to the vessel wall, absence of any side-branch crossing, and no obvious vessel tear (**c**). Following bilateral stent placement, the surgeon has flared the proximal stent struts (*arrows*) to facilitate future catheter reentry (**d**)

While this is a fairly simple technique, several words of caution are worth mentioning. If being performed in the operating room and not in a hybrid suite, this procedure puts the interventional team in an unfamiliar environment without the aid of fluoroscopy or angiography. This requires excellent communication and cooperation with the surgical team and careful pre-procedural planning. A thorough review of the pre-procedural angiography and careful calibration to ensure accurate measurements are essential. The use of floppy-tipped guidewires and avoiding rigid high-pressure balloons are important safety measures to prevent vessel damage, particularly from the distal balloon catheter tip which is not seen during inflation with this technique.

37.4.1.1 Institutional Experience

Between 1998 and 2008, this approach was utilized to implant 41 stents into the PAs of 34 patients in our program. Median age and weight at the time of implant were 36 months (5 days–31 years) and 13.8 kg (2.9–67 kg), respectively. There was one procedural failure in a child with previously implanted stents that were incompletely removed at a prior operation, which resulted in rupture of the implantation balloon and prevented hybrid stent placement. Technical success rate is 97 %. During a median follow-up of 94 months (22 months–11.5 years), 19 patients (22 stents) underwent follow-up catheterization. Angiographic assessment of vessel size showed a statistically significant improvement in mean minimal luminal diameter and the consistent ability to further expand these stents to keep up with patient growth. There were four cases of side-branch crossing resulting in the stenosis of that branch; however, only one resulted in complete occlusion. Late distal stent migration occurred in one case without clinical sequelae and that stent has remained in place with good flow around and through it. Four patients have undergone unremarkable surgical enlargement (longitudinal splitting) of their hybrid-placed stents during a subsequent operation.

37.4.2 Stent Implantation Via Surgically Provided Vascular Access

A second, more common hybrid approach to PA stent implantation involves the provision of surgical access to deliver stents to otherwise difficult or impossible to reach areas. In general, this technique has evolved to treat three distinct patient populations: (1) infants and neonates who are critically ill in the early postoperative period, often with open chests, (2) more stable patients presenting with unusual lesions or limited vascular access making percutaneous stent implantation difficult or impossible, or (3) planned elective hybrid PA stent implantation as part of a more extensive surgical procedure such as a bidirectional cavopulmonary anastomosis.

While the clinical scenario may differ, the approach in all of these scenarios is similar; surgical access for sheath placement is obtained (e.g., RVOT after tetralogy Fallot repair, innominate vein or superior vena cava after cavopulmonary anastomosis, carotid artery after systemic-PA shunt placement) and secured with a purse-string suture (Figs. 37.2, 37.3, and 37.4). Importantly, the location of this incision must allow enough distance between the tip of sheath and the target lesion, so the proximal portion of the stent delivery balloon can be inflated outside of the sheath. Angiography is performed through the side arm of the sheath, and quantitative measurements are made to determine stent diameter and length. A floppy-tipped directional guidewire is directed across the stenosis and to a distal posterior PA branch with or without the use of a catheter as needed. An appropriate-sized stent, usually with adult-size potential, is chosen and hand crimped onto a balloon catheter. Under fluoroscopic guidance the balloon/stent complex is advanced over the wire, across the target lesion. Owing to the short and simple catheter course, it is typically not necessary to protect the stent within the bloodstream by advancing the sheath. Serial hand injections performed via the side arm of the sheath are used to aid in precise positioning of the stent, after which it is deployed in the typical fashion. As with a standard stent deployment, follow-up angiography and hemodynamics are performed, after which the surgical team reenters the field to remove the sheath and repair the incision in the right ventricular outflow tract.

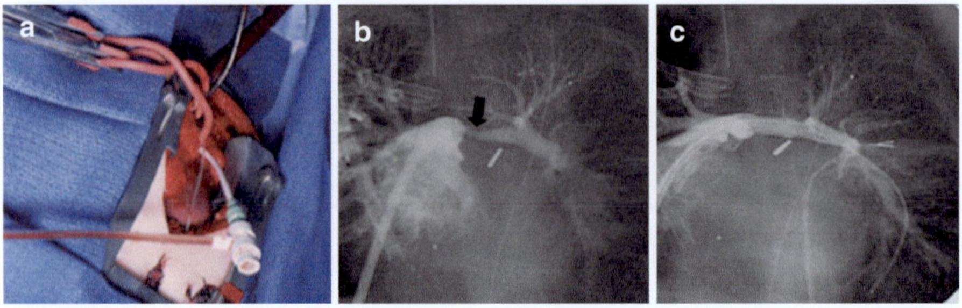

Fig. 37.2 Hybrid adult-sized pulmonary artery stent implantation via the right ventricular outflow in a critically ill infant after repair of pulmonary atresia and ventricular septal defect in association of hypoplastic PAs. An intraoperative photograph showing the delivery sheath within the outflow tract (**a**). An angiogram performed through the side arm of the sheath demonstrates severe left pulmonary artery branch pulmonary stenosis (**b**). Following the placement of an adult-sized left pulmonary artery stent, there was marked improvement in the vessel caliber and patient's clinical condition (**c**)

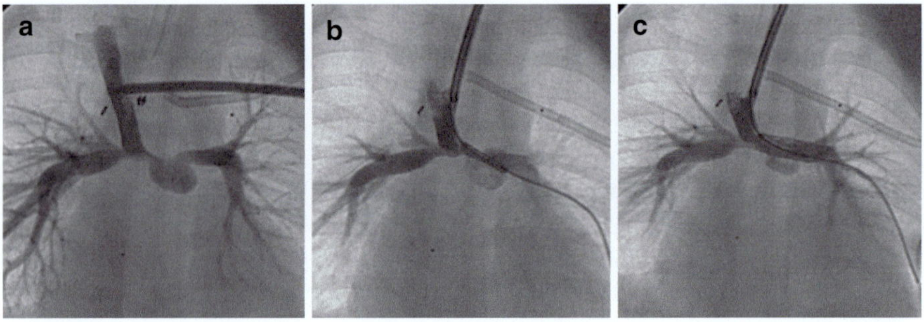

Fig. 37.3 Hybrid placement of a left pulmonary artery stent capable of adult dimension via the innominate vein in a 4-month-old infant at the time of his cavopulmonary anastomosis. (**a**) Angiography via the side arm of the short delivery sheath is used to demonstrate the stenosis and chose stent dimensions as well as for accurate positioning (**b**). After stent implant, repeat angiography (**c**) confirms vessel diameter improvement

37.4.2.1 Institutional Experience

Between 1999 and 2011, 10 infants underwent placement of 12 PA stents using direct RVOT access technique at our institution. Median weight was 6 kg and all were critically ill. Several were on mechanical cardiopulmonary support. There were no procedural complications or deaths. All stents were successfully placed (as judged by standard criteria and by clinical improvement). In follow-up, all stents placed using this technique have been further expanded via percutaneous routes with no cases of late complications. One patient, who did not have "adult-sized" stents placed at the time of the procedure, has undergone successful surgical enlargement (longitudinal splitting) of the stents during a subsequent operation.

During that same time period, 12 patients underwent stent implantation via a surgical carotid artery approach to treat an aortopulmonary shunt or pulmonary

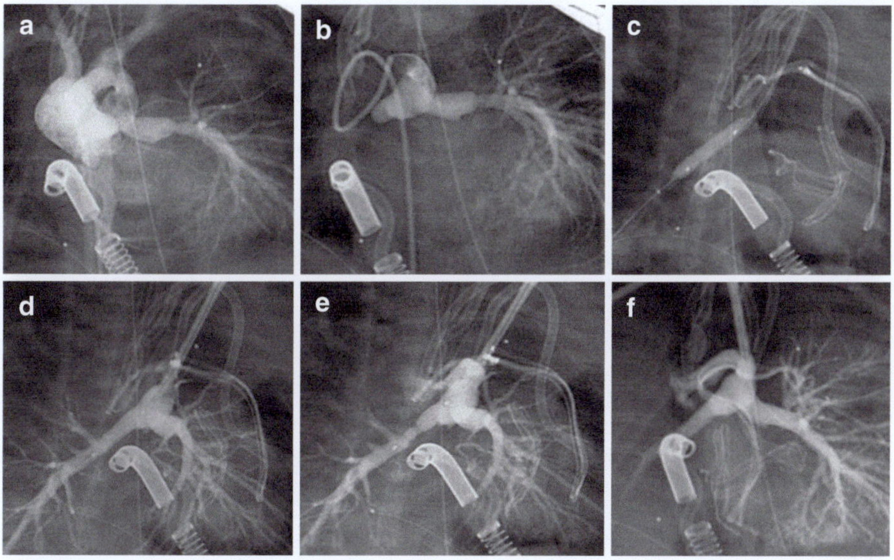

Fig. 37.4 (**a**) A newborn with a complex single ventricle and discontinuous pulmonary arteries underwent a central shunt from the ascending aorta and was profoundly cyanotic. (**b**) A selective injection into the shunt revealed a completely occluded left pulmonary artery and a significantly stenotic right pulmonary artery as well as a tortuous catheter route to access the shunt from a retrograde aortic approach. (**c**) Utilizing a right carotid cutdown hybrid approach, direct access to both branch pulmonary arteries was simple and allowed for effective stent implantation to the right (**d**) and left (**e**, **f**)

artery stenosis (via a shunt). Stent implantation was successful in all cases, and there were no instances of shunt thrombosis or procedural deaths.

Conclusions

While most pulmonary artery stents can be placed via a percutaneous approach, there are clear advantages to hybrid stent placement in certain settings. Our decade-long experience would suggest that these procedures are simple to do, safe, and effective in a variety of clinical settings and anatomies.

References

1. O'Laughlin MP, Perry SB, Lock J, et al. Use of endovascular stents in congenital heart disease. Circulation. 1991;83(6):1923–39.
2. O'Laughlin MP, Slack MC, Grifka RG, et al. Implantation and intermediate-term follow-up of stents in congenital heart disease. Circulation. 1993;88(2):605–14.
3. Pass RH, Hsu DT, Garabedian CP, et al. Endovascular stent implantation in the pulmonary arteries of infants and children without the use of a long vascular sheath. Catheter Cardiovasc Interv. 2002;55(4):505–9.
4. Stanfill R, Nykanen DG, Osorio S, Whalen R, Burke RP, Zahn EM. Stent implantation is effective treatment of vascular stenosis in young infants with congenital heart disease: acute implantation and long-term follow-up results. Catheter Cardiovasc Interv. 2008;71(6):831–41.

5. McMahon CJ, El Said HG, Vincent JA, et al. Refinements in the implantation of pulmonary arterial stents: impact on morbidity and mortality of the procedure over the last two decades. Cardiol Young. 2002;12(5):445–52.
6. Houde C, Zahn EM, Benson LN, et al. Intraoperative placement of endovascular stents. J Thorac Cardiovasc Surg. 1992;104(2):530–2.
7. Ungerleider RM, Johnston TA, O'Laughlin MP, et al. Intraoperative stents to rehabilitate severely stenotic pulmonary vessels. Ann Thorac Surg. 2001;71(2):476–81.
8. Bockencamp R, Blom NA, De Wolf D, Francois K, Ottenkamp J, Hazekamp MG. Intraoperative stenting of pulmonary arteries. Eur J Cardiothorac Surg. 2005;27:544–7.
9. Mendelsohn AM, Bove EL, Lupinetti FM, et al. Intraoperative and percutaneous stenting of congenital pulmonary artery and vein stenosis. Circulation. 1993;88:II210–7.

Literature and Results

38

Jacqueline Kreutzer and Sara M. Trucco

38.1 Historic Background

Efforts to combine catheterization and surgical techniques in a hybrid manner to treat pulmonary artery stenosis started in the early 1990s, with the first report by Houde et al. in 1992 from Toronto Sick Children's Hospital [1]. Since then, the experience has grown to now become a standard approach considered for management of specific conditions throughout the world. Although over the years major technological advances in stent profile and delivery methods have increased the feasibility of percutaneous stent implantation in small patients, it still is not always possible to implant a stent capable of achieving adult diameters in the future in a small child or within difficult anatomic substrates. Thus, the use of hybrid approaches for stent delivery continues to grow, particularly as the collaboration between surgeons and interventional cardiologists improves and more hybrid cardiac catheterization laboratories and either hybrid operating rooms or those with angiographic capability are being built. Over the last 20 years, numerous reports have demonstrated the feasibility of the technique and encouraging acute results. Table 38.1 summarizes the literature and illustrates the specifics of the experience over time. Not surprisingly, all reports refer to balloon expandable stents, as these are almost always the ones used for treatment of congenital stenotic lesions.

J. Kreutzer, MD (✉) • S.M. Trucco, MD
Pediatric Cardiology, Children's Hospital of Pittsburgh of UPMC,
4401 Penn Avenue, Pittsburgh, 15224 PA, USA
e-mail: Jacqueline.Kreutzer@chp.edu

G. Butera et al. (eds.), *Fetal and Hybrid Procedures in Congenital Heart Diseases*, DOI 10.1007/978-3-319-40088-4_38

Table 38.1 Summary of literature

First Author	Journal/year	*N*	Technique	Outcome	Complications	Mortality	F-up	Other details
Mendelsohn [2]	*Circulation* 1993	13	DV/CPB	Significant PA diameter increase and gradient reduction	None stent related	0 (0 %)	<2 m	3 pts f-up cath at mean 8.7 m no restenosis
Coles [3]	*JTCVS* 1995	11	DV/CPB	High rate of intervention for stent restenosis	1 acute thrombosis	3 (27 %)	9.6 m	71 % restenosis rate in survivors
Ungerleider [5]	*Ann Thorac Surg* 2001	22	DV/CPB	Improved PA diameter, reduced gradient	31 %: 3 malpositions 2 PA lacerations 1 non-expandable 1 reperfusion injury	0 (0 %)	2.8 yrs ± 1.7 yrs	5 hospital deaths unrelated to stent
Bokenkamp [9]	*Eur J of Cariothorac Surg* 2005	11	DV/CPB	36 % intervention for restenosis	Restenosis	0 (0 %)	15 m	1 hospital death from bleeding disorder
Mitropoulous [12]	*Ann Thorac Surg* 2007	22	DV/CPB	Improved PA diameter, reduced gradient	None stent related	0 (0 %)	22.8 m	No reintervention
Holzer [14]	*J Invasive Cardiology* 2008	20	15 DV/CPB, 3 OC/Perc 2 combo	90 % successful, 35 % reintervention	15 % complication: 2 migration, 1 stent fracture (resistant lesion)	0 (0 %)	1.7 yrs	Complications included the 2 unsuccessful cases
Menon [13]	*Am J Cardiology* 2008	24	DV/CPB	Decreased/improved RV pressure	16 %: 2 stent migrations, 2 incomplete inflations	0 (0 %)	18 m	18 % reintervention rate
Holzer [15]	*Cong Heart Dis* 2010	13	12 DV/CPB, 1 OP/Perc	Not studied	None stent related	0 (0 %)	None	PA interventions not analyzed separately

Angtuaco [16]	*Cath & Cardiovasc Intrv* 2011	67	61 DV/CPB, 6 OP/Perc	Concluded hybrid as effective as surgical plasty	9 %: 5 PA rupture, 1 embolization	0 (0 %)	7.6 yrs	49 % reintervention rate
Sridnar [17]	*Indian Heart Journal* 2013	10	DV	Improved PA diameter, reduced RV pressure	None stent related	0 (0 %)	14.8 m	2 deaths and 1 stroke not stent related
Lynch [18]	*I Card Thor Surg* 2015	7	DV	Improved PA diameter	1 PA tear	0 (0 %)	55.6 m	No reintervention

DV/CPB under direct vision on cardiopulmonary bypass, *OP/Perc* open chest via midline sternotomy and direct percutaneous access via cardiac or pulmonary artery direct puncture, *PA* pulmonary artery, *TOF* tetralogy of Fallot, *RV* right ventricle, *m* months, *yrs* years

38.2 Experience 1992–2003

Early publications refer mainly to intraoperative pulmonary artery stenting in small number of patients, typically infants [1, 2]. These were performed because of either limited vascular access, which precluded percutaneous stenting, or as adjunct to other cardiac surgery. In 1993 Mendelsohn AM and colleagues [2] from the University of Michigan reported intraoperative stenting of pulmonary arteries in nine patients without mortality or serious adverse events related to stenting. Preoperative angiographic evaluation with the testing of vessel distensibility had been performed in all. All patients were either undergoing concomitant surgery under 10 kg weight or did not have vascular access adequate for percutaneous stenting. There was a significant increase in vessel diameter and gradient reduction post-intervention in all cases.

Following that, the report by Coles et al. from Toronto Sick Children's Hospital [3] demonstrated the experience with 11 patients, a 27 % mortality, and a high rate of neointimal proliferation during follow-up. However, subsequent publications showed a much improved and different outcome. Ohye et al. [4] described in 1999 the quantitative use of preoperative angiography to determine landmarks to guide intraoperative stent implantation. They used the technique for successful implantation of 12 stents in 10 patients. Ungerleider et al. reported in 2001 [5] the experience with 22 patients, with significant gradient reduction in all implants. They pointed to the significant advantages of achieving a relatively large diameter vessel in diminutive pulmonary arteries for which patch augmentation may be technically, extremely difficult (1–2 mm vessels), plus indicated that surgical implant allows to avoid overlapping a contralateral branch and that flaring of the proximal stent is easily done and can ensure stability as well as facilitate reentry in future catheter procedures. Subsequent redilation of the surgically implanted stents was successful to expand the vessels further according to body growth during follow-up. In this report, there were no deaths related to stent implantation, but there were eight complications among 31 procedures particularly early in their experience, related to technical aspects of how to deploy the stent under direct vision. These included laceration of the pulmonary artery with balloon dilation of the stent in two patients, following which they recommended limited dissection around the pulmonary artery to be stented.

Several reports exist in the literature [6, 7] of individual cases or small series of hybrid procedures where successful pulmonary artery stenting is performed in one to five patients undergoing concomitant surgical repair.

38.3 Experience 2004–2015

Zahn et al. reported in 2004 [8] the stent placement in the early postoperative period performed in 62 patients. Some of these procedures were pulmonary artery implants via direct puncture of the right ventricle or main pulmonary artery or homograft conduit in a hybrid manner in order to gain access for implantation through an open chest, with or without circulatory support. These procedures were performed in the cardiac catheterization laboratory with the use of angiography for guidance. Success rate for stent implantation was 87 %.

In 2005 Bokenkamp et al. [9] reported 11 patients, including 7 who had elective stenting during concomitant heart surgery as well as 4 who had emergent stenting postoperatively. All these were implanted in the OR relatively blind, without fluoroscopic guidance. In the same year, Ing [10] pointed out several technical tips of intraoperative pulmonary artery stenting, indications, and advantages. Among these, intraoperative implantation would allow to avoid the hemodynamic instability related to stiff sheaths and wires, minimizing stent malposition and improved control of a potential vascular tear. He also brought up the importance of better apposition to the endothelial lining with the option to flare or fold back the proximal struts to the edge of the main pulmonary artery as well as tailoring the length of the stent to the need by cutting the stent when necessary. Disadvantages discussed included imprecise distal end positioning in particular the risk of jailing of a side branch. In order to improve accurate implantation, a recommendation to have C arm fluoroscopy with video recording was made.

Contemporary to these reports, Bacha et al. [11] published the overall experience at the University of Chicago Children's Hospital with hybrid pediatric cardiac surgery, defined as combined catheter-based and surgical interventions in either one setting or in a planned sequential fashion within 24 h. Among these patients there were three with intraoperative pulmonary artery stenting and five who underwent hybrid balloon angioplasty of branch stenosis or preexisting stents. All these patients were undergoing additional open heart surgery at the time. No guidewire was used. The implantation of stents was done under direct vision. No surgical dissection around the implantation site was performed so as to maintain the supportive tissue surrounding the vessel. Fluoroscopy was not used. There was no operative mortality. The authors concluded that hybrid cardiac surgery performed in tandem by surgeons and cardiologists is safe and effective in reducing or eliminating cardiopulmonary bypass and pointed that intraoperative pulmonary artery stenting is a valuable addition to the surgeon's armamentarium.

Mitropoulos FA reported in 2007 [12] the UCLA experience with intraoperative pulmonary artery stenting in 22 patients as adjunct to surgical repair, under direct surgical inspection, with a good intermediate follow-up outcome (no intervention at 22.8 months follow-up), with no early or late mortality. The technique was effective as assessed by the mean diameter on follow-up echocardiography and reduction in the gradient. One of the concerns brought up by live discussion at the end of the manuscript related to the lack of knowledge about the precise distal positioning of the balloon or stent when this is implanted under direct surgical vision without intra-procedural angiography and thus the risk of injury to a branch pulmonary artery branch upon the expansion of the balloon with resulting tear or jailing of branches.

Menon et al. reported in 2008 [13] the Mayo Clinic experience with intraoperative pulmonary artery stenting in 24 patients, 2 of which were done in an emergency basis due to the complication of percutaneous intervention. The technique used was direct surgical inspection after careful review of preoperative angiography. A guidewire was advanced into the distal pulmonary artery, and implantation was performed over the wire under direct inspection without the use of fluoroscopy. The proximal end was flared in some cases. Stent migration occurred in two patients. The authors suggested suturing of the stent to the vessel wall to avoid this complication. Although they recognize that ideally such procedures would be best done in a hybrid suite with capability for biplane fluoroscopy and angiography, they concluded that in experienced hands intraoperative pulmonary artery stenting can be performed safely and effectively without fluoroscopy.

The novel approach of using direct vascular puncture via an open chest was reported by Holzer et al. in 2008 [14]. Among 20 patients, 15 were done under direct vision on cardiopulmonary bypass, 3 underwent stent implantation via vascular puncture and angiographic guidance, and 2 were implanted via a combined approach.

The only multi-institutional report on hybrid procedures in the literature is that by Holzer et al. [15], who reported the results from the C3PO registry on hybrid procedures. Pulmonary artery hybrid interventions including stenting and balloon angioplasty occurred in 16 patients (among 128 total having hybrid procedures), 2 of which were done in the hybrid cardiac catheterization laboratory, while the remaining 14 were performed in the operating room. Pulmonary artery interventions were not analyzed separately with regard to outcomes and complications. However, among the description of the complications, there were none for the patients undergoing pulmonary artery hybrid stent implantation.

Angtuaco et al. [16] published in 2011 long-term outcomes of intraoperative pulmonary artery stenting in 67 patients using 96 stents. Almost half of the patients received more than one stent. At a median follow-up of 7.6 ± 4.5 years, 49 % of patients required reintervention, as expected in a growing pediatric population receiving stents at a young age. Reintervention was more common in children less than 2 years of age and diagnosis of tetralogy of Fallot or truncus arteriosus.

Sridhar et al. [17] expanded the published experience in 2013 reporting hybrid intraoperative pulmonary artery stenting at the time of concomitant congenital heart surgeries in ten patients with a total of 11 stents. All procedures were performed under cardiopulmonary bypass. Preoperative angiography or computed tomography was reviewed prior to surgery for definition of size, location, and length of the stenosis. The surgeon advanced a wire through the lesion, and the stent was implanted by direct vision. There was no use of fluoroscopy. The proximal end of the stent was flared, and the stent was sutured to the wall to avoid migration. There were two early postoperative deaths but not related to stent implantation. During a relatively brief follow-up period of 12–26 months, stent patency was satisfactory, and no reintervention was required. The authors pointed the multiple advantages of intraoperative stenting, particularly for patients with absent or difficult vascular access, those with severe pulmonary conduit obstruction, tortuous or distorted branches, presence of previously implanted tricuspid or pulmonary prosthesis, marginal hemodynamics, or ventricular dysfunction which may not allow for safe manipulation or positioning of a long sheath across the RVOT, bilateral ostial stenosis of the branches, and critically stenotic, nearly occluded vessels which are difficult to cross percutaneously. They also indicated the many difficulties of surgical patch angioplasty in these patients, including dissection and access issues, related to prior adhesions, scarring, compression, bleeding, or excessive collateral flow, all of which can lead to longer duration of cardiopulmonary bypass and potential need for circulatory arrest. In addition, the presence of fibrous scarring can be an advantage for stenting, as it provides support during stent expansion. Since with hybrid stenting dissection around the pulmonary artery is not necessary, some of the complications of redo surgeries, such as injury to the phrenic nerve, lymphatics, or other vascular structures, can be avoided. They also emphasized the fact that complications related to stenting can be better handled in the operating room while under cardiopulmonary bypass.

Most recently, Lynch et al. [18] reported hybrid branch pulmonary artery stenting in adults with congenital heart disease, pointing out that the technique can also be of benefit to larger patients. Although there was one serious complication (right pulmonary artery tear), it was managed successfully intraoperatively.

38.4 Technical Tips

The initial experience reported included intraoperative stenting guided by direct visualization or videoscopic assisted, with open heart bypass. This technique is particularly attractive in patients who require concomitant cardiac surgical procedures. The second technique, which has become common in the last ten years, is direct vascular puncture to access the stenotic vessel off cardiopulmonary bypass. In this approach access is obtained surgically via sternotomy and direct vascular puncture, and percutaneous techniques and fluoroscopy plus angiography are used to place the stents in position.

Technical tips supported by literature are as follows:

- Best to minimize or avoid surgical dissection around the pulmonary artery to be stented to maintain surrounding tissue integrity and minimize incidence of vascular tear [5, 6, 19].
- Preoperative angiographic mapping of the lesion to choose optimal stent characteristics and avoid jailing of branches [2–6, 8, 19].
- Importance of having C-arm fluoroscopy and angiography for implantation guidance [8, 10, 13].
- During open heart implantation, flare of the proximal end of the stent for improved apposition to the endothelial lining, or fold back the proximal struts to the edge of the main pulmonary artery [5, 8, 10, 17, 18].
- Consider "tailoring" the length of the stent to the need by cutting the stent when necessary [10].
- Consider suturing the stent to the vessel wall to minimize the risk of stent migration [5, 13].
- Open heart can be avoided or minimized by direct vascular puncture via open chest and angiographic guidance [5, 14, 19].

38.5 Complications

In Table 38.1, Column 6 summarizes complications related to hybrid pulmonary artery stenting, which range from 0 to 31 %. Most significant complications reported as directly related to hybrid stent implantation include stent migration/malposition and pulmonary artery tear. The need for reintervention which is commonly reported during follow-up, and sometimes listed as a complication, is inherent to pulmonary artery stenting in small growing children and thus is not attributable to the implant method. The real incidence of jailing of branches is not well reported as most of the literature includes very limited follow-up data. It is likely that those stents implanted without angiographic visualization of branching points would be associated to a higher incidence of side-branch jailing, although at this point this is speculative. Multiple technical tips have been described in the literature to minimize the incidence of these complications and are referenced above.

Conclusion

Over the past 20 years, reports of hybrid pulmonary artery stenting have demonstrated its feasibility, success, and safety, becoming a recognized therapeutic option in congenital heart disease. Novel approaches to optimize stent implant accuracy and minimize complications have been described in the literature and rely on the close collaboration between the interventional cardiologist and cardiothoracic surgeon, as well as the availability of optimal imaging technology in the operating room and hybrid cardiac catheterization suites.

References

1. Houde C. Intraoperative placement of endovascular stents. J Thorac Cardiovasc Surg. 1992;104:530. 8–92.
2. Mendelsohn AM, Bove EL, Lupinetti FM, et al. Intraoperative and percutaneous stenting of congenital pulmonary artery and vein stenosis. Circulation. 1993;88:II210–7.
3. Coles JG. Experience with repair of congenital heart defects using adjunctive endovascular devices. J Thorac Cardiovasc Surg. 1995;110:1513.
4. Ohye RG, Cohen DM, Wheller JJ, Allen HD. Quantitative digital angiography as an adjunct to the intraoperative placement of endovascular stents in congenital heart disease. J Card Surg. 1999;14(3):181–4.
5. Ungerleider RM, Johnston TA, O'Laughlin MP, Jaggers JJ, Gaskin PR. Intraoperative stents to rehabilitate severely stenotic pulmonary vessels. Ann Thorac Surg. 2001;71:476–81.
6. Bacha EA, Hijazi ZM, Cao QL, Starr JP, Waight D, Koenig P, Agarwala B. New therapeutic avenues with hybrid pediatric cardiac surgery. Heart Surg Forum. 2004;7(1):33–40.
7. Hjortdal VE, Redington AN, de Leval MR, Tsang VT. Hybrid approaches to complex congenital cardiac surgery. Eur J Cardiothorac Surg. 2002;22(6):885–90.
8. Zahn EM, Dobrolet NC, Nykanen DG, Ojito J, Hannan RL, Burke RP. Interventional catheterization performed in the early postoperative period after congenital heart surgery in children. J Am Coll Cardiol. 2004;43(7):1264–9.
9. Bökenkamp R, Blom NA, De Wolf D, Francois K, Ottenkamp J, Hazekamp MG. Intraoperative stenting of pulmonary arteries. Eur J Cardiothorac Surg. 2005;27(4):544–7.

10. Ing FF. Delivery of stents to target lesions: techniques of intraoperative stent implantation and intraoperative angiograms. Pediatr Cardiol. 2005;26:260–6.
11. Bacha EA, Hijazi ZM, Cao QL, Abdulla R, Starr JP, Quinones J, Koenig P, Agarwala B. Hybrid pediatric cardiac surgery. Pediatr Cardiol. 2005;26(4):315–22.
12. Mitropoulos FA, Laks H, Kapadia N, Gurvitz M, Levi D, Williams R, Plunkett M. Intraoperative pulmonary artery stenting: an alternative technique for the management of pulmonary artery stenosis. Ann Thorac Surg. 2007;84(4):1338–41; discussion 1342.
13. Menon SC, Cetta F, Dearani JA, Burkhart HA, Cabalka AK, Hagler DJ. Hybrid intraoperative pulmonary artery stent placement for congenital heart disease. Am J Cardiol. 2008;102(12):1737–41.
14. Holzer RJ, Chisolm JL, Hill SL, Olshove V, Phillips A, Cheatham JP, Galantowicz M. "Hybrid" stent delivery in the pulmonary circulation. J Invasive Cardiol. 2008;20(11):592–8.
15. Holzer R, Marshall A, Kreutzer J, Hirsch R, Chisolm J, Hill S, Galantowicz M, Phillips A, Cheatham J, Bergerson L. Hybrid procedures: adverse events and procedural characteristics – results of a multi-institutional registry. Congenit Heart Dis. 2010;5(3):233–42.
16. Angtuaco MJ, Sachdeva R, Jaquiss RD, Morrow WR, Gossett JM, Fontenot E, Seib PM. Long-term outcomes of intraoperative pulmonary artery stent placement for congenital heart disease. Catheter Cardiovasc Interv. 2011;77(3):395–9.
17. Sridhar A, Subramanyan R, Premsekar R, Chidambaram S, Agarwal R, Manohar SR, Cherian KM. Hybrid intraoperative pulmonary artery stenting in redo congenital cardiac surgeries. Indian Heart J. 2014;66(1):45–51.
18. Lynch W, Boekholdt SM, Hazekamp MG, de Winter RJ, Koolbergen DR. Hybrid branch pulmonary artery stent placement in adults with congenital heart disease. Interact Cardiovasc Thorac Surg. 2015;20(4):499–503.
19. Bacha EA, Marshall AC, McElheninney DB, del Nido PJ. Expanding the hybrid concept in congenital heart surgery. Semin Thorac Cardiovasc Surg Pediatr Card Surg Annu. 2007;10:146–50.

Part IX

Ventricular Septal Defect

Hybrid Closure of Muscular Ventricular Septal Defects: Anatomy, Clinical Scenarios, and Techniques

39

Kiran K. Mallula and Zahid Amin

39.1 Anatomy

Congenital ventricular septal defects (VSDs) can exist as isolated defects or may be associated with other cardiac anomalies, such as tetralogy of Fallot, double outlet right ventricle (DORV), D-transposition of great arteries (D-TGA), truncus arteriosus, or interrupted aortic arch. To date, there is no consensus on the best way to classify such defects, nor even on the curved surface that is taken to represent the defect [1]. Muscular VSDs (mVSDs) are the second most common type of VSD after perimembranous defects based on most series and account for 10–15 % of all VSDs [2, 3]. These have exclusively muscular borders and can have gross malalignment between their caudal and cranial borders. In addition to this malalignment, they can open into different parts of the right ventricle. They can be further subclassified based on their geographical location whether they open centrally, apically, anteriorly, or to the right ventricular inlet or outlet components [1]. The left ventricular view shows fewer overlying trabeculae, and multiple defects frequently coalesce to form a single defect on the left side. Occasionally such apical defects are quite large [4, 5].

The central defect is posterior to the trabecula septomarginalis (septal band of the crista) and in the midportion of the septum. Commonly, it is partially hidden by

K.K. Mallula, MD
Division of Pediatric Cardiology, Children's Hospital, Louisiana State University,
200 Henry Clay Ave, New Orleans, LA 70118, USA

Z. Amin, MD, FAAP, FSCAI, FACC (✉)
Division of Pediatric Cardiology, Children's Hospital of Georgia, Georgia Regents University,
1120 15th Street, Augusta, GA 30912, USA
e-mail: zamin@gru.edu

G. Butera et al. (eds.), *Fetal and Hybrid Procedures in Congenital Heart Diseases*, DOI 10.1007/978-3-319-40088-4_39

overlying trabeculae when viewed from the right ventricle and can give the impression of multiple defects. From the left ventricular view, this usually appears as a single rounded-off defect well away from the apex and the anterior and posterior left ventricular walls.

Small muscular defects near the septal free wall margins have been termed marginal or anterior defects. These defects are usually multiple, small, tortuous, and distributed along the ventricular septal free wall margins. Muscular defects can occur in combination with other muscular or nonmuscular defects, producing a Swiss cheese appearance of the septum.

Acquired muscular VSDs, on the other hand, are either traumatic or occur post-myocardial infarction. They complicate 0.2 % of post-MI infarcts [6].

39.2 Evolution of the Hybrid Approach

Unsuitable location for a classic surgical closure of mVSDs can be challenging in congenital heart surgery. In such situations it is not uncommon that residual shunts are still present despite several attempts to close multiple muscular defects [3]. This results in higher mortality and morbidity [7, 8]. Surgical repair via right atrial or right ventricular approaches provides suboptimal visualization of the defects due to heavy right ventricular trabeculations. Left ventriculotomy can provide better exposure; however, it is associated with apical aneurysms and with ventricular dysfunction sometimes necessitating heart transplantation [7, 9, 10]. In addition, the rate of residual defects is significant after surgical repair with a reoperation rate as high as 10 % in infants [8, 9]. This is even more significant when the defects are multiple, as in Swiss cheese mVSDs. Hence, device closure of mVSDs has become a valuable alternative to surgical patch closure, with encouraging results, particularly with the percutaneous transcatheter approach [11]. However, percutaneous closure requires the use of large venous sheaths, which may be associated with significant risk of vascular injury in children. In addition, it remains a highly challenging procedure in infants. Thus, perventricular closure of mVSDs with a device deployed intraoperatively has emerged as an alternative approach in these cases. It was first reported by Amin et al. in 1998 [12, 13], and since then, several approaches have been described. Perventricular muscular VSD closure is now an effective strategy in small children with suitable muscular defects and may avoid the morbidity associated with cardiopulmonary bypass and conventional surgical repair [14].

It is also used in older patients after trauma or post-MI [6]. Surgical repair carries a mortality as high as 40 %, since most of these patients present with rapid hemodynamic deterioration and cardiogenic shock. Transcatheter approach is also fraught with high morbidity and mortality due to the evolving nature of these defect and high residual shunting rates. The perventricular approach facilitates the use of large devices as well as plication of RV free wall to the VSD margin to prevent residual shunting. This is done by deploying the RV disk on the exterior surface of the RV.

39.3 Advantages

The main advantages of this technique include the following:

1. Avoiding CPB in the absence of associated cardiac lesions and reducing CPB time in patients with additional cardiac anomalies requiring surgical repair. This is particularly important in patients who had or might need long cross clamp time or those who already have the evidence of myocardial dysfunction.
2. The procedure only requires a minimal incision in patients without additional lesions.
3. The avoidance of ventricular incisions and the avoidance of transection of RV muscle bundles.
4. Unlike the percutaneous approach, it is not limited by weight or need for vascular access [15].
5. It also avoids possible complications of rhythm disturbances and injury to the cardiac valves from passing wires and large sheaths in repeated percutaneous techniques.
6. The procedure time is also relatively short (estimated in some studies to be less than 20 min) which compares very favorably to the percutaneous approach.
7. In addition, in cases of unusual orientation of the muscular septum as in DORV and TGA, it provides a much easier approach at crossing the VSD than the percutaneous technique by avoiding potential kinking of wires and sheaths.
8. The technique allows the immediate confirmation of adequate closure, since it is done under echo guidance, and any additional mVSDs can be easily detected and closed in the same sitting.
9. In small children, the procedure time is short, and so prolonged exposure to radiation can be avoided [16].

39.4 Patient Selection [17]

It is ideal to employ the perventricular technique in patients with significant mVSDs, who meet the following criteria:

(i) Small infants (<5.0 kg), in whom using large sheaths would be associated with significant morbidity
(ii) Patients with poor vascular access
(iii) Patients with mVSDs requiring concomitant surgical repair (DORV, TGA) for other associated anomalies as part of a single or staged approach [18].
(iv) Patients with multiple or Swiss cheese VSDs in whom surgical repair would provide suboptimal results and in whom percutaneous closure is highly challenging
(v) Patients with multiple mVSDs who have previously undergone pulmonary artery (PA) banding until they gain enough weight to have their VSDs closed

39.5 Devices

Various devices have been used for perventricular mVSD closure including the modified Rashkind double umbrella device [19], the Clamshell Septal Occluder (C.R. Bard, Inc, Billerica, MA, USA) [20], and the CardioSEAL device (NMT Medical, Boston, MA, USA) [20], all of which were placed intraoperatively under cardiopulmonary bypass and are no longer used. Other devices like the Amplatzer Ductal Occluder I [17] and II [16] and the Amplatzer Muscular VSD Occluder (AGA Medical, Plymouth, MN, USA) [21] have been used off bypass and are still used currently.

The Amplatzer Muscular VSD Occluder was designed specifically for the muscular septum. It is made of nitinol wire with polyester mesh. The self-expandable disks are connected via a central waist, and the diameter of which determines the size of the device. It carries the inherent properties of nitinol and hence is a self-expanding, malleable, shape memory device. The waist is 7 mm long, and the disks are 8 mm larger than the connecting waist except for 4 mm device whose waist is 5 mm larger than the waist. The device is available in sizes ranging from 4 to 18 mm in 2 mm increments, and it requires 6–9 Fr delivery sheath depending on its size. This device gained FDA approval in September 2007 for use in patients at high risk for surgical closure. It has several advantages that make it ideal for use in children. The disks are round, and so the potential of impingement of the valves and/or the chordae is significantly low. Another advantage is the small profile of the delivery sheath through which the device is placed. These are mainly helpful for the transcatheter technique, but advantageous for the perventricular approach as well [21].

The Amplatzer Duct Occluder I has also been used for closing mVSDs using the perventricular approach [17, 22]. This mushroom-shaped device may be advantageous in cases where the RV muscle bundles, especially at the apex, prevent the expansion of the RV disk of the Amplatzer Muscular VSD Occluder.

The use of Amplatzer Duct Occluder II has been reported as well [16] as it can be safely used in preterm and low birth weight infants.

39.6 Techniques

1. Right ventricular free wall approach [21]: This standard approach (see Fig. 39.1) is usually performed in the operating room or in a hybrid suite, if available. In the event of complex anatomy with multiple or Swiss cheese mVSDs, the procedure can be performed in the catheterization laboratory, which allows the additional use of fluoroscopy (if the operating room is not equipped with fluoroscopy) to help guide crossing additional VSDs. If the VSD is the only lesion, the procedure is performed without CPB. In case additional surgical intervention is needed to repair associated cardiac lesions, then CPB cannulas are inserted, but bypass is not initiated until after the closure of the VSD. The heart is approached via a median sternotomy or a subxiphoid minimally invasive incision without sternotomy. By epicardial or trans-esophageal echocardiography, the VSD size can

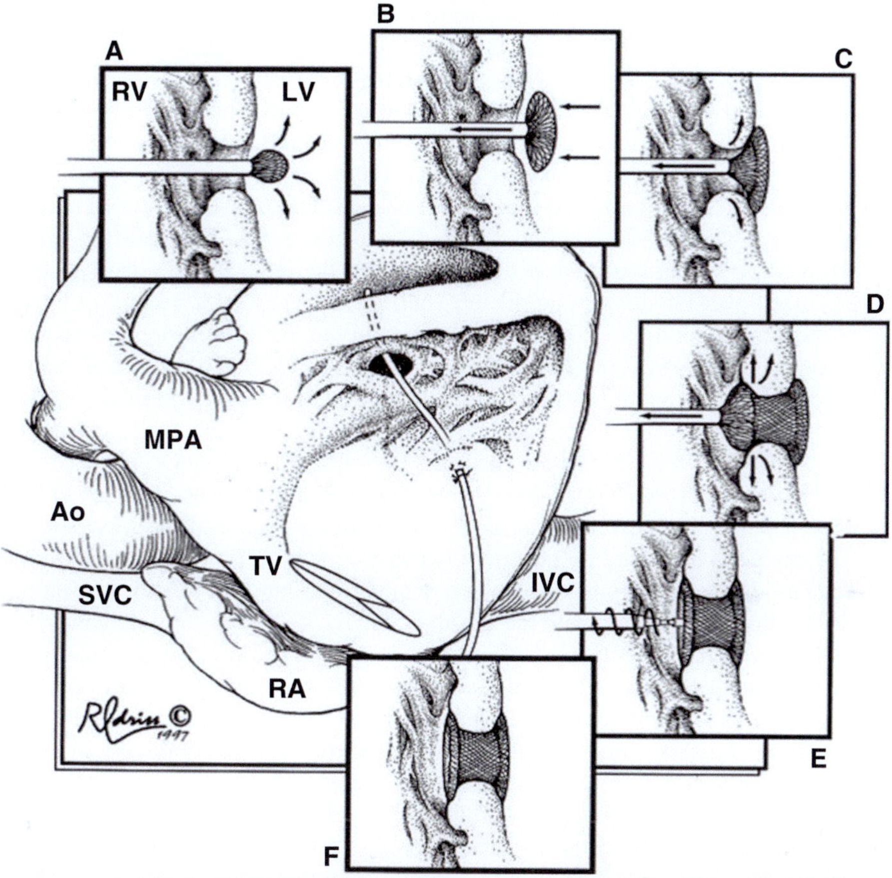

Fig. 39.1 Schematic diagram demonstrating the steps involved in device deployment through the RV free wall. *RV* right ventricle, *LV* left ventricle, *MPA* main pulmonary artery, *Ao* aorta, *SVC* superior vena cava, *TV* tricuspid valve, *RA* right atrium, *IVC* inferior vena cava. *A* Sheath Across the defect and device being advanced, *B* Left disc is being deployed, *C* Left disc completely deployed and waist is being deployed, *D* Waist and right disc deployed, *E* Delivery cable unscrewed from the device, *F* Device released

be estimated in diastole. The location of puncture on the free wall of the right ventricle is determined by applying a gentle push on the RV free wall by a finger or a forceps toward the defect guided by echocardiography. A purse-string suture is placed on the free wall of the RV. The site of the purse-string suture depends upon the location of the VSD and should be in a location the right ventricular free wall, which is opposite to the VSD and allows the sheath to remain perpendicular to the ventricular septum. An 18–20 gauge needle (angio-catheter or metal) is inserted through the purse-string suture on the RV free wall into the RV cavity. An appropriate-sized soft wire (e.g., Terumo glide wire) is inserted through the angio-catheter after removing the stylet or directly through the metal needle. This wire is maneuvered toward the VSD and the VSD is crossed. Occasionally, it may be difficult to advance the glide wire through the defect; a short J-tip Benson wire may be used in such circumstances. Once the wire is in the left ventricle (LV), a sufficient amount of the wire is advanced in the LV, and the angio-catheter/needle is removed. A short sheath dilator is used to predilate the RV free wall. Usually a dilator that is 1 F larger than the sheath that is being planned to be used for device deployment is ideal. This, however, is not a mandatory step. The dilator is removed, and an appropriate-sized short sheath is advanced over the wire. Once the dilator is in the left ventricle, the sheath is advanced over the dilator into the left ventricle. It is crucial to recognize the tip of the dilator and the sheath to prevent any injury to the left ventricular free wall. Once the sheath is in the left ventricle, its tip can be verified by echo and also by flushing small amount of saline or contrast through the side arm of the sheath. Microbubbles in the left ventricle will not only verify the tip but also confirm that the sheath is in the LV. An appropriate-size Amplatzer mVSD Occluder Device is washed in saline, screwed onto the delivery cable, and loaded into the loader. The loader is then advanced through the hemostasis valve of the short sheath. The device is advanced by pushing the cable. Under TEE or TTE or epicardial echo guidance or a combination of these modalities, and with the heart beating, the left disk is deployed; with the sheath pulled back, the waist is deployed in the VSD itself. The right disk is deployed after ensuring the left disk is approximating the septum. Before release, the position of occluder disks and potential impingement of the device on adjacent cardiac structures are carefully evaluated, including the assessment of residual shunt, aortic regurgitation, and atrioventricular valve function. After releasing the device, the loader is pulled in the sheath, and the sheath is gently withdrawn from the RV. The purse-string suture is tied. The same procedure can be repeated in case of multiple mVSDs. If the patient has other associated cardiac malformations requiring surgical repair, CPB is then initiated, and surgical repair is performed. Otherwise, if the mVSD is the only lesion, the chest is closed in the usual fashion.

2. Combined perventricular and percutaneous approaches: In patients with multiple mVSDs without additional cardiac lesions requiring repair, it is sometimes advantageous to perform the procedure in the catheterization laboratory as, on occasions, it is difficult to cross other defects after deploying the first device. In such cases, combining steps from both percutaneous and perventricular techniques may be particularly helpful to close the remaining VSDs. Percutaneous access is obtained, and additional VSDs can be crossed percutaneously under fluoroscopic guidance from the LV side. A wire is advanced into the pulmonary artery. Then, the surgeon places a short sheath in the pulmonary artery from the RV free wall. Under fluoroscopic guidance, a snare (Amplatz Snare, ev3, Plymouth, MN, USA) is used to snare the wire from the pulmonary artery and exteriorize it out of the RV free wall. Once this loop is established, a short delivery sheath is advanced over the wire to the mid-LV cavity. The remaining steps are then carried out as in the routine perventricular approach described earlier for a single defect.

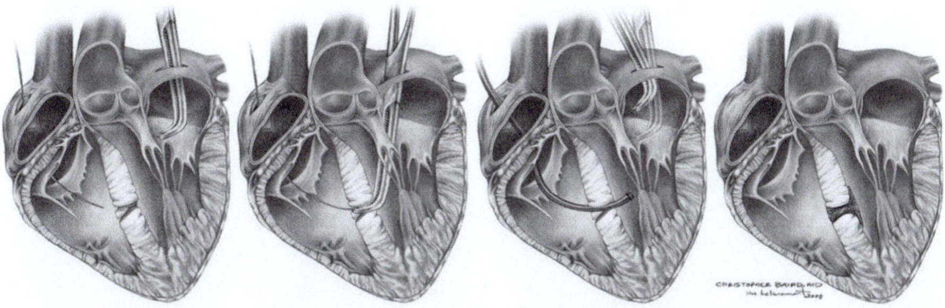

Fig. 39.2 Sequential steps in closure via the transatrial approach. *RA* right atrium, *LA* left atrium, *LV* left ventricle, *RV* right ventricle. **A** A right angle forcep introduced in the left ventricle, **B** Forcep tip cacross the VSD, **C** Wire advanced and extruded through the right atrial free wall, **D** Device deployed

3. Transatrial approach (see Fig. 39.2): Neukamm et al. [22] described this for closure of mVSDs using Amplatzer ADO I. Since the device has a tapered shape of the core, it would fit better in the narrow trabeculae on the right side. The right side of the device was attached to the myocardium with a ProleneVR suture. Based on echocardiographic measurements, the biggest diameter of the core of the PDA device is chosen 2 mm larger than the smallest end of the wedge of the VSD. A 7-French delivery sheath from the Amplatzer PDA delivery systems is chosen which can be shortened to decrease the length. The device is front-loaded into the shortened, regular delivery sheath and pulled back some millimeters to allow the forceps to grab the wall of the sheath on one side. No special shape of the sheath is needed. In cooperation with the surgeon during open heart surgery under visual and tactile control, a right-angled forceps is introduced into the left ventricle through the oval foramen and mitral valve. The tip of the forceps is manipulated through the VSD from the left ventricle, so it could be seen in the right ventricle. The sheath is then placed into the mouth of the forceps. The surgeon pulls the forceps and the clamped sheath wall into the left ventricle, releasing the delivery sheath and removing the forceps. To avoid entanglement in the mitral valve apparatus, the sheath is only pulled as much as needed into the left ventricle. The interventionist then pushes the device out of the sheath until the disk is formed. The distal disk and sheath are pulled back as one unit until it tugs the septum. Only then the sheath is pulled back to let the core develop within the defect. The end of the device that is visible just outside the right ventricle's trabeculae, still under tension from the attached delivery cable, is then secured with a Prolene suture.
4. Superior left atrial approach (see Fig. 39.3): Baird et al. [23] described this technique in patients with associated lesions that require CPB. After cardioplegia, the RV is inspected through a right atriotomy. A right angle from the LV through the VSD into RV. An anterior superior left atriotomy provides an excellent angle to pass a right angle through the VSD without torquing the mitral valve apparatus. A 0.035 in. exchange guidewire is passed through the tricuspid valve to the right

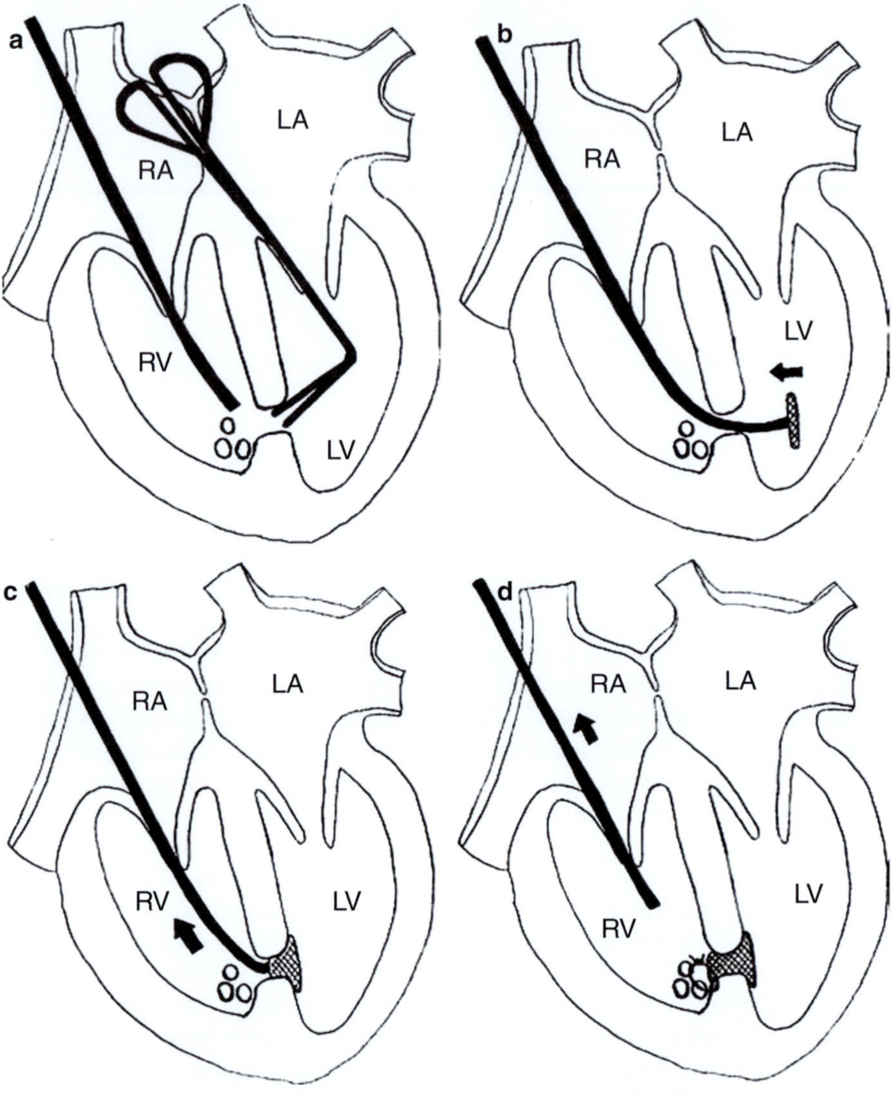

Fig. 39.3 Superior left atrial approach for hybrid closure of a muscular ventricular septal defect

angle and pulled up through the mitral valve and out the left atriotomy. Based on echocardiogram, the device size is chosen. A 6 F/7 F flexor sheath is passed over the wire from the RA through the mVSD into the LV, and the wire and dilator are removed. The device is deployed under direct vision, and the RV side is secured with sutures. Subsequently, associated lesions are repaired.

5. Trans-semilunar valve approach [24]: This hybrid surgical technique (see Fig. 39.4) may be beneficial in patients with complex tunnel like mVSD from the LV apex to the RV infundibulum anteriorly. The advantages include the

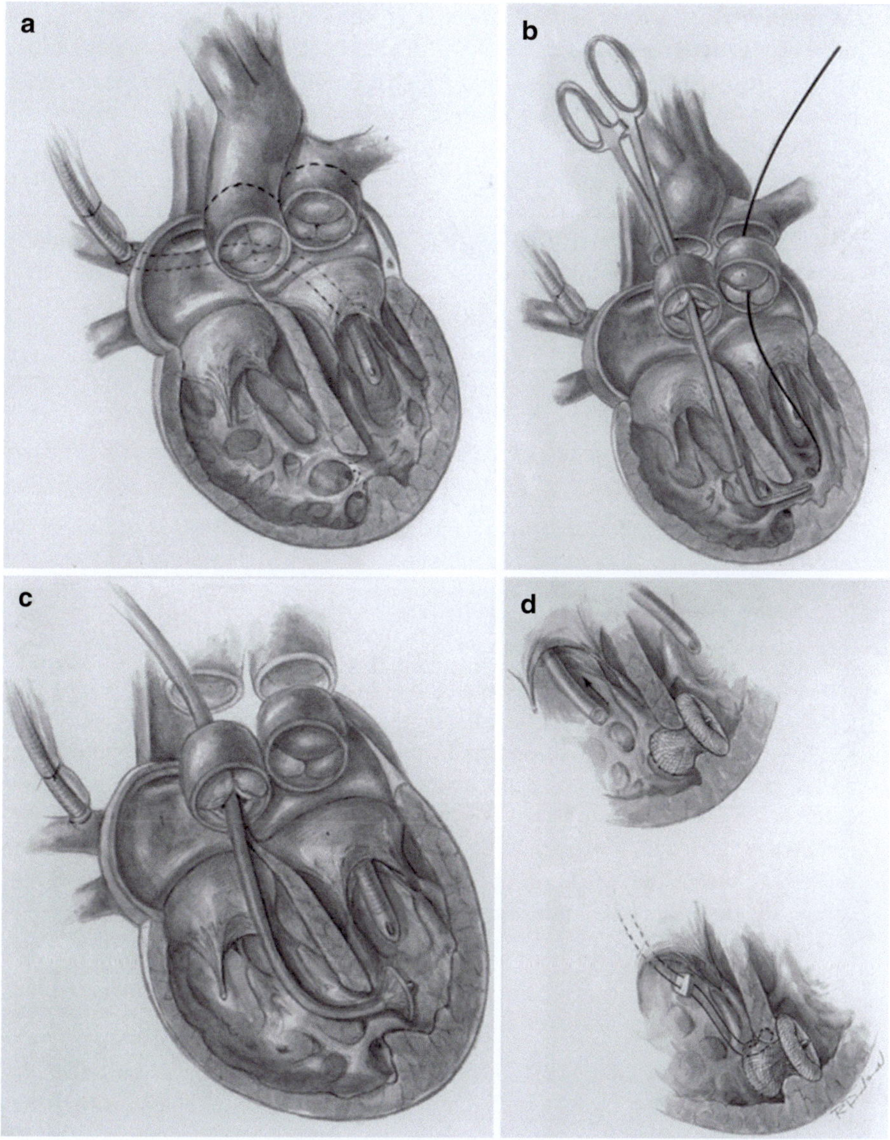

Fig. 39.4 Trans-semilunar approach for complex apical muscular VSDs. (**a**) Transposed great arteries and complex apical mVSDs. (**b**) Right angle clamp across the mVSD to snare a soft tip wire. (**c**) Partially deployed ductal occlude device across the mVSD. (**d**) Released ductal occlude device wedged in the mVSD and secured by a pledgeted suture

avoidance of left atriotomy, right and left ventriculotomy, and any associated muscle resection, especially when a midline sternotomy and CPB are required for the correction of other associated defects. The technique was described in the setting of a D-TGA patient with apical VSDs. On CPB, after the transection of the great arteries, a right angle clamp was advanced from the anterior semilunar valve across the VSD into the LV. The wire was exteriorized and swapped out for a stiffer J-tip wire with the tip secured with a forceps in the LV from the posterior semilunar valve. After crossing the VSD with an appropriate-sized sheath, the sheath tip is secured with a forceps from the posterior semilunar valve. An appropriate-sized ADO I device is then advanced to the LV apex, and the aortic retention skirt is deployed on the LV side under direct vision. The rest of the device is released on the RV side of the tunnel VSD, and this end is securely anchored to the RV septum by a single suture placed through the tricuspid valve. After this is done, the ASO operation is performed.

39.7 Complications

Major complications include:

1. Cardiac perforation: Perforation is a rare but serious complication of the percutaneous technique and could occur with the perventricular approach, although it has not been reported to date. It may occur when introducing the delivery sheath and its dilator across the VSD into the LV as the dilator is stiff enough to puncture the LV if pushed too far. This is preventable by making sure the delivery sheath is positioned in the LV cavity not too close to the LV free wall by monitoring its position with TEE or epicardial echocardiography.
2. Device embolization: This could occur if the device is released prematurely or in an inappropriate position. The device can then embolize to the LV, ascending aorta, RV, or pulmonary arteries. This may be preventable by using the appropriately sized device and by evaluating the device position by echo prior to device release. If such a complication occurs, the surgeon can proceed with CPB and surgically close the VSD after removing the device.

Minor complications include:

1. Unsuccessful closure: This may result from the inability to deploy the RV disk of the device, when there is an apical mVSD and there are heavy RV trabeculations. This problem may be avoided by using the mushroom-shaped Amplatzer Duct Occluder device. Thus, it is helpful to have these occluder devices available when planning perventricular closure, especially for apical mVSDs.
2. Valvular regurgitation: This can occur if the device impinges on the valve apparatus especially in high posterior mVSDs close to the atrioventricular valves. Therefore, it is essential to measure the distance from the defect to the various valvar structures in order to select the appropriate device size and to monitor valve function by echo prior to device release. Minimal valve regurgitation that is not hemodynamically significant can be followed up medically; however, if the device causes significant impingement on the valve apparatus after release, it should be removed surgically.

3. Hemolysis is rare and could potentially occur with the perventricular technique, as it results from residual shunting. By using the appropriate device size and avoiding under sizing, this complication should be avoidable. If hemolysis is significant, the residual shunt should be closed by implanting another additional device if possible, or the device should be removed and the defect closed surgically.
4. Air embolism is another serious complication. As in the percutaneous approach, the device should be loaded onto the delivery cable under water or blood seal to prevent such rare complications.

References

1. Spicer DE, Hsu HH, Co-Vu J, Anderson RH, Fricker FJ. Ventricular septal defect. Orphanet J Rare Dis. 2014;9:144.
2. Soto B, Becker AE, Moulaert AJ, Lie JT, Anderson RH. Classification of ventricular septal defects. Br Heart J. 1980;43(3):332–43.
3. Becker AE, Anderson RH. Classification of ventricular septal defects – a matter of precision. Heart Vessels. 1985;1(2):120–1.
4. Wenink AC, Oppenheimer-Dekker A, Moulaert AJ. Muscular ventricular septal defects: a reappraisal of the anatomy. Am J Cardiol. 1979;43(2):259–64.
5. Anderson RH, Wilcox BR. The surgical anatomy of ventricular septal defect. J Card Surg. 1992;7(1):17–35.
6. Love BA, Whang B, Filsoufi F. Perventricular device closure of post-myocardial infarction ventricular septal defect on the beating heart. J Thorac Cardiovasc Surg. 2011;142(1):230–2.
7. Kirklin JK, Castaneda AR, Keane JF, Fellows KE, Norwood WI. Surgical management of multiple ventricular septal defects. J Thorac Cardiovasc Surg. 1980;80(4):485–93.
8. Kitagawa T, Durham 3rd LA, Mosca RS, Bove EL. Techniques and results in the management of multiple ventricular septal defects. J Thorac Cardiovasc Surg. 1998;115(4):848–56.
9. Wollenek G, Wyse R, Sullivan I, Elliott M, de Leval M, Stark J. Closure of muscular ventricular septal defects through a left ventriculotomy. Eur J Cardiothorac Surg. 1996;10(8):595–8.
10. McDaniel N, Gutgesell HP, Nolan SP, Kron IL. Repair of large muscular ventricular septal defects in infants employing left ventriculotomy. Ann Thorac Surg. 1989;47(4):593–4.
11. Holzer R, Balzer D, Cao QL, Lock K, Hijazi ZM. Device closure of muscular ventricular septal defects using the Amplatzer muscular ventricular septal defect occluder: immediate and mid-term results of a U.S. registry. J Am Coll Cardiol. 2004;43(7):1257–63.
12. Amin Z, Berry JM, Foker JE, Rocchini AP, Bass JL. Intraoperative closure of muscular ventricular septal defect in a canine model and application of the technique in a baby. J Thorac Cardiovasc Surg. 1998;115(6):1374–6.
13. Amin Z, Gu X, Berry JM, Titus JL, Gidding SS, Rocchini AP. Perventricular [correction of Periventricular] closure of ventricular septal defects without cardiopulmonary bypass. Ann Thorac Surg. 1999;68(1):149–53. discussion 153–4.
14. Kang SL, Tometzki A, Caputo M, Morgan G, Parry A, Martin R. Longer-term outcome of perventricular device closure of muscular ventricular septal defects in children. Catheter Cardiovasc Interv. 2015;85(6):998–1005.
15. Pedra CA, Pedra SR, Chaccur P, Jatene M, Costa RN, Hijazi ZM, Amin Z. Perventricular device closure of congenital muscular ventricular septal defects. Expert Rev Cardiovasc Ther. 2010;8(5):663–74.

16. Haponiuk I, Chojnicki M, Jaworski R, Steffek M, Juscinski J, Sroka M, Fiszer R, Sendrowska A, Gierat-Haponiuk K, Maruszewski B. Hybrid approach for closure of muscular ventricular septal defects. Med Sci Monit. 2013;19:618–24.
17. Diab KA, Cao QL, Hijazi ZM. Perventricular closure of muscular ventricular septal defects: how do I do it? Ann Pediatr Cardiol. 2008;1(1):27–33.
18. Elhmidi Y, Hoerer J, Lange R, Schreiber C. Muscular ventricular septal defect in a newborn with truncus arteriosus communis: perventricular transcatheter closure under echocardiographic guidance only, a case report. World J Pediatr Congenit Heart Surg. 2014;5(4):589–91.
19. Chaturvedi RR, Shore DF, Yacoub M, Redington AN. Intraoperative apical ventricular septal defect closure using a modified Rashkind double umbrella. Heart. 1996;76(4):367–9.
20. Okubo M, Benson LN, Nykanen D, Azakie A, Van Arsdell G, Coles J, Williams WG. Outcomes of intraoperative device closure of muscular ventricular septal defects. Ann Thorac Surg. 2001;72(2):416–23.
21. Amin Z, Cao QL, Hijazi ZM. Closure of muscular ventricular septal defects: transcatheter and hybrid techniques. Catheter Cardiovasc Interv. 2008;72(1):102–11.
22. Neukamm C, Bjornstad PG, Fischer G, Smevik B, Lindberg HL. A novel method of hybrid intraoperative catheter-based closure of ventricular septal defects using the Amplatzer(R) PDA occluder. Catheter Cardiovasc Interv. 2011;77(4):557–63.
23. Baird CW, Stern H, Watts L. Left atrial hybrid closure of muscular ventricular septal defects with the Amplatzer device. J Thorac Cardiovasc Surg. 2009;137(3):779–80.
24. Veeram Reddy SR, Brenes JE, Forbess JM. Trans-semilunar valve hybrid technique for Amplatzer device closure of complex muscular ventricular septal defects during arterial switch operation. J Thorac Cardiovasc Surg. 2013;146(2):483–5.

Hybrid Muscular Ventricular Septal Defect Closure: Literature and Results

40

Gianfranco Butera, Nicusor Lovin, and Massimo Chessa

Ventricular septal defects (VSDs) are the most common congenital cardiac malformation at birth, with an incidence reported in literature between 15 and 40 % of total congenital heart diseases. They are usually an isolated finding; however, they can be also associated to complex congenital heart diseases [1, 2]. VSDs may be also a mechanical complication of myocardial infarction, with an incidence reported in literature of 0.26 % [3].

Nowadays, the treatment of choice is surgical repair, but in suitable cases (muscular or perimembranous VSDs), the percutaneous closure is a feasible alternative [1].

However, both surgery and transcatheter approaches may be associated to complications and limitations. In these cases the hybrid approach may provide a valuable alternative. In fact, Haponiuk showed an increased rate of hybrid therapy from 0 % in 2008 to 8.5 % in 2013 [4].

In particular, hybrid approach may be an interesting option in the following cases:

1. Residual VSDs after surgical closure [5]
2. Multiple VSDs, with some of them inapproachable by surgery such as defects under saepto-marginalis trabecula [6, 7] or apical [8, 9]
3. Intraoperative treatment during surgical correction:
   (a) Before de-banding of the pulmonary artery
   (b) Before the repair of aortic coarctation, during arterial switch for d-transposition of great arteries, or atrial septal defect surgical closure [4, 7, 9]

G. Butera (✉) • M. Chessa
IRCCS Policlinico San Donato Milanese, San Donato Milanese, Italy
e-mail: Gianfranco.Butera@grupposandonato.it

N. Lovin
Institutul de Boli Cardiovasculare "Prof. Dr. George I. M. Georgescu", Iasi, Romania

G. Butera et al. (eds.), *Fetal and Hybrid Procedures in Congenital Heart Diseases*, DOI 10.1007/978-3-319-40088-4_40

(c) When it is expected from a suboptimal result of individual percutaneous/surgical treatment [4, 7, 10]
(d) To reduce the interventional related trauma, especially in high-risk patients as in small babies less than 5 kg or under 6 months of life
(e) Concomitant correction of other abnormalities [4, 7, 10, 11]
(f) Very high-risk patients because of prematurity, cyanosis, intolerance to drug therapy, failed interventional treatment prior to admission, chronic respiratory failure, mechanical ventilation prior to the procedure, association to noncardiac malformation (e.g., diaphragmatic hernia), or acquired health issues (renal failure, cerebral hemorrhage) [12]

There are several advantages of these techniques when compared to both percutaneous interventions and surgical treatments taken alone [7, 10–12].

In fact, it is possible to avoid ventriculotomy, the risks associated to cardiopulmonary bypass, cardioplegia, and the better accessibility for apical or saepto-marginalis VSDs. Compared to transcatheter treatment alone, there are no limitations related to vascular access or sheath size, less technical difficulties and hemodynamic instability related to arterio-venous circuit, and a more perpendicular approach of the VSD with the delivery system.

The main disadvantage of a hybrid treatment for VSDs is the need of a special hybrid operating theater that involves more expensive infrastructures, trained team, and the peculiar risks of complications related to this therapy. Furthermore, the devices and tools are not especially designed for this approach.

Since the first description in 1998, by Amin et al. [13, 14] in a child with postoperative residual VSD, the most frequent technique of hybrid closure of VSD is the perventricular approach, by the puncture of the free wall of the right ventricle. Success rate of the procedure ranges between 88 and 100 % [4, 6–16].

The hybrid procedure is performed under general anesthesia and echocardiographic guidance, in most cases transesophageal [9]. However, there are cases where the procedure was performed by using transthoracic guidance through the subcostal views, with similar procedural outcome [14], epicardial echocardiography [5–7, 12, 14], or intracardiac echocardiography [3, 14], both in bidimensional and tridimensional views [6].

The dose of anticoagulation is 50 % what needed for cardiopulmonary bypass (1.5 mg/kg/body weight) and has to be continued 48 hours after the procedure [4, 7, 9].

The heart is approached usually by a median sternotomy; however, there are cases described in literature through a lateral thoracotomy or subxiphoid access for apical VSDs [7, 9, 12].

The place of the cardiac puncture is chosen by tipping the right ventricle wall in order to have a perpendicular route over the VSD and to avoid the coronary arteries, major chordae, or papillary muscles [9]. For apical VSDs, the puncture is performed at 1.5 cm by the apex, for the best angle to approach the defect [6].

After the puncture, with fluoroscopy and echocardiographic guidance, the VSD is passed with a guidewire in the left ventricle, and the occluder is placed. The Amplatzer muscular VSD occluder is the more frequently used device.

However, there are cases reported in literature where the Shanghai Shenzhen occluders [14] or the Cardi-O-Fix [11] was used successfully. Another possible approach is by using an atrial puncture access [4, 9, 10].

Although transient arrhythmia and hypotension are common during the procedure [14], there are other complications reported in literature including late malposition of the device [14], immediate embolization [8, 11], aortic regurgitation [14], progressive mitral regurgitation [9], puncture of the left ventricle with pericardial leakage [9], late right ventricle pseudoaneurysm [8], prolonged QRS, or total atrioventricular block [11].

Hybrid treatment of the VSD is an important option in selected cases. Trained team and infrastructure are mandatory. Data from literature are very encouraging.

References

1. The Task Force on the Management of Grown-up Congenital Heart Disease of the European Society of Cardiology (ESC). ESC Guidelines for the management of grown-up congenital heart disease (new version 2010). Eur Heart J. 2010;31:2915–57.
2. Ginghina C, et al. Mic tratat de cardiologie. Romania: Editura Academiei Romane; 2010. p. 563–5.
3. Jorge C, et al. Hybrid closure of postinfarction ventricular septal rupture enlargement after transcathether closure with Amplatzer occluder. Eur Heart J. 2012;1(1):57–9.
4. Haponiuk I, et al. Hybrid cardiovascular procedures in the treatment of selected congenital heart disease in children: a single-centre experience. Kardiol Pol. 2014;72(4):324–30.
5. Chojnicki M, et al. Intraoperative imaging of hybrid procedure for muscular ventricular septal defects closure with Amplatzer Duct Occluder II. Kardiol Pol. 2011;69(12):1280–1.
6. Mroczek T, et al. Hybrid, perventricular closure of muscular ventricular septal defects. Kardiol Pol. 2012;70(12):1280–2.
7. Haponiuk I, et al. Hybrid approach for closure of muscular ventricular septal defects. Med Sci Monit. 2013;19:618–24.
8. Rao K, et al. Epicardial deployment of right ventricular disk during perventricular device closure in a child with apical muscular ventricular septal defect. Ann Pediatr Cardiol. 2013;6(2): 176–8.
9. Kim SJ, et al. The hybrid perventricular closure of apical muscular ventricular septal defect with Amplatzer duct occluder. Korean J Pediatr. 2013;56(4):176–81.
10. Haponiuk I, et al. Inflammatory marker levels after hybrid treatment of selected congenital heart disease in children. Kardiol Pol. 2014;72(9):798–805.
11. Koneti NR. Hybrid muscular ventricular septal defect closure: Surgeon or physician!! Indian Heart J. 2012;64:568–9.
12. Haponiuk I, et al. Alternative hybrid and staged interventional treatment of congenital heart defects in critically ill children with complex and non-cardiac problems. Videosurgery Miniinv. 2015;10(2):244–56.
13. Amin Z, et al. Perventricular closure of ventricular septal defects without cardiopulmonary bypass. Ann Thorac Surg. 1999;68:149–54.
14. Zhang GC, et al. Minimally invasive perventricular device closure of ventricular septal defect in infants under transthoracic echocardiograhic guidance: feasibility and comparison with transesophageal echocardiography. Cardiovasc Ultrasound. 2013;11:8.
15. Bacha E, et al. Multicenter experience with perventricular device closure of muscular ventricular septal defects. Pediatr Cardiol. 2005;26:315–22.
16. Michel-Behnke I, et al. Device closure of VSD by hybrid procedures. Catheter Cardiovasc Interv. 2011;77:242–51.

Perimembranous VSD

41

Xiangbin Pan

41.1 Anatomy and Clinical Scenarios

Perimembranous ventricular septal defect (VSD) (pmVSD) is one of the most common congenital cardiac malformations. It is located within the membranous septum under the tricuspid valve septal leaflet (Fig. 41.1) allowing blood to shunt from left to right ventricle.

PmVSDs may vary from small defects usually asymptomatic associated only to a loud murmur to large ones. In the latter case, subjects may have troubles in feeding and growing at a normal rate and might develop pulmonary arterial hypertension with decreased exercise tolerance. In case of persistent shunting at high pressure, pulmonary vascular obstructive disease (Eisenmenger's syndrome) with cyanosis and clubbing may develop.

At evaluation, left ventricular and occasionally left atrial hypertrophy may be apparent by electrocardiography, while chest radiography reveals cardiomegaly and increased pulmonary vascular markings reflecting increased pulmonary blood flow. Defect number, size, type, and exact location can be identified by two-dimensional and Doppler echocardiography. PmVSDs are better seen in the left ventricular outflow tract just under the aortic valve in apical and subcostal "five-chamber" views and adjacent to the tricuspid valve in parasternal short-axis view at the aortic valve level.

Traditional treatment methods for VSD include open-heart surgery and percutaneous interventional closure. In open-heart surgery, the VSD is directly repaired under cardiopulmonary bypass, with shortcomings of significant trauma, and slow recovery. Percutaneous interventional closure does not require thoracotomy or cardiopulmonary bypass and therefore is associated with reduced myocardial injury

X. Pan
Department of Cardiovascular Surgery, National Center for Cardiovascular Disease, Fuwai Hospital, Chinese Academy of Medical Sciences and Peking Union Medical College, 167 Beilishi Road, Beijing 100037, China
e-mail: xiangbin428@hotmail.com

G. Butera et al. (eds.), *Fetal and Hybrid Procedures in Congenital Heart Diseases*, DOI 10.1007/978-3-319-40088-4_41

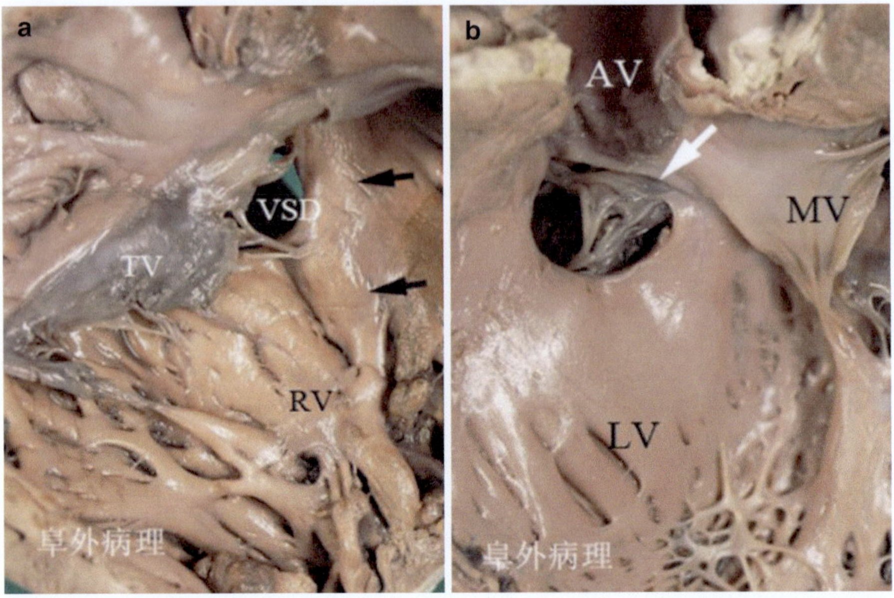

Fig. 41.1 Location of perimembranous ventricular septal defect. *Right* (**a**) and *left* (**b**) ventricular surfaces

incidence, blood transfusion requirements, recovery time, hospital stay, and medical expenses. However, it has the drawback of x-ray exposure and the potential for development of complications including complete aortic valve (AV) block.

In recent years, transesophageal echocardiogram (TEE)-guided minimally invasive perventricular device closure has emerged as a safe and effective treatment option for pmVSDs. Compared with conventional approaches, the advantages include less surgical trauma, avoidance of cardiopulmonary bypass, no radiation, and compared to percutaneous VSD occlusion expanded age and weight range.

Perventricular pmVSD device closure is indicated in patients with (1) age $\geq$2 months and weight $\geq$4 kg; (2) clinical manifestations including heart failure symptoms, recurrent respiratory infection, developmental delay, or history of bacterial endocarditis; and (3) pmVSD diameter >3 and <10 mm as determined in transthoracic echocardiography.

Exclusion criteria are (1) predominant right-to-left shunt, (2) more than trivial aortic regurgitation, and (3) active infective endocarditis.

41.2 Technique(s)

41.2.1 Devices and Delivery System

The pmVSD occluders are self-expandable, double-disk devices made of 0.005-in. nitinol wire meshes and fabric. They have a waist diameter that ranges from 4 to 10 mm in 1-mm increments and from 10 to 20 mm in 2-mm increments. The waist height is 4 mm.

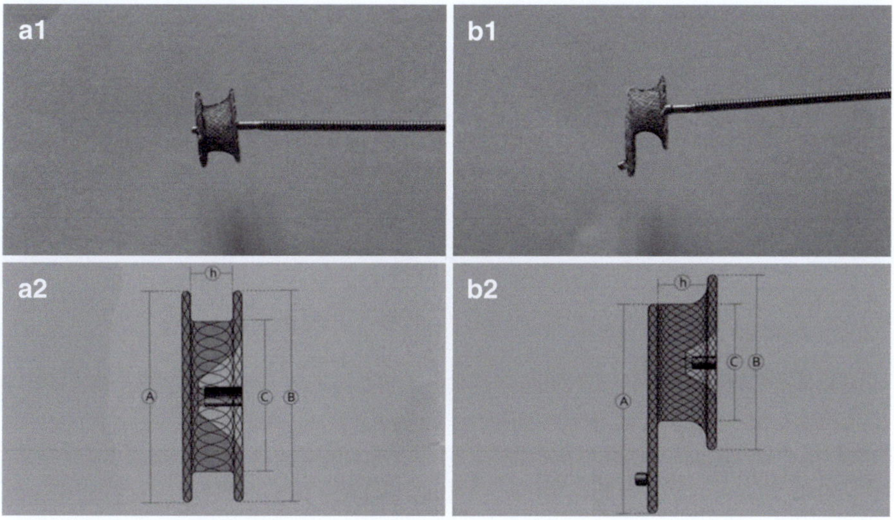

Fig. 41.2 Occluders used in perventricular closure of pmVSDs. Images (**a1, b1**) schematic diagrams (**a2**, **b2**) of symmetric and asymmetric occluders, respectively

There are two pmVSD occluders available:

1. Symmetric (Fig. 41.2a1, a2), which is used for pmVSDs at >2 mm from the aortic valve and are 2 mm larger than the waist of both the left and right ventricular disks.
2. Asymmetric (Fig. 41.2b1, b2), which is used for pmVSDs <2 mm from the aortic valve with left ventricular disk partially edgeless and 6 mm larger than the waist with a platinum marker at one end. Right ventricular disk is the same as the symmetric occluder.

The entire delivery system includes a trocar, a 0.035-in. guidewire, dilator, delivery sheath, and a loading sheath (Fig. 41.3). The size of the delivery sheath (6–12 Fr) is chosen according to the size of the occluders (Table 41.1). Thoracoscopic instruments, including a retractor and a knotter, are used for the procedures through a 1–2 cm surgical incision.

41.2.2 Procedure

Procedures are performed with patients under general anesthesia with endotracheal intubation in a standard operating room. The TEE probe is inserted, and the procedure is performed under TEE guidance. The location, size, flow direction of the pmVSD, valvular regurgitation, and distance between the pmVSD and the aortic valve are measured intraoperatively by TEE. Antibiotics and heparin (80 IU/kg) are administered intravenously before the operation.

The commonest surgical approach is via a partial median inferior sternotomy (Fig. 41.4). A 2–3 cm median incision is created over the lower sternum and xiphoid bone prior to approach the sternum. The pericardium is opened and suspended, and

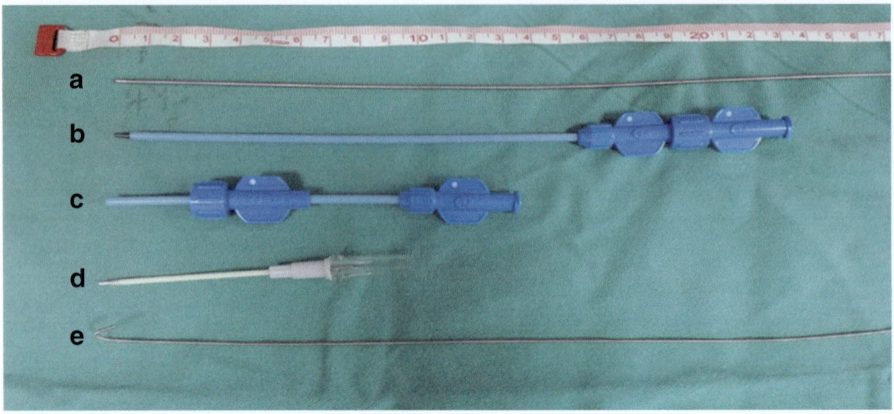

Fig. 41.3 Entire delivery system used in perventricular closure of pmVSDs including delivery cable (*A*), dilator and delivery sheath (*B*), loading sheath (*C*), trocar (*D*), and 0.035-in. guidewire (*E*)

Table 41.1 Recommended delivery sheath sizes according to type and size of occluders

A \ B \ C	4	5	6	7	8	9	10	12	14	16	18	20
symmetric	6	7	7	8	8	8	9	9	10	10	12	12
asymmetric	7	7	7	8	8	9	9	10	10	12	NO	NO

A Type of occluders, *B* Recommended delivery sheath size (Fr), *C* Size of occluders (mm). *NO* No 18 and 20 mm asymmetric occluders are available

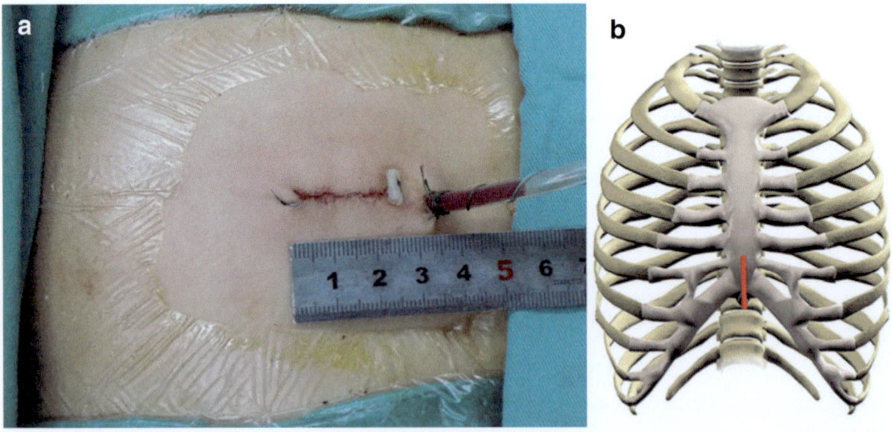

Fig. 41.4 Inferior partial median sternotomy approach. (**a**) The median skin incision (about 2 cm). (**b**) An ideograph of the lower sternum and xiphoid bone incision

then the free wall of the right ventricle is exposed for puncture. A purse-string suture is placed on the right ventricular free wall directly facing the direction of the pmVSD shunt. The right ventricle is punctured within the purse-string suture with a

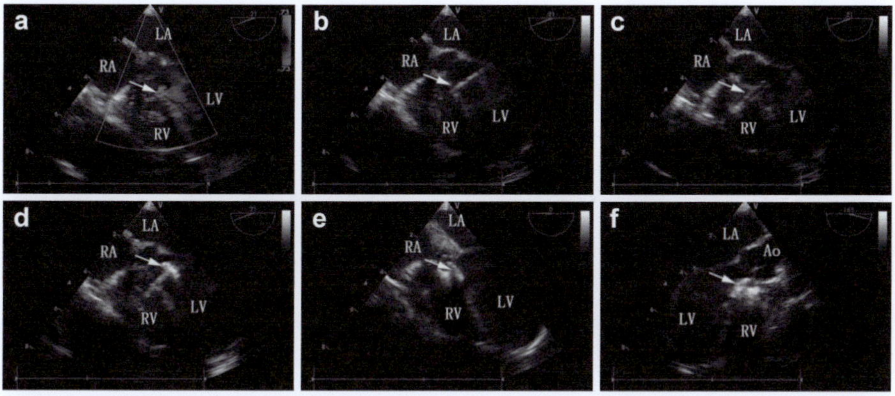

Fig. 41.5 TEE views of the procedures. (**a**) Doppler view of pmVSDs (*arrow*). (**b**) The guidewire (*arrow*) was inserted through the pmVSD. (**c**) The delivery sheath (*arrow*) was inserted through the pmVSD. (**d**) The left ventricle disk of the occluder (*arrow*) was deployed. (**e**) The occluder (*arrow*) was deployed under four-chamber view guidance. (**f**) Occluder (*arrow*) and aortic valve in the long axis view of the aorta. *RA* right atrium, *RV* right ventricle, *LA* left atrium, *LV* left ventricle, and *AO* aorta

trocar. A 0.035-in. guidewire is placed in the trocar. The guidewire is passed through the pmVSD, then the trocar is removed, and the dilator and delivery sheath are advanced through the pmVSD to the left ventricle along the guidewire. The size of the occluder is chosen 1–2 mm larger than the diameter of the pmVSD. After removing the guidewire and dilator sheath, the selected occluder is deployed through the delivery sheath under TEE guidance.

TEE is used to reassess the shape and position of the occluder, the presence of a residual shunt, and the valvular regurgitation before and after occluder release (Fig. 41.5). Finally, the delivery sheath is withdrawn, and the purse-string suture is tied using the knotter. After the procedure, a drainage tube is placed in the mediastinum.

Another common surgical approach is via the left fourth parasternal intercostal space incision. After placing patients in supine position, a 1–2 cm median thoracic skin incision is made. The subcutaneous tissue is dissected up to the left fourth parasternal intercostal space. The intercostal muscles are dissected to establish the procedural approach.

The two approaches have differential advantages. The inferior partial median sternotomy provides better surgical exposure and facilitates incision extension. The parasternal intercostal approach is less traumatic and precludes the use of a drainage tube.

Potential complications of TEE-guided perventricular pmVSD device closure include valve regurgitation, malignant arrhythmia, device dislocation, and residual shunt. In patients with tricuspid regurgitation before the procedure, it is very important to verify the absence of worsening tricuspid regurgitation. If severe atrioventricular block develops after the release of the occluder, the patient must be converted immediately to conventional surgical closure, ideally in the same operation room after extending the incision. In case of device dislocation, an absorbable insurance

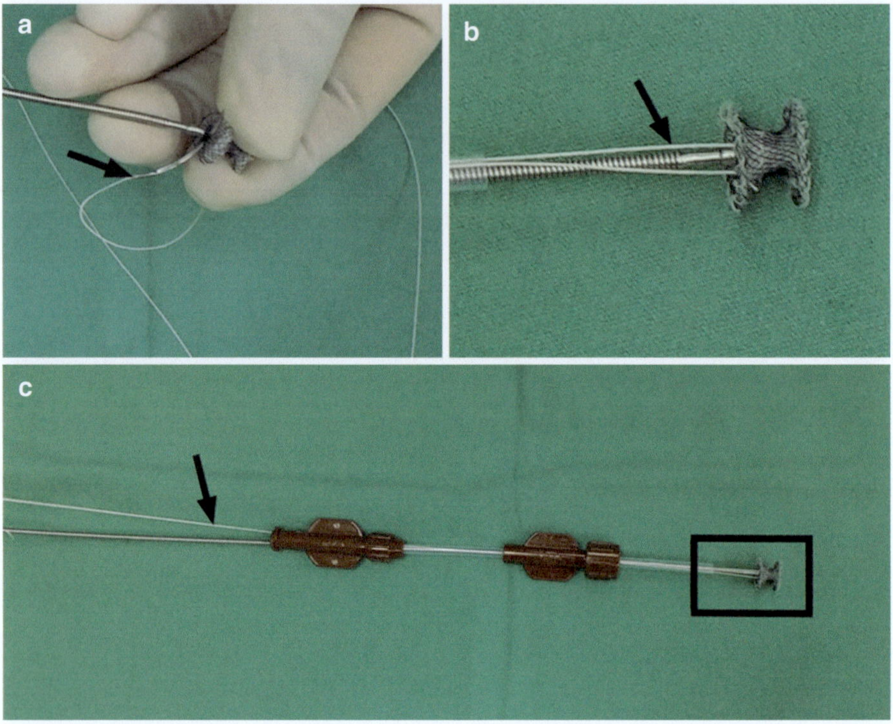

Fig. 41.6 Intraoperative insurance line. (**a**) The absorbable insurance line is stitched into the occluder. (**b**, **c**) The absorbable insurance line is fixed in the delivery sheath

stitch can be sutured on the right side of the occluder, after being delivered together with the occluder from the delivery sheath and knotted with the purse-string suture (Fig. 41.6).

41.2.3 Postoperative Management

After procedure completion, patients are transferred to an intensive care unit where the endotracheal tube is removed. Echocardiography, chest radiography, and electrocardiography are used for postoperative evaluation. After operation, all patients receive aspirin (3–5 mg/kg body weight, orally) daily for 6 months, and undergo transthoracic echocardiography and electrocardiography evaluation at 1, 3, 6, and 12 months and annually thereafter.

41.3 Literature and Results

Perventricular device pmVSD closure can be used in patients as young as 2 months old [1, 2]. First attempted in 1999 [2–4], perventricular device closure was developed to overcome the drawbacks of transfemoral device occlusion and conventional surgical repair [1, 5, 6], achieving a current success rate of 88.9–100 % in most studies [1, 5–8], as summarized in Table 41.2. Perventricular device pmVSD closure is a simple procedure with almost no blood loss, minimal physical injury, quick recovery and lower mean mortality than that of percutaneous and surgical repair approaches.

Complete atrioventricular block (cAVB) is one of the most serious complications of conventional transcatheter occlusion of pmVSD with a reported incidence of 1–8 % [9] and even up to 22 % in one report [10]. Compared with open-heart surgery, cAVB occurrence in patients with transcatheter occlusion is unpredictable, and late-onset cAVB has drawn much attention [11–13] driving many cardiac centers to discontinue the use of this method in patients with pmVSDs.

In contrast, perventricular device pmVSD closure appears to provide a differential advantage in terms of cAVB occurrence. In a group of 1630 pmVSDs patients (Table 41.2), heart block was a rare complication with no cAVB developing during over 12 months follow-up in three studies [5, 14, 15], only one case of delayed cAVB that reverted to sinus rhythm after glucocorticoid treatment in another study [1], and seven cases of cAVB, five cases of Mobitz type II AVB, and 23 cases of incomplete right bundle branch block in another nine studies (Table 41.2).

Xing et al. [5] showed that cAVB incidence associated with perventricular device pmVSD closure is significantly lower with modified occluders (0–1.3 %) [13, 16, 17] than conventional procedure with Amplatzer occluders (2.0–20 %) [10, 13].

This could be explained by the following hypothesis:

(1) Inflammation and edema of tissues around pmVSDs resulting from compression of the occluder might play an essential role in the occurrence of early postoperative cAVB, modified occluders with a waist height of 4 mm and a waist diameter 1–2 mm larger than pmVSD diameter appear to reduce the compression of tissues around pmVSDs. (2) The basic principle in occluder selection is that the occluder should not exceed VSD diameter by more than 2 mm, which may reduce the possibility of cAVB caused by an oversized occluder. (3) In perventricular device pmVSD closure, a short and flexible delivery device is used with no need to operate on the left ventricle or to establish an arteriovenous circuit across the tricuspid annulus. The conduction systems lay under the left ventricular endocardium; therefore, perventricular approach produces less stimulation to the left ventricular endocardium and the defect's surrounding tissue. (4) Familiarity with cardiac anatomy together with skillful manipulation of the easily controlled delivery could obviously reduce the stimulation of defect edges and its surrounding tissues.

Valve regurgitation is another important complication due to the short subaortic rim of pmVSDs and close proximity of the closure device to valves or the subvalvular apparatus. According to published studies (Table 41.2), the most common valve dysfunction is device-induced tricuspid regurgitation (61 cases, 4.2 %), followed by aortic regurgitation (15 cases, 1.0 %). Most cases of regurgitation were asymptomatic and improved spontaneously during follow-up. Compared to the 9.2 % rate of tricuspid and aortic regurgitation reported with the percutaneous approach [18], the perventricular approach is less likely to induce valve complications because the sheath approaches the defect directly, without passing through the valves. The simplicity and controllability of perventricular technique can avoid damage to the valves and subvalvular.

Table 41.2 Studies on perventricular device closure of pmVSDs

Author/year	Sample size	Age	Weight (kg)	VSD size (mm)	Device size (mm)	Successful/complete closure rate	Complication	Follow-up length
Pan/2015 [1]	187	8.2 ± 10.2 years	Not reported	5.31 ± 2.86 mm	6.68 ± 3.07 mm	95.7 %	Trivial residual shunt (8/187) iRBBB (6/187) cAVB(1/187)	(12.6 ± 10.4) months
Xing/2015 [5]	458	11.4 ± 6.73 m	9.82 ± 5.88	5.21 ± 2.95	No reported	96.29 %	No deaths or major complications Minor complications: New iRBBB or cRBBB(41/441) New trace to mild TR (26/441) Trace to mild AR(7/441) Trivial to small residual shunting (27/441)/(11/441) at follow-up	6-78 months (47.31 ± 19.69) months
Zhu/2013 [6]	40	2.1 ± 0.9 years (0.4–3.5)	12.7 ± 3.4 (5.5–19)	5.8 ± 1.7 (3–10.5)	7.3 ± 2.0 (4–12)	77.5 %/83.9 % postop 96.8 % at follow-up	Failure in establishing track (3/40) > mild TR (2/40) > mild AR (2/40) cAVB(1/40)	1–1.5 years (1.2 ± 0.2) years
Wang/2013 [7]	61	2.1(0.5–11) years	12.1 (6–25)	4.2 (2.5–7)	5.3 (4–8)	100 %/100 %	Mild AR (1/61)	1–21 months (13.5 ± 8.2) months
Zhang/2012 [8]	18	12.0 ± 7.4 months	10.2 ± 3.6	6.5 ± 1.0 (5–9)	8.1 ± 0.9 (7–10)	88.9 %/88.9 %	Residual shunt to reoperate (1/18) Transient arrhythmia (1/18) Mild AR (1/18)	Not reported

Xing/2009 [15]	21	3.6 years	15.8 ± 6.4 kg	3–12	4–13	100 %/100 %	No residual shunt, noticeable aortic or tricuspid regurgitation, or significant arrhythmias developed	>5 months
Xing/2010 [20]	408	3.1 ± 1.7 years	13.6 ± 5.5 (4.5–26)	5.3 ± 1.6 (3–12)	Not reported	96.3 %/100 % at follow-up	Device-induced TR (13/408) (5 months–15 years) IRBBB (11/408)	(14.6 ± 6.2) months
Luo/2015 [19]	172	3.7 ± 5.5	14.9 ± 13.0	4.5 ± 1.6	Not reported	94.8 %/99.4 %	CAVB (2/172) Mobitz II AVB (1/172) Large residual shunt(1/172) Minor residual shunt (10/172)/(1/172) at follow-up Failure to establish the occluder conveying rail (1/172) Failure to achieve a suitable or stable occluder position (4/172)	>2 years
Zhang/2015 [14]	265	14.15 ± 8.01	8.94 ± 3.06	7.05 ± 2.42	Not reported	96.23 %	Residual arrhythmia (82/265) Residual AR (14/265) Residual T R (20/265) Residual MR (18/265)	>12 months

Data are presented as mean ± SD (range) when available

IRBBB incomplete right bundle branch block, *cAVB* complete atrioventricular block, *TR* tricuspid regurgitation, *AR* aortic regurgitation, *PR* pulmonary regurgitation

Residual shunting is a common complication in most studies; however, minor residual shunting (<2 mm) can spontaneously disappear after the procedure, with rate of residual shunting decreasing significantly from 6.12–2.58 % at follow-up [19, 20]. Midterm results showed a successful closure rate of 100 % (3–24 months) without significant complications [20]. The long-term (6 years) clinical outcomes are also promising [3]. Perventricular device closure of pmVSDs on a beating heart therefore appears to be a safe and effective alternative to conventional treatments.

In terms of technical considerations, passing the guidewire and the delivery sheath across the defect is a crucial step for successful closure. It is mandatory to check the delivery sheath tip as it passes through the defect. In fact, when the delivery sheath enters the left ventricle, bright red blood is obtained from the proximal end of the delivery sheath. Surgeons and ultrasound specialists should always be cautious in order to avoid any damage of cardiac structures such as aortic or mitral valves. Finally, involvement of the patient's parents in deciding on the most appropriate choice of pmVSDs closure procedure is mandatory.

In conclusion, the perventricular device VSD closure can be performed successfully and with satisfied outcomes under echocardiography while avoiding radiation and contrast agent exposure. With a combination of strict indications, procedural specifications, and rigorously trained medical staff, this technology has broad potential for further development and applications.

References

1. Ou-Yang WB, Li SJ, Wang SZ, et al. Echocardiographic guided closure of perimembranous ventricular septal defects. Ann Thorac Surg. 2015;100(4):1398–402.
2. Xing Q, Zhuang Z, Pan S, et al. Minimally invasive transthoracic device closure of perimembranous ventricular septal defect with a newly designed delivery system in 11 children. Chin J Exp Surg. 2007;24(9):1135–36.
3. Amin Z, Danford DA, Lof J, et al. Intraoperative device closure of perimembranous ventricular septal defects without cardiopulmonary bypass: preliminary results with the perventricular technique. J Thorac Cardiovasc Surg. 2004;127:234–41.
4. Amin Z, Gu X, Berry JM, et al. Periventricular closure of ventricular septal defects without cardiopulmonary bypass. Ann Thorac Surg. 1999;68:149–53; discussion 153–4.
5. Xing Q, Wu Q, Shi L, et al. Minimally invasive transthoracic device closure of isolated ventricular septal defects without cardiopulmonary bypass: long-term follow-up results. J Thorac Cardiovasc Surg. 2015;149:257–64.
6. Zhu D, Gan C, Li X, et al. Perventricular device closure of perimembranous ventricular septal defect in pediatric patients: technical and morphological considerations. Thorac Cardiovasc Surg. 2013;61:300–6.
7. Wang S, Zhuang Z, Zhang H, et al. Perventricular closure of perimembranous ventricular septal defects using the concentric occluder device. Pediatr Cardiol. 2014;35:580–6.
8. Zhang GC, Chen Q, Chen LW, et al. Transthoracic echocardiographic guidance of minimally invasive perventricular device closure of perimembranous ventricular septal defect without cardiopulmonary bypass: initial experience. Eur Heart J Cardiovasc Imaging. 2012;13:739–44.
9. Butera G, Carminati M, Chessa M, et al. Percutaneous closure of ventricular septal defects in children aged <12: early and mid-term results. Eur Heart J. 2006;27:2889–95.
10. Predescu D, Chaturvedi RR, Friedberg MK, et al. Complete heart block associated with device closure of perimembranous ventricular septal defects. J Thorac Cardiovasc Surg. 2008;136:1223–8.

11. Zhou K, Hua Y, Qiao L. A case of late-onset sustained ventricular tachycardia following deployment of Amplatzer-type perimembranous VSD occluder. Catheter Cardiovasc Interv. 2014;83:256–60.
12. Li X, Li L, Wang X, et al. Clinical analysis of transcatheter closure of perimembranous ventricular septal defects with occluders made in China. Chin Med J (Engl). 2011;124:2117–22.
13. Carminati M, Butera G, Chessa M, et al. Transcatheter closure of congenital ventricular septal defects: results of the European Registry. Eur Heart J. 2007;28:2361–8.
14. Zhang X, Xing Q, Wu Q. Treatment of perimembranous ventricular septal defect in children weighing less than 15 kg: minimally invasive periventricular device occlusion versus right subaxillary small incision surgical repair. Thorac Cardiovasc Surg. 2015;63(5):409–18.
15. Quansheng X, Silin P, Zhongyun Z, et al. Minimally invasive perventricular device closure of an isolated perimembranous ventricular septal defect with a newly designed delivery system: preliminary experience. J Thorac Cardiovasc Surg. 2009;137:556–9.
16. Jin Y, Han B, Zhang J, et al. Postimplant complications with transcatheter closure of congenital perimembranous ventricular septal defects: a single-center, longitudinal study from 2002 to 2011. Catheter Cardiovasc Interv. 2013;2013(81):666–73.
17. Wang L, Cao S, Li J, et al. Transcatheter closure of congenital perimembranous ventricular septal defect in children using symmetric occluders: an 8-year multiinstitutional experience. Ann Thorac Surg. 2012;94:592–8.
18. Holzer R, de Giovanni J, Walsh KP, et al. Transcatheter closure of perimembranous ventricular septal defects using the amplatzer membranous VSD occluder: immediate and midterm results of an international registry. Catheter Cardiovasc Interv. 2006;68:620–8.
19. Luo YK, Chen WH, Xiong C, et al. Comparison of effectiveness and cost between perventricular device occlusion and minimally invasive surgical repair for perimembranous ventricular septal defect. Pediatr Cardiol. 2015;36:308–13.
20. Xing Q, Pan S, An Q, et al. Minimally invasive perventricular device closure of perimembranous ventricular septal defect without cardiopulmonary bypass: multicenter experience and mid-term follow-up. J Thorac Cardiovasc Surg. 2010;139:1409–15.

Part X

Other Hybrid Procedures

Hybrid Atrial Septal Defect Closure

42

Ziyad M. Hijazi

Secundum atrial septal defect (ASD) is one of the most common congenital heart diseases (CHD) accounting for approximately 6–10 % of all CHD in children [1]. In general, the recommendation for elective ASD closure is after 4 years of age [2] as many of these defects have a high rate of spontaneous closure and these patients are largely asymptomatic in the first few years of life [3–6]. Occasionally, however, patients with ASD present in infancy with signs and symptoms of congestive heart failure [7], frequent respiratory infections [8], and failure to thrive [9]. This can necessitate earlier intervention.

Since 1975, when King et al. [10] attempted the first transcatheter closure of a secundum ASD in a patient using a double-umbrella device, device closure became a widely acceptable alternative to surgery in most patients with ASD [11–13]. It is, however, still considered technically challenging in some cases, particularly in infants and in patients with deficient rims or large defects. Despite many studies showing that transcatheter ASD closure in small children is highly successful [14–18], some reported significantly higher complication rates [19]. Indeed, several factors make this procedure challenging in these patients including a small left atrial (LA) cavity, deficient atrial rims, floppiness of the inferior rim, and the orientation of the interatrial septum which makes it challenging to keep the ASD device parallel to the plane of the septum [20, 21].

The hybrid technique, also called peratrial or percardiac technique, for ASD closure is a relatively recent alternative approach to closure of ASDs. This approach combines the advantages of percutaneous intervention and open-chest surgery without the trauma of cardiopulmonary bypass (CPB) and has been increasingly used for various additional lesions [22–25].

This technique is usually performed in pediatric patients in whom size is a limiting factor, particularly infants less than 3.5 kg, those who are at high risk for

Z.M. Hijazi
Department of Pediatrics, Weill Cornell Medical College, Doha, Qatar
e-mail: zhijazi@sidra.org

G. Butera et al. (eds.), *Fetal and Hybrid Procedures in Congenital Heart Diseases*, DOI 10.1007/978-3-319-40088-4_42

surgical closure or exposure to CPB or those with significant ASDs in addition to other cardiac lesions necessitating hybrid procedures (e.g., perventricular ventricular septal defect (VSD) closure). In addition, the technique has been shown to be also advantageous in young adults with deficient rims or large defects [26–30]. It provides several advantages to either surgical or transcatheter closure techniques.

First, it avoids CPB and its systemic inflammatory response and potential neurologic sequelae, particularly in young infants. There is no need for chest tube drainage or blood transfusion and it results in less pain, faster recovery, shorter hospital stay, and a better cosmetic result [26, 28].

Second, the hybrid approach allows preservation of the femoral vessels and avoidance of the challenge in patients with femoral venous obstruction or interrupted inferior vena cava and avoidance of inserting large sheaths into the jugular or hepatic veins. This can be particularly advantageous in small children.

Third, it can help avoid exposure to radiation and contrast agents, which can be especially important in vulnerable infants.

Lastly, this technique provides an easier and more stable approach to closing the atrial defect with a device because of the perpendicular angle to the atrial septum that helps avoid prolapse of the LA disk into the right atrium (RA). In the hybrid procedure, the position of the left disk is easier to adjust with the short sheath being used compared to the long delivery sheath system used in the transcatheter approach. This can also be particularly helpful in patients with ASDs with a deficient rim as well as in those with large ASDs where the device could be unstable [30].

42.1 Peratrial Closure Protocol

This procedure is done under transesophageal echocardiogram (TEE) guidance and can be performed either in the catheterization laboratory or in the operating or hybrid room. The ASD is first assessed fully by TEE noting the number and size of ASD(s) and the adequacy of the atrial rims as is done for the percutaneous transcatheter procedure ASD closure. Following this assessment, a minimal 2.5–3 cm lower sternotomy incision is typically performed. Some operators have opted to approach the septum through a mini or a lateral thoracotomy incision to expose the RA [26, 27, 29]. Heparin is then administered at 100 units/kg to achieve an activated clotting time of greater than 200 s at the time of device deployment. The RA wall is then punctured with an 18-gauge needle through which a 0.035 wire is passed to the LA [alternatively, a micropuncture needle (0.021'0 can be used and a coaxial dilator is used)]. The delivery sheath, together with the dilator, is then passed over the wire into the mid LA. The correct position of the sheath is then verified by TEE by injecting agitated saline bubbles into the LA. Extreme care should be exercised how far to pass the dilator/sheath assembly. Therefore, TEE imaging is crucial and measurement of the distance between the cavity of the left atrium and the free wall of the right atrium is done so that the dilator/sheath won't be advanced more than this distance.

The appropriately sized device as determined by echocardiography is then loaded into the sheath as is done with the standard percutaneous approach. There is no need for balloon sizing during this procedure. We usually choose a device about 1–2 mm larger than the ASD as measured by color Doppler. The left disk of the device is deployed first and retracted against the atrial septum and then the sheath is retracted to allow deployment of the right disk. The position of the device is then confirmed by TEE in multiple planes in order to ensure stability of the device, no significant residual shunt, no AV valve regurgitation, and no pulmonary vein obstruction before the device is released. There is little risk of device embolization with this technique; however, in the event of such complication, the device can be retrieved through the same sternotomy incision, after going on CPB. Figure 42.1 demonstrates the steps of a closure in a 4 kg infant with large atrial septal defect.

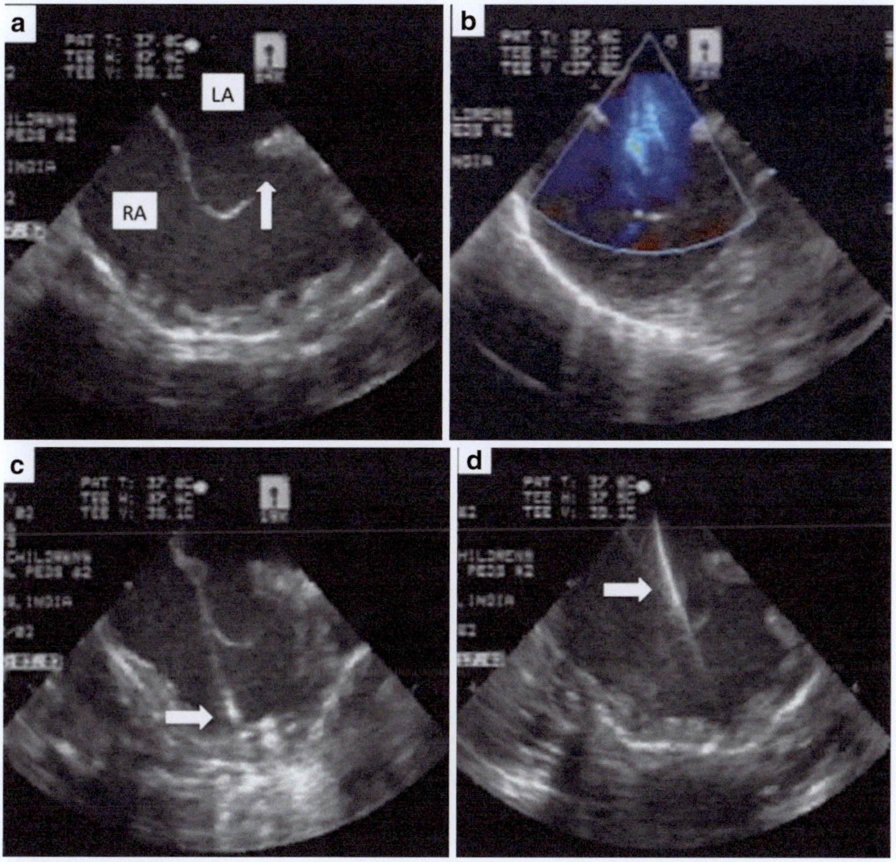

Fig. 42.1 Transesophageal echocardiographic (TEE) images in 2.5 month female infant, 4 kg in weight with a large muscular ventricular septal defect (VSD) and a large atrial septal defect (ASD) measuring 10 mm with aneurysm formation, who underwent a hybrid closure of her VSD followed by hybrid (peratrial) device closure of her ASD. (**a**, **b**) TEE images without and with color Doppler showing the large ASD with aneurysm formation (*white arrow* in (**a**)) and the color jet in (**b**). LA, left atrium; RA, right atrium. (**c**, **d**) TEE images during puncture of the right atrial free wall with a 0.035" needle (*white arrow* in (**c**)), then passage of the guidewire into the left atrium via the defect (*white arrow* in (**d**)). (**e**, **f**) TEE images in four chamber view (**e**) showing the tip of the sheath (*white arrow*). Then the left atrial desk of a 11 mm Amplatzer septal occlude (*white arrow*) positioned on the atrial septum as seen in (**f**). (**g**, **h**) TEE images after deployment of the two desks, while the device still attached to the delivery cable (*white arrow* in (**g**)), then image (**h**) after the device was released showing good device position

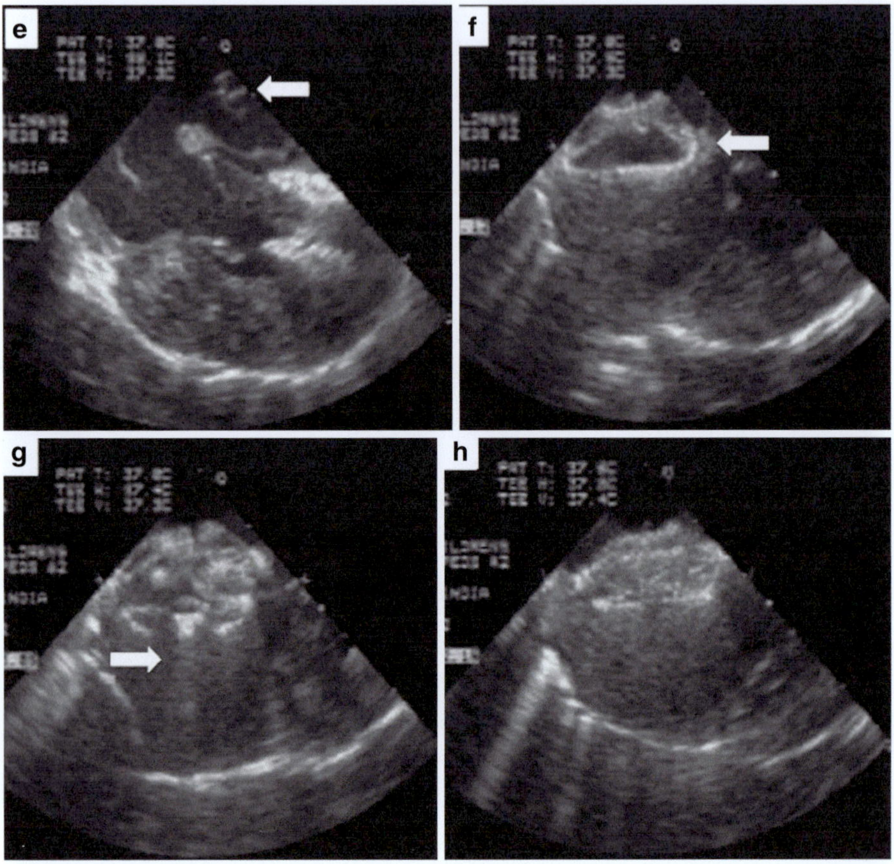

Fig. 42.1 (continued)

42.2 Results

Several studies have recently documented the efficacy, safety, and advantages of the hybrid approach to ASD closure. One large study by Hongxin et al. [27] reported on the successful use of intraoperative device closure of secundum ASDs in 100 patients ranging in ages from 5 to 71 years (mean 29 ± 16 years) and with a weight range of 16–94 kg (mean weight, 54 ± 18 kg). The procedure was done through a right minithoracotomy incision without CPB or fluoroscopy. It was successful in all patients including five patients with double ASDs that were successfully occluded with one device. Of note, 61 patients had an ASD measuring more than 20 mm (range 5–37 mm) and the implanted devices ranged in size from 8 to 36 mm. Residual shunts were uncommon with complete occlusion rates of 95 % at discharge, 99 % at the 3-month follow-up, and 100 % at the 1-year follow-up, and no late complications during the follow-up period.

Zeng et al. [29] reported on the use of a modified Amplatzer device for peratrial closure of ASD in a series of 96 ASDs in 83 patients with an age range of 2–61 years (mean 25.6 ± 14.6) and a weight of 10–80 kg. The ASD size ranged from 10 to 39 mm (mean 25.5 ± 8.4 mm). The closure was done through a minithoracotomy under TEE guidance. All ASDs were successfully closed with device size ranging from 12 to 46 mm. There were ten cases of hemothorax but no major morbidity.

Another study compared a series of 115 children with secundum ASDs who underwent peratrial device closure through a small sternotomy under TEE guidance and without CPB to a group of 54 children who underwent surgical ASD closure with CPB [31]. They had successful closure in 114 cases and showed that the duration of the operation, mechanical ventilation, intensive care, and hospitalization and the rate of blood transfusion were significantly lower in the peratrial group compared to the bypass group.

Similar encouraging results were reported after hybrid closure of ASD in infancy and small children [16, 22, 31–36]. Li et al. [33] reported their 5 years experience of intraoperative hybrid procedure with neonates and young children with CHD. They had 43 patients undergoing device closure including perventricular VSD and transatrial ASD closure with only two failed ASD cases.

Zhao et al. [22] reported the use of TEE guidance of percardiac closure of intracardiac defects in 42 patients with low weight including 19 with ASDs. Patients ranged in ages from 2 months to 5 years (median, 18.4 months) and weighed from 4 to 10 kg (median, 8.9 kg). The ASDs ranged in size from 7 to 24 mm (mean 13.4 ± 4.6 mm). They had successful occlusions and low rate of complications with one patient developing first degree heart block and early pericardial effusion that resolved later.

We have also previously reported on the safety and outcome of device closure of ASDs with the Amplatzer septal occluder in infants in a series of 15 patients with three cases being deployed through the peratrial technique [16]. The approach was selected owing to the size of the infant (<3.5 kg) in two cases and because of simultaneous perventricular VSD closure in the third case. The size of the defects ranged from 2 to 8 mm with a case with three defects. All had successful closure with one minor complication with intermittent heart block in one case.

Additional case reports also documented the efficacy of the peratrial approach to ASD closure in infants [34–36]. The technique was used for various reasons including blocked femoral access, the risk of neurological injury from exposure to CPB due to neurological factors such as cerebral arteriovenous malformation, and the risk of complications from CPB particularly in patients with chronic lung disease and pulmonary hypertension.

The protocol for peratrial closure under TEE guidance is straightforward and does not require balloon sizing. Some authors have argued that a key issue for the success of the procedure is the site for puncturing the right atrial wall at the base of the right atrial appendage [36] which provides the straightest course to the LA allowing to cross the atrial septum in a perpendicular fashion and to orient the LA disk as parallel as possible to the septum. This would help avoid prolapse of the device if there is any deficient rims.

Conclusion

The hybrid or peratrial approach to ASD closure is feasible and provides an effective alternative approach for ASD closure in small and high risk infants and those with limited access. It also allows avoidance of CPB and provides an attractive approach to treating children with multiple congenital cardiac shunt lesions as well as in some adults. Long-term follow-up will further help assess the safety and effectiveness of these procedures as alternatives to conventional therapy.

References

1. Dickinson DF, Arnold R, Wilkinson JL. Congenital heart disease among 160480 live-born children in Liverpool 1960 to 1969. Implications for surgical treatment. Br Heart J. 1981;46:55–62.
2. Castaneda AR, Jonas RA, Mayer JE, Hanley FL. Atrial septal defect. In: Cardiac surgery of the neonate and infants. Philadelphia: WB Saunders; 1994.
3. Cockerham JT, Martin TC, Gutierrez FR, Hartmann AF, Goldring D, Strauss AW. Spontaneous closure of secundum atrial septal defect in infants and young children. Am J Cardiol. 1983;52:1267–71.
4. Fukazawa M, Fukushige J, Ueda K. Atrial septal defects in neonates with reference to spontaneous closure. Am Heart J. 1988;116:123–7.
5. Radzik D, Davignon A, Van Doesburg N, Fournier A, Marchand T, Ducharme G. Predictive factors for spontaneous closure of atrial septal defects diagnosed in the first 3 months of life. J Am Coll Cardiol. 1993;22:851–3.
6. Saxena A, Divekar A, Soni NR. Natural history of secundum atrial septal defect revisited in the era of transcatheter closure. Indian Heart J. 2005;57:35–8.
7. Phillips SJ, Okies JE, Henken D, Sunderland CO, Starr A. Complex of secundum atrial septal defect and congestive heart failure in infants. J Thorac Cardiovasc Surg. 1975;70:696–700.
8. Hunt CE, Lucas Jr RV. Symptomatic atrial septal defect in infancy. Circulation. 1973;47:1042–8.
9. Dimich I, Steinfeld L, Park SC. Symptomatic atrial septal defect in infants. Am Heart J. 1973;85:601–4.
10. King TD, Thompson SL, Steiner C, Mills ML. Secundum atrial septal defect. Nonoperative closure during cardiac catheterization. JAMA. 1976;235:2506–9.
11. Du ZD, Hijazi ZM, Kleinman CS, et al. Comparison between transcatheter and surgical closure of secundum atrial septal defect in children and adults: results of a multicenter nonrandomized trial. J Am Coll Cardiol. 2002;39:1836–44.
12. Visconti KJ, Bichell DP, Jonas RA, et al. Developmental outcome after surgical versus interventional closure of secundum atrial septal defect in children. Circulation. 1999;100(19 Suppl):II145–50.
13. Thomson JDR, Aburawi EH, Watterson KG, Van Doorn C, Gibbs JL. Surgical and transcatheter (Amplatzer) closure of atrial septal defects: a prospective comparison of results and cost. Heart. 2002;87:466–9.
14. Vogel M, Berger F, Dahnert I, Ewert P, Lange PE. Treatment of atrial septal defects in symptomatic children aged less than 2 years of age using the Amplatzer septal occluder. Cardiol Young. 2000;10:534–7.

15. Butera G, De Rosa G, Chessa M, et al. Transcatheter closure of atrial septal defect in young children: results and follow-up. J Am Coll Cardiol. 2003;42:241–5.
16. Diab KA, Cao QL, Bacha EA, Hijazi ZM. Device closure of atrial septal defects with the Amplatzer septal occlude: safety and outcome in infants. J Thorac Cardiovasc Surg. 2007;134:960–6.
17. Fischer G, Smevik B, Kramer HH, Bjornstad PG. Catheter-based closure of atrial septal defects in the oval fossa with the Amplatzer device in patients in their first or second year of life. Catheter Cardiovasc Interv. 2009;73:949–55.
18. Bishnoi RN, Everett AD, Ringel RE, Owada CY, Holzer RJ, Chisolm JL, Radtke WA, Scott Lim D, Rhodes Jr JF, Coulson JD. Device closure of secundum atrial septal defects in infants weighing less than 8kg. Pediatr Cardiol. 2014;35(7):1124–31.
19. Bartakian S, Fagan TE, Schaffer MS, Darst JR. Device closure of secundum atrial septal defects in children <15 kg. JACC Cardiovasc Interv. 2012;5:1178–84.
20. Varma C, Benson LN, Silversides C, et al. Outcomes and alternative techniques for device closure of the large secundum atrial septal defect. Catheter Cardiovasc Interv. 2004;61:131–9.
21. Nagm AM, Rao PS. Percutaneous occlusion of complex atrial septal defects. J Invasive Cardiol. 2004;16:123–5.
22. Zhao T, Yang Y, Xu X. Transesophageal echocardiographic guidance of percardiac device closure of intracardiac defects in patients weighing less than 10 kg. J Card Surg. 2012;27:740–4.
23. Wen Z, Xu M, Chun Z, Yan L. Transthoracic occlusion for patent ductus arteriosus. J Cardiovasc Pulm Dis. 2011;30:325–7.
24. Xuezeng X, Shiqiang Y, Jincheng L. Comparison between totally thoracoscopic and transthoracic occlusion surgery in treatment of arterial septal defect for children. Chin J Clin Thorac Cardiovasc Surg. 2007;14:338–40.
25. Quansheng X, Zhongyun Z, Sijin P. Minimally invasive device closure of perimembranous ventricular septal defect with a new delivery system. Chin J Exp Surg. 2007;24:1135–6.
26. Yoshimura N, Yamaguchi M, Oshima Y, Oka S, Ootaki Y, Yoshida M. Repair of atrial septal defect through a right posterolateral thoracotomy: a cosmetic approach for female patients. Ann Thorac Surg. 2001;72:2103–5.
27. Hongxin L, Wenbin G, Lijun S, Zhengjun W, Hao L, Chengwei Z, et al. Intraoperative device closure of secundum atrial septal defect with a right anterior minithoracotomy in 100 patients. J Thorac Cardiovasc Surg. 2007;134:946–51.
28. Liang T, Xiangjun Z, Xiaojing M, Yun L, Leng CY. New minimally invasive technique to occlude secundum atrial septal defect in 53 patients. Ann Thorac Surg. 2006;81:1417–9.
29. Zeng XJ, Chen XF, Cheng D, Ma XJ, Hu XS, Tao L. Peratrial closure of atrial septal defects without cardiopulmonary bypass. Asian Cardiovasc Thorac Ann. 2007;15:191–3.
30. Tao KY, An Q, Gan CP, Tang H, Feng Y, Song HB. Give the patient another chance: peratrial device closure of a secundum atrial septal defect that failed percutaneous device closure. J Thorac Cardiovasc Surg. 2009;137:1024–7.
31. Yin N, Zhao T, Yang Y, Xu X, Wang X, Wu Q, Gao L, Chen J. Evaluation of minimally invasive peratrial device closure of secundum atrial septal defects in children. Zhong Nan Da Xue Xue Bao Yi Xue Ban. 2011;36:576–80.
32. Hu S, Yang Y, Zhu Y, Wu Q, Muhoozi R, Wei S, Huang X, Zhao T. Experience with percardiac interventions for multiple congenital heart diseases in children. Interact CardioVasc Thorac Surg. 2014;19:812–5.
33. Li SJ, Zhang H, Sheng XD, Yan J, Deng XC, Chen WD, et al. Intraoperative hybrid cardiac surgery for neonates and young children with congenital heart disease: 5 years of experience. Ann Thorac Cardiovasc Surg. 2010;16:406–9.
34. Sheth K, Jain S, Joshi S, Dalvi B. Hybrid closure of atrial septal defect: a modified approach. Ann Pediatr Cardiol. 2015;8:74–7.
35. Delaney JW, Thorell WE, Hammel JM. Hybrid peratrial double device closure of a patent foramen ovale and sinus venosus defect in an infant with vein of Galen malformation. Catheter Cardiovasc Interv. 2011;78:1045–50.
36. Pedra SF, Jatene M, Pedra CA. Hybrid management of a large atrial septal defect and a patent ductus arteriosus in an infant with chronic lung disease. Ann Pediatr Cardiol. 2010;3:68–73.

Treatment of RV Outflow Tract Dysfunction: New Valve Technologies

43

John P. Cheatham

Approximately 22 % of all congenital heart disease patients have an abnormality of the right ventricular outflow tract. During the course of surgery for this condition, approximately 23 % of the patients will receive some form of a valved RV to PA conduit. These patients are candidates for the Medtronic Melody transcatheter pulmonary valve (TPV) (Medtronic, Minneapolis, MN) or, in some parts of the world, the Edwards SAPIEN pulmonic valve (Edwards Lifesciences Corp., Irvine, CA). However, approximately 77 % of patients will have surgical correction of the RV outflow tract with patch enlargement, with or without pulmonary valvectomy, and many will have a transannular patch placed. Most of these patients will be left with significant pulmonary regurgitation (PR) resulting in RV volume overload and potential RV dysfunction later in life. Developing a transcatheter pulmonary valve to fit this complex anatomy was much more challenging than the design of the Melody TPV for RV-PA conduit dysfunction.

Eventually, Medtronic worked with Professor Philipp Bonhoeffer, similar to the Melody TPV, in designing and testing the Native Transcatheter Pulmonary Valve. This resulted in the first inhuman (FIH) implant at Great Ormand Street Hospital (GOSH) in January 2009 in a very complex adult who was an extreme high risk for surgical repair [1]. After ethical committee approval, the implant occurred with a successful outcome. Unlike the Melody TPV, which is a bovine jugular vein valve sewn to a platinum-iridium stent frame, NuMED CP stent (NuMED, Inc., Hopkinton, NY), and is balloon expandable, the Native Transcatheter Pulmonary Valve is a porcine pericardial valve sewn within a self-expandable nitinol frame covered with a polyester cloth and was manufactured in only one size to fit the patient in question. However, after the successful FIH implant, the development of this product was delayed while further design and testing was performed at Medtronic.

J.P. Cheatham, MD, FAAP, FACC, MSCAI
The Heart Center, Nationwide Children's Hospital, Pediatrics & Internal Medicine, Cardiology, The Ohio State University, Columbus, OH, USA
e-mail: John.Cheatham@nationwidechildrens.org

G. Butera et al. (eds.), *Fetal and Hybrid Procedures in Congenital Heart Diseases*, DOI 10.1007/978-3-319-40088-4_43

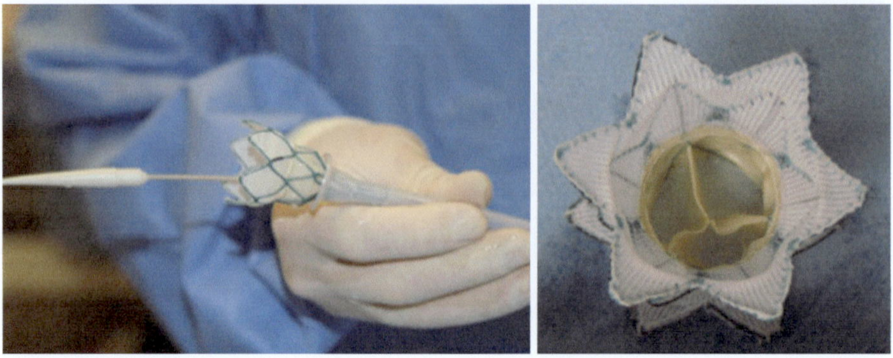

Fig. 43.1 The *left panel* shows the white "nose cone" and the funnel loading technique of the valve frame. The panel to the right demonstrates the porcine pericardial valve sewn into the polyester fabric frame

Finally in 2012, Medtronic submitted an early feasibility study (EFS) to the FDA for the Native Transcatheter Pulmonary Valve and was the first EFS to be approved in the USA. The research clinical study involved three sites: Nationwide Children's Hospital (NCH) for the USA, Toronto Sick Kids Hospital (TSK) for Canada, and Munich Heart Institute for Europe. There were regulatory issues in Germany that prevented the EFS from being performed there, so the third site was offered to Boston Children's Hospital (BCH). This particular study was unlike any other device trial involving congenital heart disease. The primary endpoint was to assess "in vivo" loading conditions of the device for product development specifications and to summarize clinical outcomes over 5 years of follow-up. In other words, it was primarily an "engineering study" of device design and development. In addition, a "screening committee" comprised of interventional cardiologists, CT surgeons, and imaging experts from North America and Europe was formed with a charge to assess every potential candidate for device implant.

This Native Transcatheter Pulmonary Valve had an asymmetric frame, unlike the symmetric frame used in the FIM implant at GOSH in 2009. The porcine pericardial tissue valve used is AOA treated, similar to the commercialized Medtronic CoreValve for Transcatheter Aortic Valve Replacement. The valve is mounted on a self-expandable nitinol frame covered in polyester fabric. It is attached to a coil-loading catheter and requires a loading funnel to collapse the valve prior to sheathing (Fig. 43.1). The entire valve and delivery system requires a 25 Fr crossing profile. The intended patient population is patients with surgically repaired right ventricular outflow tract and severe pulmonary regurgitation incident (PR) and who do not have an RV-PA conduit. Either echocardiography or cardiac MR was used to assess the pulmonary regurgitation with the severity graded according to established criteria. The patients must be a candidate for surgical RV-PA conduit or bioprosthetic pulmonary valve replacement. It was a non-randomized study with competitive enrollment involving 20 patients in the three investigative sites and was consented for follow-up for 5 years at the site of implantation.

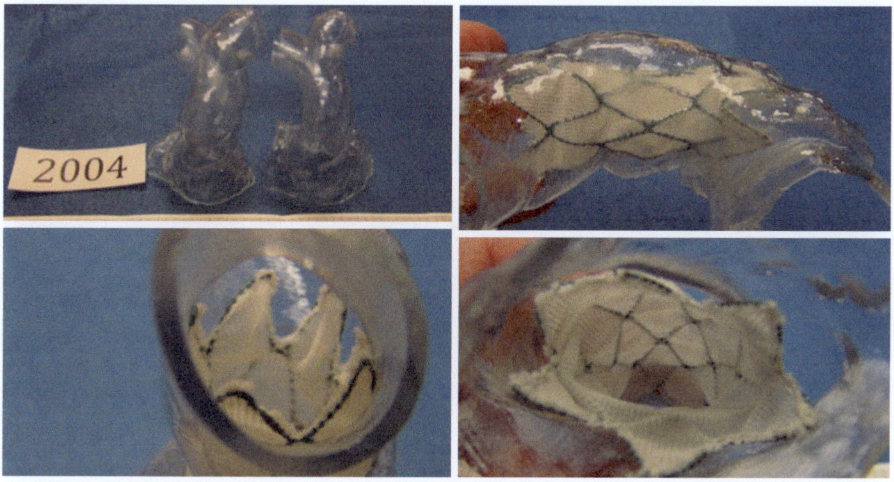

Fig. 43.2 The SLA models in systole and diastole are sown in the top left panel. The valve frame, without the valve, is shown inside the SLA model to simulate a "virtual implant"

Because this was primarily an "engineering study," after entry into the study according to New York Heart Association classification, echo and CMR criteria being met, a dual source CT scan was performed with the data set sent to Medtronic engineering so stereolithography (SLA) models of the RV outflow tract in systole and diastole could be created. The SLA models were then sent to the implanting physician and to Medtronic. The physician then placed a replica of the self-expandable frame, without the valve, in the optimal position in the SLA models and photographed and filmed the "virtual implant" and sent it back to Medtronic (Fig. 43.2). The Medtronic engineering team then generated "perimeter plots" of the valve implant within the SLA model to assess proper fit according to the criteria set forth by the engineering team (Fig. 43.3). Then, the patient's history, physical exam, echo and CMR results, and the" virtual SLA implants" were presented to the screening committee, investigative sites, and Medtronic staff, which met every 2 weeks. A vote of the screening committee members to accept, deny, or defer was made, with the final decision of whether to implant left up to the implanting physician. If accepted, the patient was then scheduled for implant with representatives from the investigative sites, screening committee, and Medtronic in attendance. However, the real challenge was how could the image from the CMR translate into what is seen with the dual source CT scan. Our Heart Center imaging team described a new technique for this correlation (Fig. 43.4).

The first implant was performed successfully at Nationwide Children's Hospital in May of 2013. By May of 2015, the final 20th implant was performed at Toronto Sick Kids Hospital and the study was closed. There were ten patients implanted at Nationwide Children's Hospital, seven patients implanted at Boston Children's Hospital, and three patients implanted at Toronto Sick Kids Hospital. All patients implanted had a follow-up dual source CT scan within 4 days of implant for

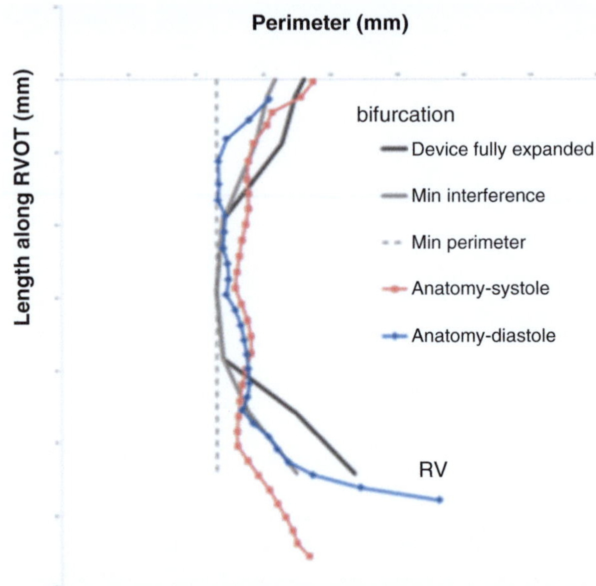

Fig. 43.3 After the valve frame is implanted in the SLA models, the engineering team manufactures a perimeter plot to assess the "fit" of the valve in a given patient

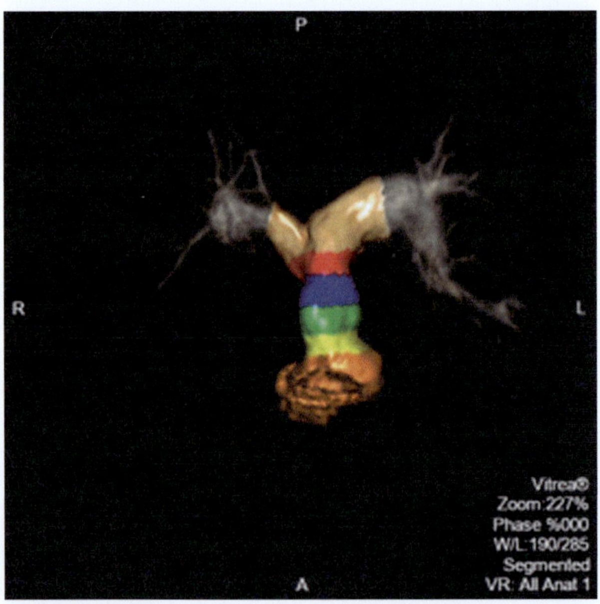

Fig. 43.4 The 3D CMR of the RVOT is reconstructed in five color schemes to represent the landing areas of the valve frame. The NCH imaging team came up with this method to help correlate the CMR and the dual source CT findings of the RVOT

comparison with the pre-implant study. We also performed intracardiac echocardiography (ICE) pre- and post-implant to assess the degree of PR (Fig. 43.5). As of this writing, all of the pre-implant and post-implant studies and data are being analyzed. The preliminary data will be presented at ACC 2016 in Chicago.

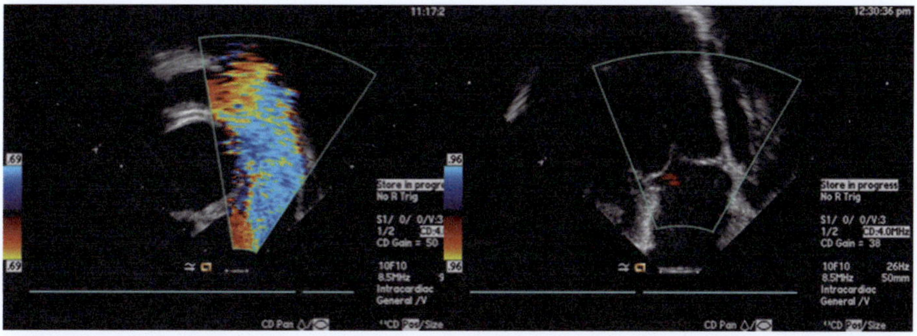

Fig. 43.5 ICE imaging before and after the Native TPV has been implanted and demonstrates severe PR before implant and no PR after. The valve leaflets are nicely seen with excellent coaptation

What are the lessons learned from the first ever early feasibility study? The 25 Fr delivery system is usually not too difficult to place at the implant site. The flexibility of the self-expandable frame allows the system to "bend" in the native RV outflow tract. Since these patients do not have an RV-PA conduit, the catheter course is favorable. Frame composition is not as easy to visualize under fluoroscopy compared to the platinum-iridium Melody transcatheter pulmonary valve frame, which is very radiopaque. Because the Native Transcatheter Pulmonary Valve frame is much longer than the Melody TPV frame, removing the long "carrot" through the implanted valve is more challenging. Also, because all the patients had severe pulmonary regurgitation with very little pulmonary stenosis, the landing zone is not as "secure" as seen with those patients with RV-PA conduit dysfunction and Melody TPV implant. Patient selection and careful anatomic screening are critical parts of the process, as RV outflow tract anatomies very widely. The dynamic nature of the RVOT and interaction with the pulsatility of the main pulmonary artery makes device design challenging and highlights the limitation of a single device design and size that was available for the study. None of the 20 patients implanted met all of the proposed engineering criteria, demonstrating our learning curve during the study. A large valve with several frame dimensions may serve more patients. Finally, although the screening process was arduous and heavily engineer-driven, the scrutiny of the screening committee and learning from the SLA models and perimeter plots were invaluable.

Outside the USA, there have been successful clinical implants in Asia and Europe with the Venus P-Valve, which also uses a nitinol self-expandable frame with a porcine pericardial valve, but the frame is covered with porcine pericardial tissue rather than polyester cloth [2, 3]. There will be further reports using this valve in the future. There is another Native TPV being developed by Beijing Med Zenith Medical Scientific Co. and is currently in animal testing as of this writing.

The future for specifically designed transcatheter pulmonary valves to be placed in the native RVOT after surgical correction will be challenging, but will serve approximately 77 % of patients and have a huge impact in future transcatheter heart valve therapies.

References

1. Schievano S, et al. First-in-man implantation of a novel percutaneous valve: a new approach to medical device development. EuroInterven J EuroPCR Collaboration Working Group Interv Cardiol Eur Soc Cardiol. 2010;5(6):745–50.
2. Cao QL, et al. Early clinical experience with a novel self-expanding percutaneous stent-valve in the native right ventricular outflow tract. Catheter Cardiovasc Interv Off J Soc Cardiac Angiograp Interv. 2014;84(7):1131–7.
3. Promphan W, et al. Percutaneous pulmonary valve implantation with the venus P-valve: clinical experience and early results. Cardiol Young. 2015;26:1–13.

Mitral Valve Replacement with Melody Valve Prosthesis

44

Sitaram M. Emani

44.1 Introduction

Mitral valve repair is the preferred approach for patients with mitral valve disease. However, extremely diseased valves can be difficult to repair, creating a risk of reoperation that is age dependent [1, 2]. Particularly in neonatal patients, the risk of reoperation is significant and contributes to mortality and morbidity, associated with nearly 50 % reoperation at 2 years. An acceptable mitral valve repair is not achievable in some patients, and mitral valve replacement is the only option.

Options for mitral valve replacement in children with irreparable mitral valve are limited, particularly for annular size less than 15 mm [3]. The options for mitral valve replacement include mechanical valves which are available at sizes larger than 15 mm, bioprosthetic valves that are generally larger than 19 mm but available at sizes as small as 12 mm (porcine valves within Dacron conduit). Homograft valves can be fashioned for use in the mitral position, and pulmonary autograft (Ross-mitral) procedure has been described [4–6]. Finally, supra-annular implantation may be necessary in patients with limited annular dimensions [7]. There are several disadvantages of these options. Importantly, mechanical valves require anticoagulation with warfarin, which can be very difficult to titrate accurately in a child. Furthermore, many of these valves have unfavorable effective orifice area (internal diameter to external diameter ratio), predisposing the valve to early stenosis as a child grows. Finally, all of these prostheses are associated with a fixed diameter frame which lacks the ability to increase in size as the patient grows. At the time of repeat valve replacement, the annulus, maintained at fixed diameter by the prosthesis, has limited ability to accept a larger-sized valve. Ultimately, frequent and early reoperation for valve replacement is expected with traditional valve replacement.

S.M. Emani, MD
Department of Cardiac Surgery, Boston Children's Hospital, Harvard Medical School, 300 Longwood Ave, Boston, MA 02115, USA
e-mail: Sitaram.Emani@CARDIO.CHBOSTON.ORG

G. Butera et al. (eds.), *Fetal and Hybrid Procedures in Congenital Heart Diseases*, DOI 10.1007/978-3-319-40088-4_44

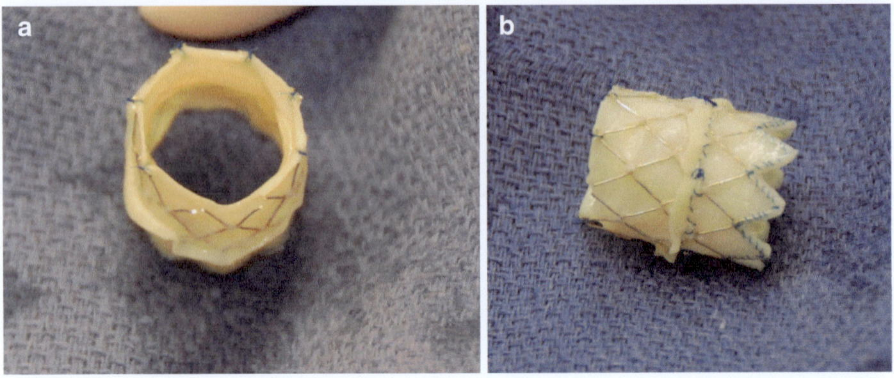

Fig. 44.1 The Melody valve demonstrates favorable internal to external orifice area dimensions due to thin housing surrounding the valve apparatus (**a**). Modification of the valve with shortening may prevent LVOT obstruction, and addition of sewing cuff assists with suture implantation and prevention of perivalvular leaks (**b**)

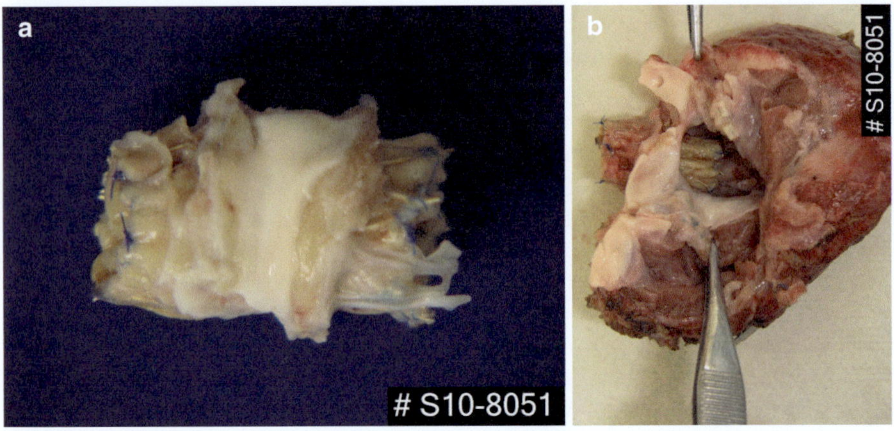

Fig. 44.2 Appearance of the melody valve following transplantation in a patient who underwent replacement for severe ventricular dysfunction. Pannus ingrowth onto the external housing is evident at the midsection, but the proximal and distal aspects are relatively spared of pannus ingrowth (**a**), which protects the underlying valve tissue from deterioration. The long length of the Melody in the mitral position is a major disadvantage of this valve as it requires protrusion into both the LV cavity and the left atrium (**b**)

The Melody valve provides several theoretical advantages over other commercially available prostheses. The valve can be implanted into neonates or infants with annuli as smaller than 12 mm. It is encased by a thin-walled conduit and stent, providing a larger effective orifice area, which is critical in neonatal and infant valve replacement (Fig. 44.1a). This is particularly critical for patients presenting with congenital mitral stenosis, in whom the native annular size may be relatively small. Encasement of the leaflets by the conduit and stent also serves to protect the underlying leaflets from pannus ingrowth Fig. 44.2a). The bovine jugular vein leaflet tissue is very thin and pliable, which is suitable for low opening and closing stress associated with neonatal circulation. The potential for valve expansion percutaneously in the catheterization laboratory as the child grows is maintained by its unique design. The Melody valve has demonstrated the ability to withstand systemic pressures [8]. The ability to enlarge the valve may delay the time to reoperation. Further advances in transcatheter valve technology and valve-in-valve insertion techniques may allow nonsurgical replacement options.

This chapter describes the off-label use of a device (Melody valve). Long-term performance of this device in the mitral position has not been established, and its use should be considered investigational. Although institutional policies regarding off-label use of a device vary, we have pursued approval from institutional review board prior to approaching families with this option. During discussions and parental consent process, a clear statement regarding the off-label use of the device is provided.

44.2 Technical Considerations

Recent experience with a bovine jugular vein graft (Melody valve) for mitral replacement has revealed several important technical considerations [9]. Certain design features of the device that makes it favorable for percutaneous implantation into the right ventricular outflow tract renders it less favorable for implantation into the mitral position.

44.2.1 Left Ventricular Outflow Tract Obstruction

The length of the Melody device (2.3–2.5 cm) predisposes it to protrusion into the left ventricle (LV), leading to left ventricular outflow tract obstruction (LVOTO) (Fig. 44.2b). This complication is of particular concern in patients with hypoplastic left ventricle and small short-axis ventricular dimensions. In these patients, protrusion of a fixed device into the ventricle may lead to cantilever effect of the distal aspect of the device with the ventricular septum, creating mid-cavitary obstruction. Additionally, when a valve of this length is fixed only in its midsection to the annulus, the potential exists for deviation toward the left ventricular outflow tract during systole (Fig. 44.3a). The hemodynamic perturbation created by the initial LVOTO predisposes to further development of subaortic membrane and obstruction as seen in Fig. 44.3a.

In order to avoid LVOTO, several modifications may be necessary. The LV short-axis dimensions measured by preoperative echocardiogram may be used to anticipate LVOTO. If left ventricular end-diastolic diameter at the level of the papillary muscles during systole is smaller than the intended diameter of the Melody valve, modification of the valve may be necessary. Shortening of the valve or excision of the stent and fabric adjacent to the LVOTO is performed in such patients, particularly in neonates and infants with LV hypoplasia (Fig. 44.1b). However, our preference is to avoid any disruption of the stent structure supporting the valve apparatus, as this may predispose the valve to early failure. Thus it is only the patient with

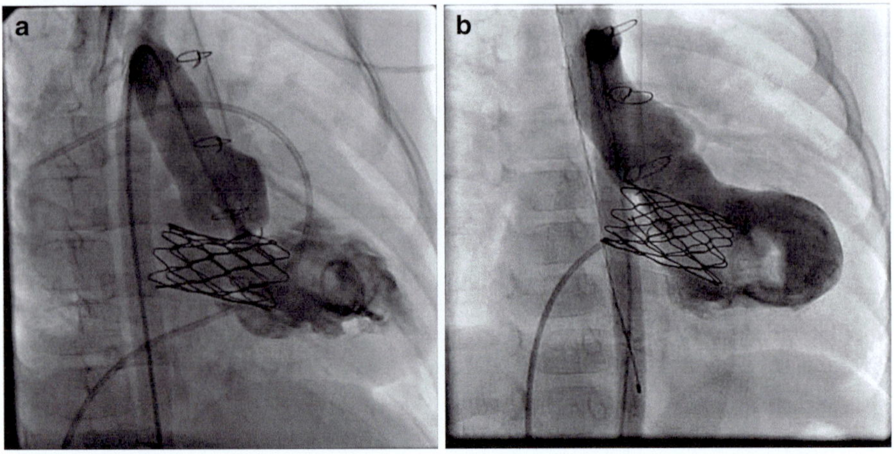

Fig. 44.3 Left ventricular outflow tract obstruction may result from tilting of the Melody valve toward the outflow tract (**a**). This is predominantly attributed to the long length of the valve protruding into the LV cavity with fulcrum located at the midsection of the valve. In order to prevent this complication, the distal aspect of the stent must be fixed to the posterior LV free wall to prevent the deviation (**b**)

severe hypoplasia of the LV (typically a neonatal patient) who should undergo valve modification.

In order to prevent deviation of the Melody valve into the LVOT during systole, the distal aspect of the stent is fixed to the endocardium of the LV free wall, pulling it away from the LVOT (Fig. 44.3b). To prevent LVOTO in a neonate or hypoplastic LV, tapered dilation can be performed by dilating the LV end of the valve with a smaller balloon that is used to dilate the atrial end of the valve.

Left ventricular outflow tract obstruction can occur late after Melody valve implantation due to progressive development of subaortic membrane. Management options include transcatheter relief of obstruction and surgical septal myectomy. Transcatheter relief includes dilation of the valve stent adjacent to the left ventricular outflow tract or perforation of the conduit material with balloon dilation of the stent cells. This approach is effective at relieving gradient acutely, but more definitive relief requires surgical management of the left ventricular outflow tract. At surgery, the septal muscle adjacent to the distal portion of the Melody valve is resected, without a need to modify the Melody valve itself. Rarely, repeat replacement of the valve may be necessary if these maneuvers are ineffective at relieving obstruction.

44.2.2 Annular Fixation

The Melody device lacks a sewing cuff to anchor the device to the mitral annulus. Several iterations of fixation technique have been utilized over the past 5 years. In the initial experience, direct suture of the stent to the annulus resulted in perivalvular leak, leading to design modification. In the most recent modifications, a sewing

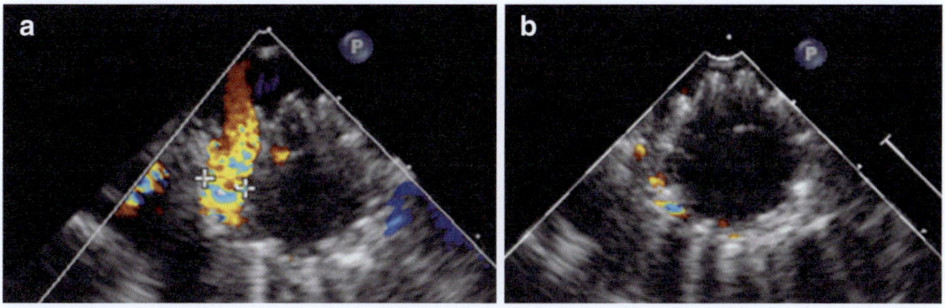

Fig. 44.4 Inadequate sizing of balloon dilation of the mitral Melody at initial implantation leads to development of perivalvular leak (**a**). This is managed by intraoperative balloon dilation at the same operative encounter, leading to resolution of the leak (**b**)

cuff is added externally to the Melody valve stent in its midsection. Although we have used bovine pericardium, any expandable material (expanded polytetrafluoroethylene (ePTFE), autologous pericardium) can be utilized (Fig. 44.1). The use of a sewing cuff minimizes the risk of perivalvular leak and allows stable fixation to the annulus. The sewing skirt is anchored to the annulus by either interrupted sutures or two separate purse-string sutures. Extreme caution must be exercised when placing sutures into the external stent/graft housing of the Melody, as inadvertent injury to the underlying leaflets is possible. This could occur either during suturing of the skirt onto the valve or if the valve is sutured directly to the annulus without addition of a skirt [9, 10].

Choice of intraoperative balloon size is critical as fixation of the device to the annulus relies significantly upon secure apposition of the stent and sewing cuff material to the annular tissue. The initial expansion size is chosen based upon preoperative measurement of the annulus size by echocardiogram and intraoperative sizing. Balloon size of 1 mm + anterior-posterior (AP) annular dimension by echocardiogram has yielded satisfactory results in our experience. Undersizing may result in perivalvular leak and valve instability, whereas oversizing may lead to LVOTO, coronary artery compression, or heart block. The balloon is carefully inserted through the central lumen of the valve which is initially kept patent by compression of the valve over a dilator or balloon. Prior to securing the knots for the anchoring purse-string suture, the balloon is inflated within the valve to the desired diameter to avoid compression of the device by the suture. Flaring of the proximal end of the stent within the left atrium has been described and may facilitate subsequent transcatheter intervention [10].

Despite careful surgical techniques, perivalvular leaks may occur. Most perivalvular leaks may be managed effectively by transcatheter balloon dilation of the valve performed either intraoperatively or postoperatively in the catheterization laboratory (Fig. 44.4). Occasionally, the perivalvular leak may occur as a result of separation of the stent housing from the underlying conduit fabric. Such leaks are not amenable to transcatheter closure, and surgical repair or repeat replacement may be necessary.

44.3 Medical Management and Follow-Up

Aspirin is the only long-term anticoagulation therapy, and the child is maintained on heparin until aspirin is initiated. Antiplatelet effect is confirmed with Verify Now or thromboelastography (TEG) platelet mapping. Surveillance echocardiograms every 4–6 months are recommended to follow the gradient across the valve. Typically, gradients across the valve as measured by echocardiogram are overestimates of the gradient as measured by catheterization. Nevertheless, an increase in the gradient should prompt consideration of catheterization to confirm the gradient and perform balloon dilation. Prosthetic valve endocarditis remains a concern with this valve, and antibiotic prophylaxis in the setting of bacterial infections is advised. The compressibility of this valve raised initial concerns of the impact of cardiac massage (either during de-airing in the operating room or in the event of CPR) upon luminal diameter of the prosthesis and thus efficacy of these maneuvers. Although this remains a concern, our experience with several patients who have undergone external cardiac compressions of post-implantation has demonstrated adequate function of the prosthesis despite these maneuvers.

44.4 Balloon Expansion of the Valve

With somatic growth, gradient may develop across the mitral Melody valve, indicating need for balloon dilation. Typically this occurs between 1 and 2 years following implantation of the device. If an increase in the gradient has not been observed by 2 years of age, we generally recommend empiric dilation of the valve to avoid fixation of the annulus at its original diameter. Although the gradient as measured by echocardiogram frequently underestimates the gradient as measured by catheterization, catheterization for hemodynamics and potential balloon dilation is warranted if the gradient increases by 3–4 mmHg on subsequent echocardiograms or if the absolute gradient exceeds 10 mmHg.

The techniques for balloon dilation of the valve have evolved over time, and care must be taken to avoid injury of the leaflets during intubation of the central portion of the valve. Since the proximal end of the valve protrudes into the left atrium, introduction of the guide wire into the valve can be challenging. Following transeptal puncture, the wire is allowed to loop within the left atrium prior to approaching the orifice of the Melody (Fig. 44.5). Wire position must be confirmed by biplane imaging, as perivalvular wire position may lead to creation of perivalvular leak following balloon dilation. Improper catheterization technique may also lead to inadvertent perforation of the gossamer venous valve leaflets (Fig. 44.6).

44.5 Valve-in-Valve Options

If the valve prosthesis is successfully expanded until a child is old enough to undergo transcatheter insertion of valve device, then reoperation for valve replacement could theoretically be avoided. Although this has not yet been performed in this clinical setting, the feasibility of valve-in-valve replacement has been demonstrated [11].

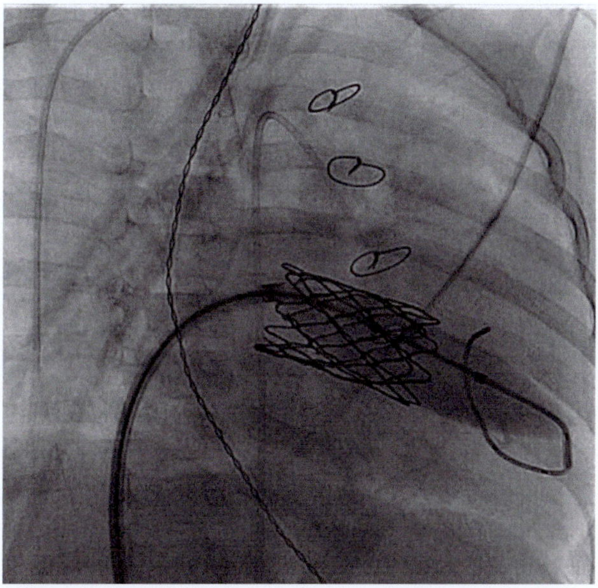

Fig. 44.5 Transcatheter balloon dilation of the mitral Melody several years following implantation. The valve maintains competence despite multiple balloon expansions

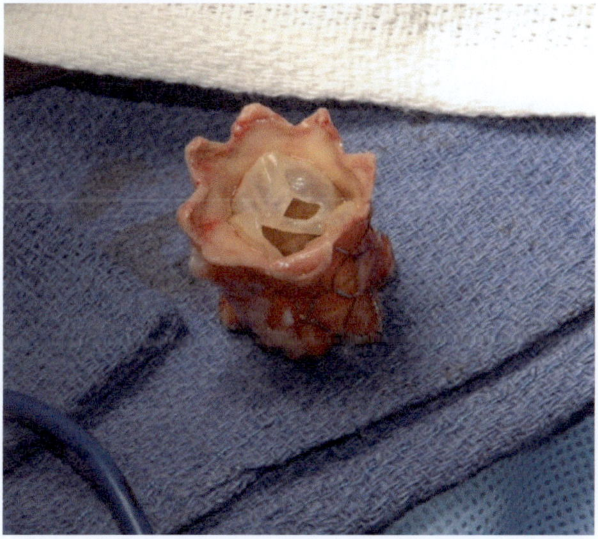

Fig. 44.6 Perforation of a leaflet of the Melody valve early following implantation. The thin leaflets of the valve are prone to injury with improper implantation or transcatheter manipulation

44.6 Results

The Melody valve appears to function well at short-term follow-up, with complications including LVOTO in 10 % of patients [10, 12]. Balloon expansion of the valve at up to 4 years following implantation has been successful at preserving valvular competence and low gradient. Reoperation for perivalvular leak and LVOTO remains a concern and requires close follow-up. Perivalvular leaks and LVOTO can be managed with transcatheter techniques, whereas severe LVOTO may require reoperation [9]. Future development of a device that is specifically designed for implantation into the mitral position with sewing cuff and shorter profile may reduce the incidence of perivalvular leaks and LVOTO.

Despite valve replacement, many patients with congenital mitral valve disease succumb to complications of associated ventricular systolic and diastolic dysfunction. Thus the morbidity and mortality remain relatively high in this population despite adequate valvular function. Thus valve replacement is an adjunct for aggressive medical management in these patients, and ongoing close follow-up is warranted.

Conclusions

Mitral valve replacement with Melody prosthesis has several potential advantages, including favorable initial hemodynamics, small size, and eventual expandability. Early experience with its use has been encouraging. Since the valve is not designed for surgical mitral application, technical modifications are necessary to prevent left ventricular outflow tract obstruction and perivalvular leaks. Close follow-up is warranted, and transcatheter dilation is performed if gradient increases.

References

1. Myers PO, Baird CW, Del Nido PJ, Pigula FA, Lang N, Marx GR, Emani SM. Neonatal Mitral Valve Repair in Biventricular Repair, Single Ventricle Palliation, and Secondary Left Ventricular Recruitment: Indications, Techniques, and Midterm Outcomes. Front Surg. 2015;2:59.
2. Caldarone CA, Raghuveer G, Hills CB, Atkins DL, Burns TL, Behrendt DM, Moller JH. Long-term survival after mitral valve replacement in children aged <5 years: a multi-institutional study. Circulation. 2001;104:I143–7.
3. Brizard CP, d'Udekem Y, Eastaugh LJ, Lane GK, Jones BO. Intra-annular mitral valve replacement in neonates and infants. J Thorac Cardiovasc Surg. 2015;149:390–2. e1.
4. Brown JW, Ruzmetov M, Rodefeld MD, Turrentine MW. Mitral valve replacement with Ross II technique: initial experience. Ann Thorac Surg. 2006;81:502–7; discussion 507–8.
5. Pace Napoleone C, Oppido G, Angeli E, Giardini A, Gargiulo G. Ross-kabbani operation in an infant with mitral valve dysplasia. Cardiol Res Pract. 2009;2009:593659.
6. Kabbani S, Jamil H, Nabhani F, Hamoud A, Katan K, Sabbagh N, Koudsi A, Kabbani L, Hamed G. Analysis of 92 mitral pulmonary autograft replacement (Ross II) operations. J Thorac Cardiovasc Surg. 2007;134:902–8.
7. Selamet Tierney ES, Pigula FA, Berul CI, Lock JE, del Nido PJ and McElhinney DB. Mitral valve replacement in infants and children 5 years of age or younger: evolution in practice and outcome over three decades with a focus on supra-annular prosthesis implantation. J Thorac Cardiovasc Surg. 2008;136:954–61, 961 e1–3.
8. Hasan BS, McElhinney DB, Brown DW, Cheatham JP, Vincent JA, Hellenbrand WE, Jones TK, Zahn EM and Lock JE. Short-term performance of the transcatheter Melody valve in high-pressure hemodynamic environments in the pulmonary and systemic circulations. Circ Cardiovasc Interv. 2011;4:615–20.
9. Quinonez LG, Breitbart R, Tworetsky W, Lock JE, Marshall AC and Emani SM. Stented bovine jugular vein graft (Melody valve) for surgical mitral valve replacement in infants and children. J Thorac Cardiovasc Surg. 2014;148:1443–9.

10. Hofmann M, Dave H, Hubler M, Kretschmar O. Simplified surgical-hybrid Melody(R) valve implantation for paediatric mitral valve disease. Eur J Cardiothorac Surg. 2015;47:926–8.
11. Cullen MW, Cabalka AK, Alli OO, Pislaru SV, Sorajja P, Nkomo VT, Malouf JF, Cetta F, Hagler DJ, Rihal CS. Transvenous, antegrade Melody valve-in-valve implantation for bioprosthetic mitral and tricuspid valve dysfunction: a case series in children and adults. JACC Cardiovasc Interv. 2013;6:598–605.
12. Abdullah I, Ramirez FB, McElhinney DB, Lock JE, del Nido PJ, Emani S. Modification of a stented bovine jugular vein conduit (melody valve) for surgical mitral valve replacement. Ann Thorac Surg. 2012;94:e97–8.

A Hybrid Approach to Aortic Stent Implantation

45

Evan Zhan

45.1 Introduction

The vast majority of aortic stent placement can be performed simply and safely using percutaneous retrograde access from the femoral artery [1]. There are, however, several settings when a hybrid approach to aortic stenting may be preferable or the only option available. Examples include:

1. Neonate or small infant with severe coarctation and contraindication for surgery and not amenable to balloon angioplasty
2. Recurrent coarctation after Stage 1 Norwood palliation at the time of the Glenn anastomosis
3. Limited or absent adequate peripheral vascular access at any age

In these scenarios there may be several advantages to hybrid aortic stenting including: avoidance of ileofemoral arterial trauma, irrelevance or sheath size allowing for placement of stents with larger "growth" potential in small children, technically direct and simple access to the target lesion facilitating precision stent placement, and avoidance of hemodynamic instability during implant and combining surgical and catheter-based procedures that serve to limit cumulative morbidity.

E. Zhan
Guerin Family Congenital Heart Program, Cedars-Sinai Heart Institute, Los Angeles, CA, USA
e-mail: Evan.Zahn@cshs.org

G. Butera et al. (eds.), *Fetal and Hybrid Procedures in Congenital Heart Diseases*, DOI 10.1007/978-3-319-40088-4_45

45.2 General Technique

These procedures can be performed in the operating room, catheterization suite, or hybrid room depending on the clinical scenario and facility availability. In general these procedures may be performed without the use of cardiopulmonary bypass. The technique involves providing direct surgical access to the aorta or large central conducting artery (e.g., carotid) for the interventional cardiologist either via a midline sternotomy (access via ascending aorta) or arterial cut down. With either technique the approach to the target lesion will typically be from an anterograde direction as opposed to percutaneous aortic stenting, which is performed from a retrograde approach. This approach allows the operator to obtain high-quality serial angiograms via the sidearm of the delivery sheath for precise stent positioning and typically results in a very simple and stable catheter course for stent delivery. In general, the vessel to be used for access is isolated by the surgeon who then places the delivery sheath into it via an arteriotomy created through a purse-string suture, similar to other hybrid stenting procedures. Care must be taken to place the sheath far enough away from the intended target lesion to allow for complete uncovering of the stent and most proximal end of the delivery balloon prior to balloon inflation. Long delivery sheaths are not needed for these procedures as the balloon-stent complex is only being advanced a few centimeters through a relatively straight catheter course. Once the sheath is in position, an angiogram is performed by performing a hand injection through the sidearm of the sheath to obtain quantitative measurements of the aorta including diameter of the transverse arch, coarctation, and aorta at the level of the diaphragm, as well as the approximate length of the vessel intended for stent delivery. Single plane angiography (versus biplane) is typically utilized due to the large number of people, small working area, and simplicity of the intervention. We size the delivery balloon in identical fashion to our percutaneous implants, attempting to match the size of the normal aortic arch and using the aorta at the level of the diaphragm as an upper diameter limit. In general we chose a stent with the shortest possible length that will treat all of the pathology present and provide maximal stent stability. The lesion is then crossed using a 0.035-inch guidewire placed through a right coronary artery catheter. The tip of the guidewire is advanced far down the descending aorta, which provides a stable "rail." The chosen stent (as large an ultimate diameter as possible) is then hand crimped onto the delivery balloon and the balloon-mounted stent is advanced over the guidewire into position. Repeat angiography via the sidearm of the sheath is performed as needed to obtain optimal positioning. A slow controlled balloon inflation is then performed to implant the stent. As the balloon-stent complex is considerably more stable during implantation when using this approach compared to a percutaneous retrograde approach, we do not typically use overdrive right ventricular pacing or balloon-in-balloon catheters for stent deployment in this setting. After stent deployment, the balloon catheter is removed and repeat angiography is performed via the sidearm of the sheath with the guidewire left in place. Should further stent expansion be needed, a different (larger or higher pressure) balloon catheter can be placed over the wire. Using a catheter with a smaller French size than the sheath, simultaneous pressure measurements above and below the stent can be performed.

When a satisfactory result has been achieved, the guidewire is withdrawn, the sheath removed, and the arteriotomy repaired by the surgeon.

A few specific scenarios involving hybrid aortic stenting are worth mentioning individually:

45.2.1 Hybrid Aortic Stent Following Stage 1 Norwood Procedure

Recurrent or residual aortic obstruction following Stage 1 Norwood procedure of HLHS is a fairly common problem with a described incidence of 11–37 % [2, 3]. Factors contributing to recurrence of obstruction include surgical technique and contraction of residual ductal tissue not resected at the time of the initial operation.

Because of the unique postoperative circulation after Stage 1 Norwood procedure, aortic obstruction usually has a profound negative impact on these infants' outcome. The effect of increased after load can result in permanent damage to the single ventricle and can negatively impact suitability for further palliative surgery. The anatomic substrate of aortic obstruction in this setting is variable, ranging from discrete lesions that angiographically resemble typical isolated aortic coarctation to more diffuse, long segment lesions that may be the result of a failure to extend the initial aortic patch far enough down the aortic isthmus. Surgical revision of the reconstructed distal aortic arch may be difficult and may not completely relieve the obstruction. Additionally, reoperation may increase morbidity and mortality when performed alone or in combination with other procedures such as bidirectional cavopulmonary anastomosis [4]. Balloon angioplasty is not always successful and may carry an increased risk compared with isolated coarctation angioplasty [5, 6]. The incidence of recurrent coarctation following balloon angioplasty in this setting is as high as 17 % and commonly occurs during the first year after initial balloon angioplasty [7]. Stent therapy while theoretically attractive in this setting poses a number of challenges not the least of which is that this issue typically occurs in young infants where arterial access for retrograde aortic stent placement limits the size stent which may be safely implanted. In an attempt to overcome this obstacle, several operators have described stent placement via a transvenous approach facilitated by the unique anatomy of this palliated circulation. While intuitively this approach makes sense, we have found that too often these infants do not tolerate placement of a rigid guidewire, delivery sheath, and balloon-mounted stent across their only functional atrioventricular (tricuspid) and semilunar (neo-aortic) valves.

For these reasons we have utilized a hybrid approach for aortic stent placement in this setting, performed at the time of cavopulmonary anastomosis [8]. In most institutions, bidirectional cavopulmonary anastomosis is performed between 3 and 6 months of age, often when recurrent arch obstruction is manifested and requires treatment. Placing a hybrid aortic stent at the time of this surgery has numerous obvious potential advantages. By avoiding repeat dissection around the distal transverse arch and isthmus, the risk of damage to recurrent laryngeal and vagal nerves as well as the thoracic duct is minimized. This is particularly important in this single ventricle population where vocal cord and diaphragmatic paresis, and chylous effusions may be poorly tolerated. By avoiding percutaneous placement, the potential for severe arterial damage is avoided. The hybrid approach allows for precise positioning of a stent capable of reaching an adult diameter in an infant, taking advantage of a simple catheter course with virtually no hemodynamic compromise during the procedure. The procedure can be performed quickly and when coupled with cavopulmonary anastomosis avoids the necessity of an additional interventional catheterization, surgical procedure, and anesthetic. We have shown that stent redilation can be performed safely and effectively in this population during subsequent catheterizations [8, 9].

45.2.1.1 Technique (Fig. 45.1)

Typically this procedure has been performed at the time of cavopulmonary anastomosis in infants who have had unsuccessful balloon angioplasty for recurrent coarctation after Stage 1 palliation. Via a median sternotomy a 6–10 F introducer sheath

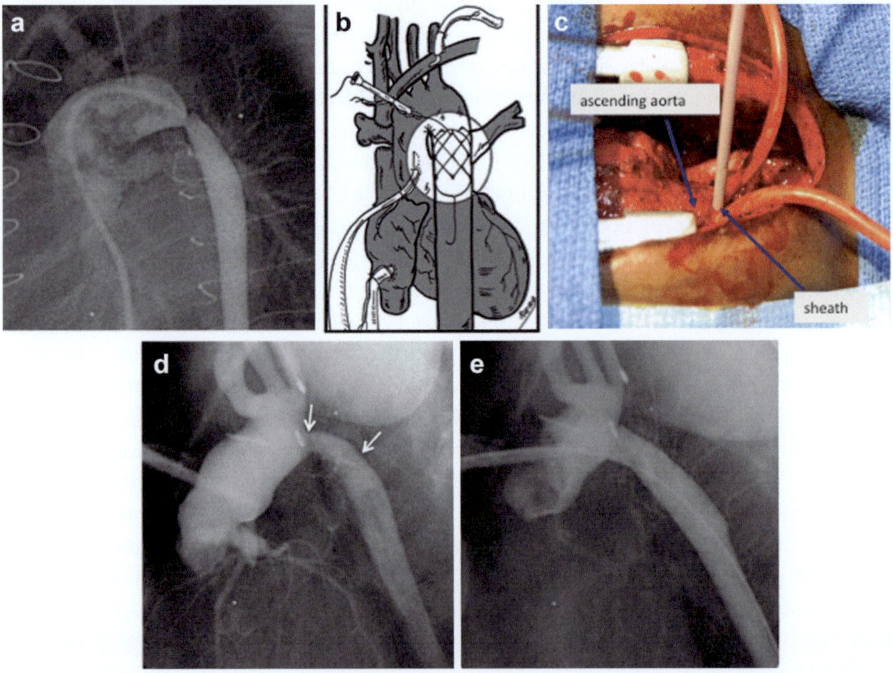

Fig. 45.1 Hybrid aortic stent placement after Norwood 1 at the time of cavopulmonary anastomosis. A 4-month-old was discovered at 3 months of age to have severe recurrent coarctation after Norwood Stage 1 (**a**). He underwent catheter-directed antegrade balloon angioplasty but continued to have significant aortic obstruction. At the time of cavopulmonary anastomosis, a 9 F sheath was placed into the ascending aorta (**b**, **c**), and angiography performed through the sidearm of the sheath (**d**) demonstrated what now appeared to be a long segment isthmal hypoplasia (*arrows*). An adult-sized stent was successfully implanted (**e**)

is advanced to the proximal transverse aortic arch via a purse-string incision in the neo-ascending aorta. The sidearm of the sheath is utilized for serial angiography and aortic pressure measurements throughout the procedure. Typically a 0.035-inch guidewire can be advanced under fluoroscopic guidance across the obstructed segment into the descending aorta using fluoroscopic guidance. A stent with adult sized potential diameter is manually crimped onto an angioplasty balloon and passed over the guidewire to the narrowed area of the distal arch without the use of a long sheath as the distance is short and the catheter course quite simple. After confirming position with angiography, the stent is deployed in typical fashion. Angiography and hemodynamic measurements are repeated after stent deployment. The guide wire and sheath are removed and the arteriotomy is repaired.

45.2.1.2 Experience

We described our experience using this approach in six consecutive infants [8] with a mean weight of 5.8 kg (2.9–7.7) and a mean age of 5.6 months (0.5–12.9) at the time of the procedure. Five patients had undergone prior balloon angioplasty at a mean age of 2.8 months (2.1–3.5), and five had moderately depressed single ventricular function prior to the hybrid procedure. The balloons used had a diameter of 7–10 mm and the introducer sheath size ranged from 6 to 10 F. The mean peak-to-peak systolic gradient across the site of aortic obstruction under general anesthesia decreased from 29 mmHg (14–46) before implantation to 1 mmHg (0–3) after the procedure ($P<0.05$). The mean diameter of the coarctation site increased from 3.5 mm (2–5.4) to 7.3 mm (5.5–10 mm) after stent implantation ($P<0.05$). The mean percentage increase in diameter after the procedure was 120 % (83–250). There were no significant immediate or late procedure related complications. One patient (youngest in the group) had transient bradycardia, hypotension, and supraventricular tachycardia during the procedure. There were no vascular complications related to the site of aortotomy. Five patients had subsequent catheterizations. The first follow-up catheterization was performed at a mean interval of 17.8 months (6.3–33.6) from the stent implant. The mean patient age was 24.5 months (13.6–39.8) and weight 11.1 kg (7.3–15.8) at the time of first catheterization. Recurrence of aortic obstruction was identified in four patients with a mean gradient of 24.5 mmHg (13–40) at the first follow-up catheterization

primarily due to luminal in growth. Stent redilation was performed in these patients for relief of obstruction and improvement of lumen diameter. Redilation was done in the fifth patient to keep pace with somatic growth. Balloons of 8–12 mm diameter were used at mean maximal inflation pressures of 10.9 atmospheres. Reduction in the mean peak-to-peak gradient to 2.8 mmHg (0–7) ($P<0.05$) and improvement in the diameter of the stented segment from 5.7 mm (3.2–8) to 9.4 mm (6.7–12) ($P<0.05$) was achieved. The mean percentage increase in diameter obtained with redilation of the stent was 80 % (25–162). In the long term only 50 % of these patients survived. The remaining three patients have undergone successful Fontan surgery and continue to have functioning hybrid stents in their aorta.

45.2.2 Hybrid Aortic Stent Due to Small Size and Limited Vascular Access

Surgical repair of coarctation of the aorta in the newborn period is the gold standard with reasonable short- and long-term outcomes. While this surgery can be performed in premature newborns, it is associated with significant morbidity and mortality in babies <1.5 kg [10–12]. A strategy of prolonged prostglandin E 1 (PGE1) infusion is typically employed to allow these low birth weight infants time to grow, but in selected cases, complications of this therapy such as high output failure with ventricular dysfunction, pulmonary overflow, and marginal systemic perfusion, which predisposes to necrotizing enterocolitis, may complicate this strategy, necessitating earlier definitive therapy. While successful percutaneous stent implantation in this situation has been described, it is not without significant risk of vascular injury [13, 14]. In this setting a reasonable palliative option which has been described is hybrid stenting of the aortic coarctation. This can be performed through either a carotid artery cutdown or midline sternotomy [15, 16]. The technique is similar to that described above with the major difference being that in these cases, owing to the small size of these patients (and their aortas), cases reported to date have involved implantation of small (coronary) stents with a dilation potential to only 5–6 mm in diameter. This strategy therefore is strictly palliative and will necessitate surgical removal or manipulation of these stents at the time of definitive surgical correction. For that reason, the shortest stent length possible is utilized and a cohesive comprehensive treatment plan must be developed in conjunction with the cardiac surgical team and patient family before embarking. That being said, this may provide life-saving therapy in selected cases of severe premature neonatal coarctation. The imminent availability of dissolvable stents and stents designed to "grow" with infants will likely alter this approach significantly.

Finally, as our surviving complex congenital heart population is surviving longer and undergoing more procedures, we have encountered rare cases of adolescents and young adults with "no vascular access" that require an aortic intervention. Employing a hybrid strategy for aortic stent implantation in this population (which we speculate is increasing in frequency), either through a midline sternotomy or carotid cutdown approach, may allow these patients to avoid a complex and high-risk reoperation (Fig. 45.2).

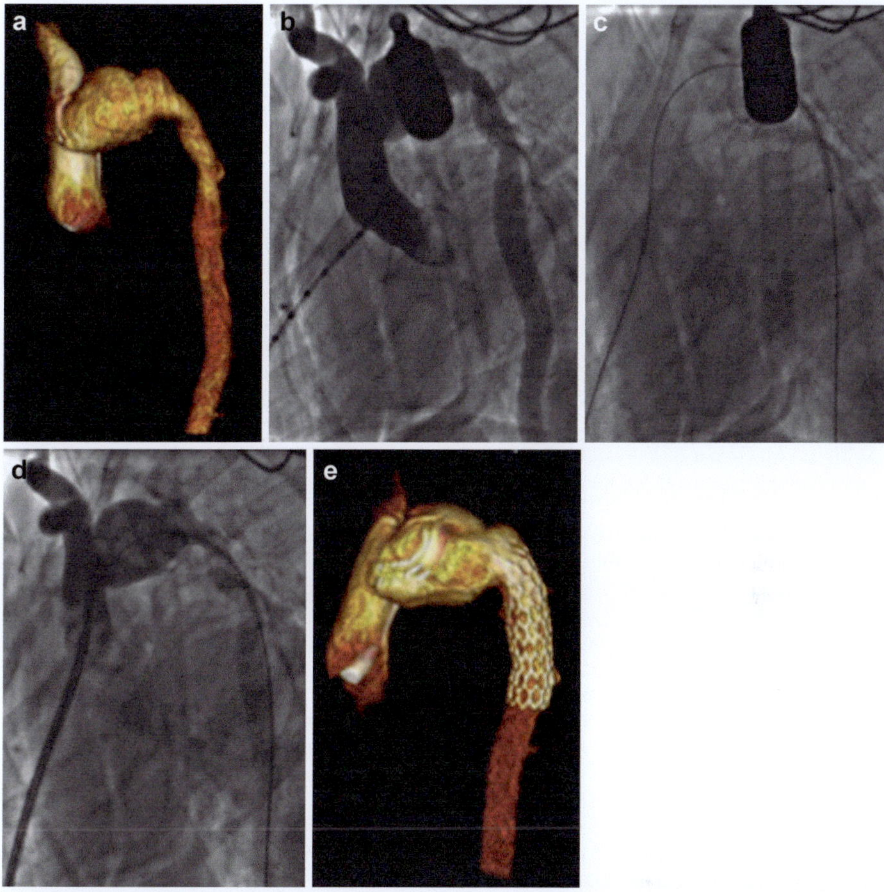

Fig. 45.2 Hybrid stent placement in a 15-year-old with severe recurrent coarctation, bilateral ileofemoral, and left common carotid arterial occlusion. A three-dimensional rotation angiogram (**a**) performed through a sheath paced in the ascending aorta through a midline sternotomy demonstrates a long segment complex coarctation, which is also seen on a corresponding two-dimensional image (**b**). After placing a standard 0.035 guidewire across the narrowed segment, a long adult-sized stent has been placed into position (**c**), and a confirmatory angiogram performed through the sidearm of the sheath confirms good positioning (**d**). Following stent implant, a repeat three-dimensional angiogram (**e**) demonstrates an improved appearance of the narrowed segment with no aortic wall damage

References

1. Forbes TJ, Kim DW, Du W, Turner DR, Holzer R, Amin Z, Hijazi Z, Ghasemi A, Rome JJ, Nykanen D, Zahn E, Cowley C, Hoyer M, Waight D, Gruenstein D, Javois A, Foerster S, Kreutzer J, Sullivan N, Khan A, Owada C, Hagler D, Lim S, Canter J, Zellers T; CCISC Investigators. Comparison of surgical, stent, and balloon angioplasty treatment of native coarctation of the aorta: an observational study by the CCISC (Congenital Cardiovascular Interventional Study Consortium). J Am Coll Cardiol. 2011.
2. Bartram U, Grunenfelder J, Van Praagh R. Causes of death after the modified Norwood procedure: a study of 122 postmortem cases. Ann Thorac Surg. 1997;64:1795–802.
3. Zellers TM. Balloon angioplasty for recurrent coarctation of the aorta in patients following staged palliation for hypoplastic left heart syndrome. Am J Cardiol. 1999;84:231–3.
4. Anderson JB, Beekman 3rd RH, Border WL, Kalkwarf HJ, Khoury PR, Uzark K, Eghtesady P, Marino BS. Lower weight-for-age z score adversely affects hospital length of stay after the bidirectional Glenn procedure in 100 infants with a single ventricle. J Thorac Cardiovasc Surg. 2009;138:397–404.
5. Chessa M, Dindar A, Vettukattil JJ, Stumper O, Wright JG, Silove ED, De Giovanni J. Balloon angioplasty in infants with aortic obstruction after the modified stage I Norwood procedure. Am Heart J. 2000;140:227–31.
6. Soongswang J, McCrindle BW, Jones TK, Vincent RN, Hsu DT, Kuhn MA, Moskowitz WB, Cheatham JP, Kholwadwala DH, Benson LN, Nykanen DG. Outcomes of transcatheter balloon angioplasty of obstruction in the neo-aortic arch after the Norwood operation. Cardiol Young. 2001;11:54–61.
7. Zeltser I, Menteer J, Gaynor JW, Spray TL, Clark BJ, Kreutzer J, Rome JJ. Impact of re-coarctation following the Norwood operation on survival in the balloon angioplasty era. J Am Coll Cardiol. 2005;45:1844–8.
8. Kutty S, Burke R, Hannan R, Zahn E. Hybrid aortic reconstruction for treatment of recurrent aortic obstruction after stage 1 single ventricle palliation. Catheter Cardiovasc Interv. 2011;78:93–100.
9. Stanfill R, Nykanen DG, Osorio S, Whalen R, Burke RP, Zahn EM. Stent implantation is effective treatment of vascular stenosis in young infants with congenital heart disease: acute implantation and long-term follow-up results. Catheter Cardiovasc Interv. 2008;71(6):831–41.
10. Sudarshan CD, Cochrane AD, Jun ZH, Soto R, Brizard CP. Repair of coarctation of the aorta in infants weighing less than 2 kilograms. Ann Thorac Surg. 2006;82:158–63.
11. Bove T, Francois K, De Groote K, Suys B, De Wolf D, Verhaaren H, Matthys D, Moerman A, Poelaert J, Vanhaesenbroeck P, Van Nooten G. Outcome analysis of major cardiac operations in low weight neonates. Ann Thorac Surg. 2004;78:181–7.
12. Karamlou T, Bernasconi A, Jaeggi E, Alhabshan F, Williams WG, Van Arsdell GS, Coles JG, Caldarone CA. Factors associated with arch reintervention and growth of the aortic arch after coarctation repair in neonates weighing less than 2.5 kg. J Thorac Cardiovasc Surg. 2009;137:1163–7.
13. Gorenflo M, Boshoff D, Heying R, Eyskens B, Rega F, Meyns B, Gewillig M. Bailout stenting for critical coarctation in premature/critical/complex/early recoarcted neonates. Catheter Cardiovasc Interv. 2010;75:553–61.
14. Sutton N, Lock JE, Geggel RL. Cardiac catheterization in infants weighing less than 1.500 grams. Catheter Cardiovasc Interv. 2006;68:948–56.
15. Davenport JJ, Lam L, Whalen-Glass R, Nykanen DG, Burke RP, Hannan R, Zahn EM. The successful use of alternative routes of vascular access for performing pediatric interventional cardiac catheterization. Catheter Cardiovasc Interv. 2008;72(3):392–8.
16. Cools B, Meyns B, Gewillig M. Hybrid stenting of aortic coarctation in very Low birth weight premature infant. Catheter Cardiovasc Interv. 2013;81:E195–8.

Other Hybrid Treatments: Tetralogy of Fallot

46

Vladimiro L. Vida, Alvise Guariento, and Giovanni Stellin

Tetralogy of Fallot (TOF) repair is nowadays a routine treatment that is achieved with a very low surgical risk in many pediatric cardiac centers. A transventricular approach combined with a transannular patching remains the most frequent repair [1]. More recently, a revival of a transatrial approach has become the preferred procedure, in many centers, yielding to excellent early and midterm results [2]. The objective of a transatrial repair is to avoid (or minimize) a structural damage to the subpulmonary pump, which has proved to be the Achilles' heel, in the long term.

Follow-up studies are showing that the use of a transannular patch results in pulmonary insufficiency with chronic right ventricular volume overload, leading inevitably to progressive right ventricular dilation and dysfunction which is associated with impaired functional capacity [3].

In the last few years, the interest in preserving the pulmonary valve (PV) function has stimulated surgeons in the last few years in devising PV-sparing techniques [4–8]. Since 2007, to our routine early transatrial/transpulmonary repair, we have combined new PV-sparing techniques, for treating a hypoplastic pulmonary annulus, by means of transcatheter balloon dilatation and additional PV reconstruction maneuvers (Fig. 46.1).

V.L. Vida (✉) • A. Guariento • G. Stellin
Pediatric and Congenital Cardiac Surgery Unit, Department of Cardiac, Thoracic and Vascular Sciences, University of Padua, Padua, Italy
e-mail: vladimirovida@yahoo.it

G. Butera et al. (eds.), *Fetal and Hybrid Procedures in Congenital Heart Diseases*, DOI 10.1007/978-3-319-40088-4_46

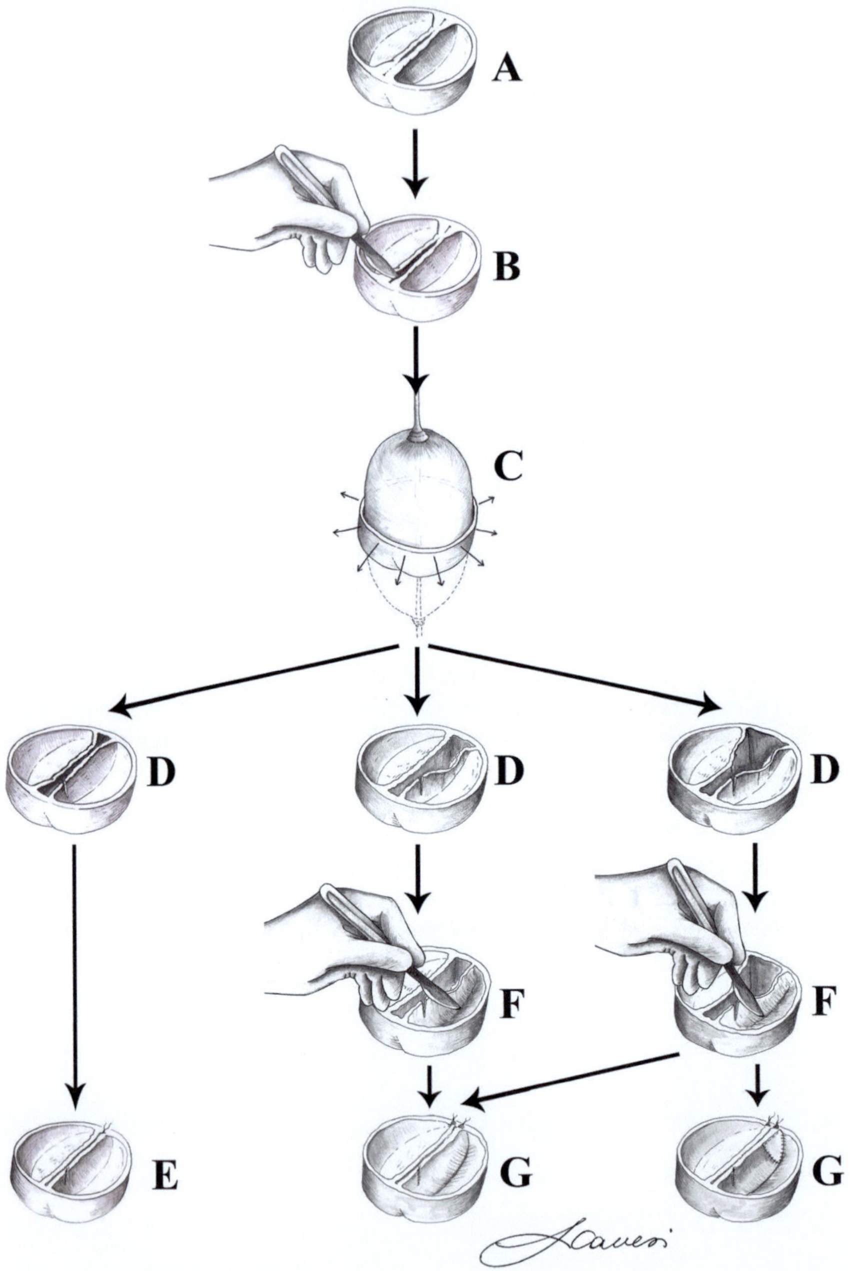

Fig. 46.1 Showing the various types of PV plasty procedures that can be performed in addition to PV balloon dilation. (**a**) Dysplastic PV with commissure fusion (effective PV opening), (**b**) PV commissurotomy (true initial PV annulus diameter), (**c**) PV balloon dilation and (**d**) final PV annulus diameter, (**e**) simple additional PV plasty (including PV leaflet repair and resuspension), and (**f**–**g**) complex additional PV plasty, including PV leaflet delamination (**f**) and patch augmentation when needed and resuspension (**g**)

46.1 Techniques for PV Preservation

At the time of repair, following a longitudinal main pulmonary artery (MPA) arteriotomy, the PV is inspected and sized to assess the effective PV orifice diameter. In the presence of a stenotic PV, a valvular commissurotomy is performed at each commissure, down to the subvalvar area. After this maneuver the valve is again sized to measure the true annular diameter. Particular care is taken to remove any possible RVOT obstruction up to the subannular level by combining transatrial, transtricuspid muscle band resection and a further transpulmonary residual muscle band excision through the PV annulus, before and after balloon dilatation.

Only after a satisfactory muscle bundle resection is achieved (by a combined myotomy/myectomy of the sub-pulmonary area), a valvuloplasty balloon catheter is introduced through the TV across the PV orifice and inflated under direct vision [4, 6–8] while securing its tip through the MPA arteriotomy until the inner pressure reaches 10 atm (Fig. 46.2). We employ short (2 cm) high-pressure (>10 atm.) noncompliant balloons, sized according to the calculated size of the PV orifice relative to the body surface area of the patient. When the PV effective orifice is particularly narrow (z-score <-3) we employ an "in-series balloon dilatation strategy," by using increasing diameters of balloons for allowing a progressive stretching and dilation of the PV annulus up to the ideal size according to the body surface area.

When the PV effective orifice is particularly narrow (z-score <-3), additional surgical maneuvers on the PV are required after dilatation for repairing any possible valve disruption, to achieve valve competence. The repair and resuspension of PV leaflet is in general sufficient (simple PV plasty) in most of them; however in more severe cases, where the balloon spreads the PV commissures apart so that the leaflets become insufficient to cover the new PV annular area, more complex PV plasty maneuvers, including the PV cusp delamination, may be required (Fig. 46.1). In these patients, we have included a shaving of the thickened PV cusps. The coaptation area is then extended by carefully delaminating the base of each PV cusp at the hinge point with a fine scalpel, extending the reconstructed leaflet area down

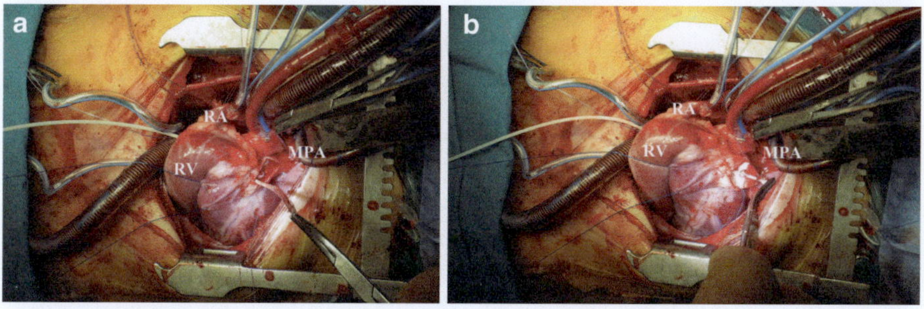

Fig. 46.2 Intraoperative image showing the intraoperative balloon dilation of the pulmonary valve. The balloon catheter is inserted through the right atrium (RA) and tricuspid valve into the pulmonary valve annulus. *RV* right ventricle, *MPA* main pulmonary artery

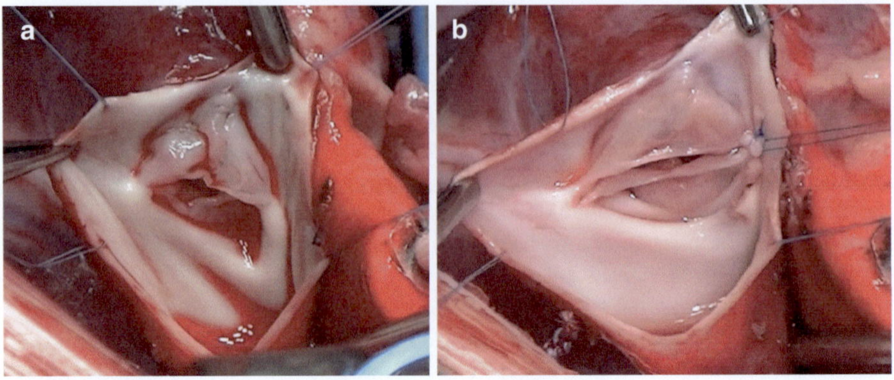

Fig. 46.3 Intraoperative images of the pulmonary valve in a 5-month-old boy with tetralogy of Fallot showing the (**a**) initial (6 mm) and (**b**) final (10 mm) diameters of the valve after preservation techniques

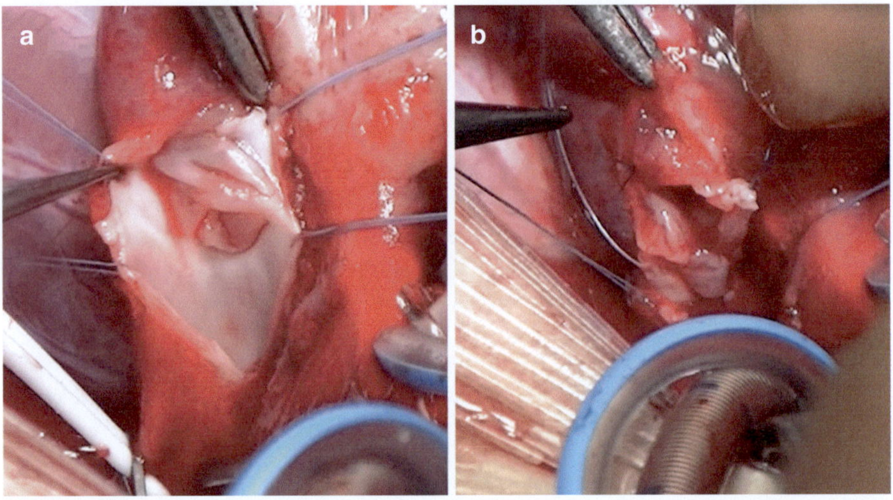

Fig. 46.4 Intraoperative images of the pulmonary valve in a 4-month-old boy with tetralogy of Fallot showing the (**a**) initial (3.5 mm) and (**b**) final (10 mm) diameters of the valve after preservation techniques

into the RV myocardium, when necessary. Subsequently, the extended cusps are resuspended creating new PV commissures. Occasionally PV cusps are augmented by using small triangles of prosthetic (biologic) patch material and then resuspended (Figs. 46.1, 46.3, and 46.4). The MPA is eventually patch enlarged, when needed, with an autologous pericardial patch, which is anchored proximally below the PV annulus, onto the RVOT epicardium, with the aim of avoiding any potential early or late constriction over the reconstructed PV apparatus.

Goals of the intraoperative PV balloon dilation are to achieve: (1) an annular PV *z*-score of zero, (2) a thorough myotomy/myectomy of the subpulmonary area, and (3) a half-systemic right ventricular pressure [4, 6–8] at the end of the procedure.

References

1. Al Habib HF, Jacobs JP, Mavroudis C, et al. Contemporary patterns of management of tetralogy of Fallot: data from the Society of Thoracic Surgeons Database. Ann Thorac Surg. 2010;90:813–9.
2. Stellin G, Milanesi O, Rubino M, et al. Repair of tetralogy of Fallot in the first six months of life: transatrial versus transventricular approach. Ann Thorac Surg. 1995;60:588–S591.
3. Lee C, Lee CH, Kwak JG, Kim SH, Shim WS, Lee SY, Jang SI, Park SJ, Kim YM. Factors associated with right ventricular dilatation and dysfunction in patients with chronic pulmonary regurgitation after repair of tetralogy of Fallot: analysis of magnetic resonance imaging data from 218 patients. J Thorac Cardiovasc Surg. 2014;148(6):2589–96.
4. Bacha E. Valve-sparing options in tetralogy of Fallot surgery. Semin Thorac Cardiovasc Surg Pediatr Card Surg Annu. 2012;15:24–6.
5. Vida VL, Padalino MA, Maschietto N, et al. The balloon dilation of the pulmonary valve during early repair of tetralogy of Fallot. Catheter Cardiovasc Interv. 2012;80:915–21.
6. Vida VL, Guariento A, Castaldi B, et al. Evolving strategies for preserving the pulmonary valve during early repair of tetralogy of Fallot: mid-term results. J Thorac Cardiovasc Surg. 2014;147:687–94; discussion 694–6.
7. Vida VL, Zucchetta F, Padalino MA, Milanesi O, Stellin G. Pulmonary valve-sparing technique in patients with tetralogy of Fallot and anomalous coronary artery crossing the infundibulum. J Heart Valve Dis. 2013;22:425–7.
8. Vida VL, Angelini A, Guariento A, Frescura C, Fedrigo M, Padalino M, Sanders SP, Thiene G, Stellin G. Preserving the pulmonary valve during early repair of tetralogy of Fallot: anatomic substrates and surgical strategies. J Thorac Cardiovasc Surg. 2015;149(5):1358–63.e1.

Other Hybrid Treatments: RV-to-PA Hybrid Conduit

47

Gianfranco Butera, Mario Carminati, and Alessandro Frigiola

Tetralogy of Fallot with pulmonary atresia may be associated to various degrees of development of pulmonary arteries. Their size is the key issue in the prognosis and treatment of this disease. In subjects with hypoplastic pulmonary arteries, surgical options include implantation of a modified Blalock–Taussig shunt or of a right ventricular outflow tract conduit. We have developed a hybrid approach for cases where the surgical alternatives are not available [1].

A 2.2 kg newborn who underwent a cardiac catheterization at 2 days of life showed pulmonary atresia, ventricular septal defect and confluent pulmonary arteries of 2.5 mm in diameter and a Nakata of 50 mm/m^2. Pulmonary arteries were supplied from a major aortopulmonary collateral from the left subclavian artery (Panel A). Oxygen saturation was around 60 %. Surgical options were considered too risky. A hybrid approach was undertaken under general anaesthesia and orotracheal intubation. Patient underwent midline sternotomy. Under direct vision and by using a 21 gauge needle, the free wall of the right ventricle was punctured and the cannula directed towards the atretic right ventricular outflow tract (RVOT) and towards the small pulmonary artery trunk (Panel B). A 0.021 inch 21 cm-long standard guidewire was advanced and then a 5 Fr paediatric sheath was placed over that wire through the atretic RVOT and the pulmonary trunk (Panels C and D). A 0.014 in. coronary guidewire was exchanged and a JOSTENT Graft Master Coronary Stent Graft 3.5 × 19 mm (Abbott Vascular Devices, Holland BV, the Netherlands) was implanted (Panel E). A final angiography showed a well-placed covered stent (Panel F). Visual inspection showed no bleeding and a satisfactory position of the stent (Panel G). Oxygen saturation increased from 60 % at the beginning of the procedure to 90 % at the end. Total procedural time was 60 min. The postprocedural course was uneventful. At a 3-month follow-up, the stent is patent

G. Butera (✉) • M. Carminati • A. Frigiola
Department of Congenital Cardiology and Surgery, Policlinico San Donato IRCCS, San Donato Milanese, MI, Italy
e-mail: Gianfranco.Butera@grupposandonato.it

G. Butera et al. (eds.), *Fetal and Hybrid Procedures in Congenital Heart Diseases*, DOI 10.1007/978-3-319-40088-4_47

(Panel H), patient's weight is 5 kg, and oxygen saturation is 85 %. During follow-up, the patient needed several cardiac catheterization procedures of pulmonary artery rehabilitation and RVOT surgical opening and she is ready for VSD closure.

Hybrid implantation of a coronary graft may be an appealing alternative in small newborns with diminutive pulmonary arteries.

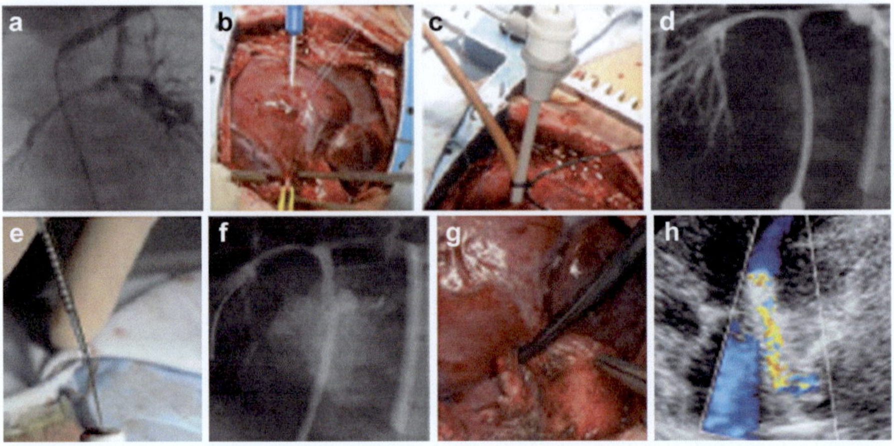

With permission from European heart Journal

Reference

1. Butera G, Abella R, Carminati M, Frigiola A. Perventricular implantation of a right ventricular-to-pulmonary artery 'conduit'. Eur Heart J. 2009;30(17):2078.

Hybrid VSD Creation or Enlargement

48

Frank F. Ing

48.1 Introduction

The need for ventricular septal defect (VSD) creation or enlargement is a relatively rare one. It usually involves a combination of what appears to be an adequate VSD for flow to the systemic circulation usually in the context of a single ventricle variant (most commonly double outlet right ventricle (DORV)) at birth or at the time of palliative surgery. As the child grows, the VSD becomes restrictive as evidenced by a significant gradient of flow across the VSD, which may be accompanied by depressed ventricular function. Treatment options include surgical or transcatheter creation or enlargement of the VSD. While surgery has been the primary option, it often carries high morbidity and risks [1, 2]. Transcatheter techniques have been developed for this rare anatomic problem. VSD enlargement is relatively straightforward involving the passage of a wire across the existing VSD, balloon septoplasty, and stent implantation. VSD creation is technically more demanding requiring a transseptal puncture across the ventricular septum and in the muscular septum, followed by positioning of a wire, septoplasty, and stent implantation [3, 4]. This technique was first reported in 2006 in a small series of eight patients from Meadows et al. [3]. In that series, five patients underwent VSD creation and three for VSD enlargement. Three of the patients had prior surgical attempts at LV decompression. Gradients across the septum decreased from 76.9 to 20.3 mmHg post intervention. At last follow-up, all stented VSDs were patent although recurrent obstruction was found in the majority of patients due to muscular hypertrophy extending beyond the stent edges. Their conclusion was that in high-risk surgical patients, transcatheter creation or enlargement of VSDs is possible with need for repeat interventions due to recurrent obstruction.

The advent of hybrid techniques has permitted a third alternative at VSD creation or enlargement for this rare lesion. This technique is particularly advantageous in infants

F.F. Ing, MD, FACC, FSCAI
Department of Cardiology, Children's Hospital Los Angeles, University of Southern California, Los Angeles, CA, USA
e-mail: fing@chla.usc.edu

G. Butera et al. (eds.), *Fetal and Hybrid Procedures in Congenital Heart Diseases*, DOI 10.1007/978-3-319-40088-4_48

and small children where transseptal puncture of the ventricular septum or passage of the delivery system and stent across the VSD is technically difficult due to the small size and/or poor ventricular function. A transcatheter technique for VSD stenting was reported in a 2.9 kg infant, but only a small premounted stent (PG1280 BPX stent, Cordis) was used which cannot be further dilated to accommodate somatic growth [4].

48.2 Hybrid Technique for Creation or Enlargement of VSD

Prior to the hybrid procedure, a diagnostic cardiac catheterization is performed to evaluate the existing VSD anatomy and the two ventricles. Careful measurements of the septal thickness adjacent to the restrictive VSD in both systole and diastole are made (Fig. 48.1). The inside dimensions of both the RV and the LV are assessed,

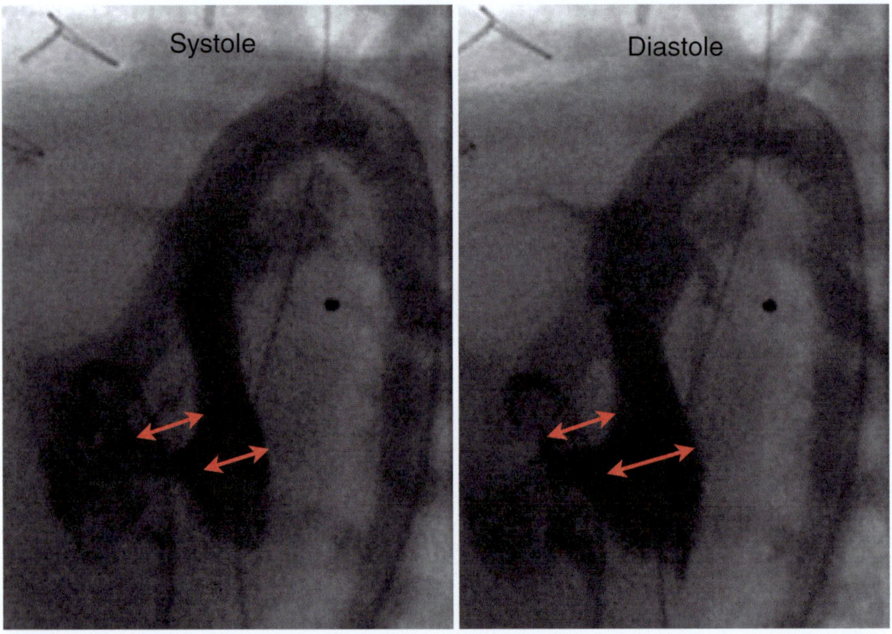

Fig. 48.1 Diagnostic catheterization revealing a rare combination of mitral atresia, hypoplastic left ventricle, normally related great arteries, normal size ascending aorta, coarctation of the aorta, and a VSD (which supplies the systemic output) as well as a diaphragmatic hernia with a hypoplastic right lung. Initially, the VSD was felt to be adequate measuring 8 mm in diameter. Initial surgery was diaphragmatic hernia repair, coarctation repair, and a PA band. By 5 weeks of age (2.9 kg), the VSD had become restrictive. Ventricular septal thickness and both RV and LV dimensions are carefully measured in both systole and diastole to determine appropriate stent diameter and length as well as ventricular dimensions to a permit safe passage of needle, sheath and wire. In this case, the interventricular septal diameter in both systole and diastole measured 9.1 mm while the distance from the septum to the backwall of the LV varies from 8.5 mm in systole to 10.6 mm in diastole (*red arrows*). The VSD diameter varies from 3.5 mm in systole to 5.7 mm in diastole. The distance from the RV freewall to septum measured 14 mm

and distance from both ventricular free walls to their respective sides of the VSD is measured carefully. A large size stent should be selected which permits further dilation (up to 18 mm diameter) to accommodate growth of the child. Unfortunately, the commercially available lengths for these stents are too long for the thickness of the infant ventricular septum and must be folded to the correct length (Fig. 48.2). The Genesis XD stent is commonly used. Next, the stent is mounted on a balloon with a predetermined diameter. In the operating room, following a standard thoracotomy, the hybrid procedure is assisted by transesophageal echocardiogram (TEE) imaging as well as fluoroscopy (Fig. 48.3). Initial needle puncture is made from the RV-free wall toward the VSD. Once inside the RV, a 0.035″ guidewire is passed from the needle across the VSD into the LV. The wire can be positioned out of the left ventricular outflow tract or curled inside the LV body depending on the space available for the balloon length. TEE is used to visualize the wire position. A 9 Fr short sheath

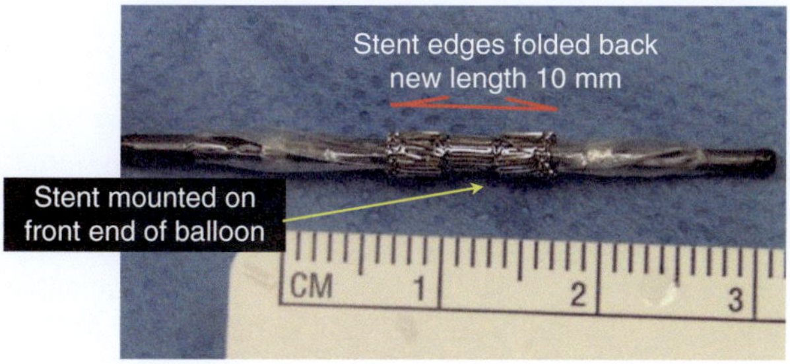

Fig. 48.2 A Genesis 1910XD stent is selected and both edges are folded back to 10 mm length and mounted on a 8 mm diameter balloon

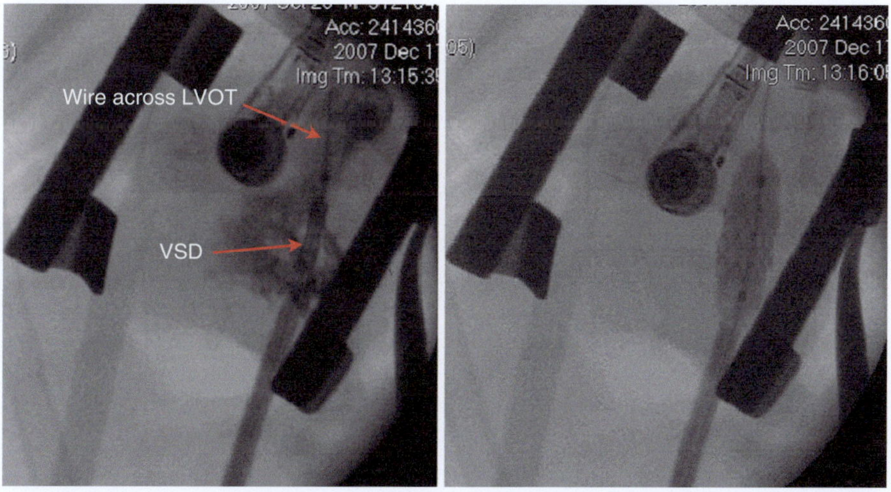

Fig. 48.3 Flouroscopic guidance of stent and balloon to straddle the VSD. The wire was positioned across the left ventricular outflow tract (LVOT) due to the small size of the LV as shown in Fig. 48.1. Once in good position, the balloon is inflated and implanted in the stent across the VSD

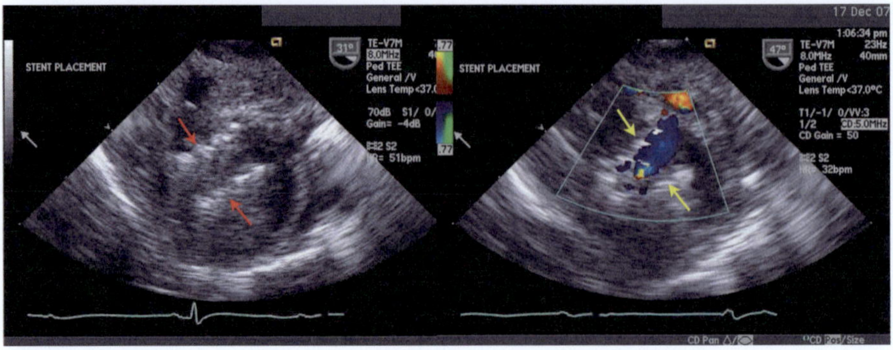

Fig. 48.4 TEE imaging demonstrates the stent in the interventricular septum after removal of the balloon, wire, and sheath (*red arrows*). Color Doppler shows nonturbulent flow across the VSD (*yellow arrows*)

is passed across the VSD over the wire under both TEE and fluoroscopic guidance. Hand injections of contrast are generally adequate to visualize the VSD and adjacent anatomy. Since the flow across the VSD is required for systemic output, blood pressure may drop once the sheath is passed into the VSD. Therefore, it is prudent to prepare the stent and balloon prior to positioning the sheath into the VSD. Once the stent is straddled across the VSD, the balloon is inflated implanting the stent and enlarging the VSD. The balloon is deflated and removed leaving the stent in place. Follow-up angiogram and TEE imaging will reveal a larger volume of blood crossing the stented VSD (Fig. 48.4). Generally, the LV function and cardiac output improve immediately since there is adequate egress of blood across the VSD. If VSD creation is required, a longer needle may be required to puncture the RV-free wall and guided through the mid-muscular septum by TEE and fluoroscopy imaging. Once the needle is positioned in the LV, the rest of the procedure is similar to what is described above.

It is important to resist the temptation of using a smaller premounted stent. While the smaller stents may be adequate for an infant or small child, the VSD has to "grow" to match the increased cardiac output for normal somatic growth. As mentioned previously, the large size stents require folding to "fit" the infant ventricular septal thickness and avoid excessive protrusion into both ventricles. This folding does require the need for a larger delivery sheath. The advantage of the hybrid approach is that the larger sheath size does not have a negative impact on the procedure. Furthermore, the folded stent actually adds more radial strength against the contracting ventricular septum to minimize stent recoil. In the infant, or when the LV size is small, the wire may need to be positioned across the outflow tract. Beware that when the balloon is inflated in this position, there may be some irritation of the conduction system which may result in transient heart block. Be prepared to pace the ventricles if complete heart block occurs.

In the paper by Meadows et al, there was important recurrent obstruction caused by muscular hypertrophy at the stent edges. This can be easily treated with further dilation and/or addition of a longer stent when the child has grown bigger. Medium term follow-up catheterization and angiography is recommended to assess the VSD stent (Fig. 48.5).

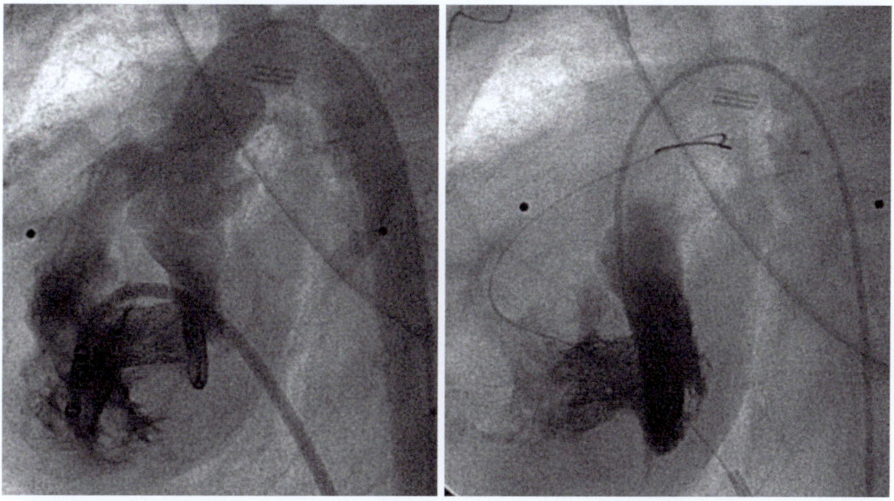

Fig. 48.5 Follow-up angiography 5 months later shows persistent patency of the stented VSD with no gradient between the two ventricles

48.3 Summary

In DORV with single ventricle palliation or other rare instances of single ventricle variants, left ventricular obstruction due to progressive restriction of the outflow VSD can rarely occur resulting in LV hypertension and depressed ventricular function as well as compromised cardiac output. While there are surgical and transcatheter options to create or enlarge the VSD, surgical risks may be high. In infants and small children, routine transcatheter techniques may be difficult and may be limited to the use of small stents which cannot be further expanded to accommodate somatic growth. The hybrid approach offers another alternative but does require advanced planning with a diagnostic catheterization and close collaboration with the cardiac surgeons. While there is little data on the long-term outcomes of this rare lesion, certainly the hybrid technique has been proven to be safe and effective in the short term. Longer follow-up with larger series is crucial to understand and improve the outcomes of this difficult anatomy.

References

1. Aoki M, Forbess JM, Jonas RA, Mayer Jr JE, Castaneda AR. Results of biventricular repair for double-outlet right ventricle. J Thorac Cardiovasc Surg. 1994;107:338–50.
2. Kleinert S, Sano T, Weintraub RG, et al. Anatomic features and surgical strategies in double-outlet right ventricle. Circulation. 1997;96:1233–9.
3. Meadows J, Pigula F, Lock J, Marshall A. Transcatheter creation and enlargement of ventricular septal defects for relief of ventricular hypertension. J Thorac Cardiovasc Surg. 2007;133: 912–8.
4. Lin H, Huddleston C, Balzer DT. Transcatheter Ventricular septal defect (VSD) creation for restrictive VSD in double outlet right ventricle. Pediatr Cardiol. 2013;34:743–7.

MIX
Papier aus verantwortungsvollen Quellen
Paper from responsible sources
FSC® C105338

If you have any concerns about our products,
you can contact us on
ProductSafety@springernature.com

In case Publisher is established outside the EU,
the EU authorized representative is:
Springer Nature Customer Service Center GmbH
Europaplatz 3, 69115 Heidelberg, Germany

Printed by Libri Plureos GmbH
in Hamburg, Germany